DR. SEBI BIBLE

10 BOOKS IN 1:

THE ULTIMATE GUIDE TO A DISEASE-FREE LIFE.

EVERYTHING YOU EVER NEED TO KNOW ABOUT DR. SEBI'S ALKALINE DIET, HERB SELECTION, TREATMENTS AND CURES FOR ANY DISEASE

By Serena Brown

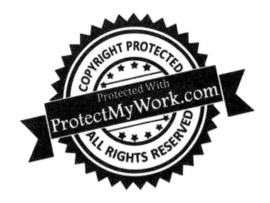

Table of Contents

❋ A FREE BOOK FOR YOU! (DOWNLOAD IT) ❋ 7

❋ WHAT TO DO NOW ❋ 8

BOOK 1: DR. SEBI DIET 12

CHAPTER 1: ABOUT DR. SEBI 14

CHAPTER 2: DR.SEBI ALKALINE DIET 25

CHAPTER 3: DETOXING YOUR BODY 28

CHAPTER 4: APPROVED FOOD LIST 30

CHAPTER 5: 7 COMMON YET DANGEROUS DISEASE YOU CAN TREAT 36

CHAPTER 6: HOW TO NATURALLY REVERSE DIABETES 39

CHAPTER 7: HOW TO NATURALLY REVERSE HIGH BLOOD PRESSURE 43

CHAPTER 8: UNDERSTANDING YOUR LUNGS HEALTH AND DISEASES 45

CHAPTER 9: EVERYTHING YOU NEED TO CLEANSE YOUR LUNGS 47

CHAPTER 10: TIPS FOR A GOOD KICKSTART AND A LONGER LIFE 50

CHAPTER 11: ALKALINE HERBS AND SPICES 52

CHAPTER 12: DR.SEBI SUPPLEMENTS 56

CONCLUSION 58

BOOK 2: DR. SEBI TREATMENTS 60

CHAPTER 1: DR. SEBI AND HIS PHILOSOPHY 62

CHAPTER 2: DR. SEBI TEACHING AND METHODS 63

CHAPTER 3: BENEFITS OF DR. SEBI TREATMENTS 67

CHAPTER 4: ASTHMA 69

CHAPTER 5: DIABETES 71

CHAPTER 6: HIV 75

CHAPTER 7: HAIR LOSS 77

CHAPTER 8: HYPERTENSION 79

CHAPTER 9: LUPUS 81

CHAPTER 10: PCOS TREATMENT 84

CHAPTER 11: STD TREATMENTS 87

CHAPTER 12: HERBAL MEDICINE 89

CHAPTER 13: FASTING TO PREVENT ALL DISEASES 92

BOOK 3: DR SEBI'S CURE FOR HERPES 97

CHAPTER 1: HERPES SIMPLEX VIRUS 99

CHAPTER 2: GENITAL HERPES 106

CHAPTER 3: HERPES AND RELATIONSHIPS 108

CHAPTER 4: DR. SEBI THOUGHTS ON HERPES 110

CHAPTER 5: DR. SEBI'S 3-STEP METHOD 115

CONCLUSION 149

BOOK 4: DR. SEBI AUTOIMMUNE SOLUTION 151

CHAPTER 1: IMMUNE SYSTEM MADE SIMPLE 153

CHAPTER 2: AUTOIMMUNE DISEASES 159

CHAPTER 3: COMPLICATIONS THAT CAN ARISE BECAUSE OF AN AD 166

CHAPTER 4: HEALING YOUR IMMUNE SYSTEM WITH DR. SEBI'S TEACHINGS ... 174

CONCLUSION 202

BOOK 5: DR. SEBI KIDNEY FAILURE SOLUTION 204

CHAPTER 1: KIDNEYS 206

CHAPTER 2: CHRONIC KIDNEY DISEASE (CKD) 211

CHAPTER 3: KIDNEY FAILURE 215

CHAPTER 4: CAUSES OF CKD 220

CHAPTER 5: SYMPTOMS OF CKD 222

CHAPTER 6: CORRELATION WITH OTHER DISEASES 224

CHAPTER 7: CONVENTIONAL TREATMENTS 227

CHAPTER 8: DR. SEBI AND KIDNEY'S HEALTH 229

CHAPTER 9: DR. SEBI METHOD TO HEAL KIDNEYS 232

CHAPTER 10: SUPPLEMENTS 255

CONCLUSION 258

BOOK 6: DR. SEBI ANXIETY SOLUTION 260

INTRODUCTION 262

CHAPTER 1: ANXIETY 263

CHAPTER 2: DEPRESSION 273

CHAPTER 3: RISK FACTORS FOR ANXIETY 279

CHAPTER 4: CONVENTIONAL TREATMENTS 282

CHAPTER 5: ANXIETY AND ALKALINE DIET 285

CHAPTER 6: ESSENTIAL OILS FOR ANXIETY RELIEF 288

CHAPTER 7: DR. SEBI'S 3-STEP SOLUTION 290

CONCLUSION 317

BOOK 7: DR. SEBI COOKBOOK 319

CHAPTER 1: BREAKFAST 320

CHAPTER 2: LUNCH 325

CHAPTER 3: DINNER 332

CHAPTER 4: SMOOTHIES 340

CHAPTER 5: SOUPS 344

CHAPTER 6: SALAD 349

CHAPTER 7: DESSERT 353

CONCLUSION 359

BOOK 8: DR. SEBI'S ALKALINE AND ANTI-INFLAMMATORY DIET 361

INTRODUCTION 362

CHAPTER 1: DR. SEBI 364

CHAPTER 2: THE ALKALINE DIET 368

CHAPTER 3: DETOXIFICATION AND CLEANSING 394

CHAPTER 4: 28-DAY DETOX PLAN 405

CHAPTER 5: SMOOTHIE RECIPES 409

CHAPTER 6: SWITCHING FROM A STANDARD DIET 420

BOOK 9: DR. SEBI'S HERB ENCYCLOPEDIA 428

CHAPTER 1: DR. SEBI'S DIET PILLARS 429

CHAPTER 2: SOURCING HERBS 432

CHAPTER 3: ALKALINE HERB LIST 439

BOOK 10: DR. SEBI'S BOOK OF REMEDIES 515

CHAPTER 1: ACIDIC BODY, MUCUS BUILD-UP AND DISEASES 517

CHAPTER 2: HARVESTING, DRY, PRESERVING AND PURCHASING HERBS 520

CHAPTER 3: ALKALINE HERBAL REMEDIES FOR COMMON AILMENTS 527

CHAPTER 4: REMEDIES FOR COMMON CHILDHOOD PROBLEMS 570

HAVE YOU LIKED IT? 574

⭐ A FREE BOOK FOR YOU! (DOWNLOAD IT) ⭐

- Are you interested in **getting rid of toxins** and nourishing your body?
- Are you curious about how Dr. Sebi used to **face disease and strengthen the immune system**?

SCAN THE QR CODE BELOW AND DISCOVER HOW TO CLEANSE YOUR WHOLE BODY IN JUST 7 DAYS!

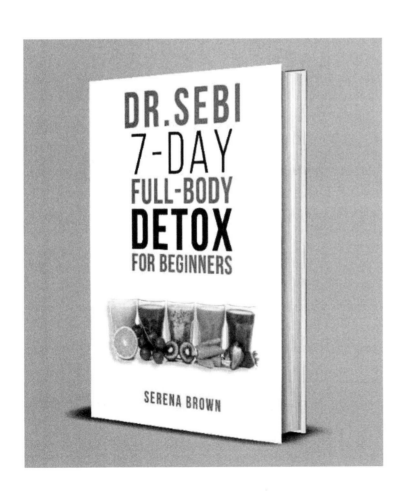

⭐ WHAT TO DO NOW ⭐

At this point, I guess you can't wait to start reading this book and learn every aspect of the true alkaline lifestyle inspired by Dr. Sebi. But first, do these two things!

STEP 1: **Scan the QR Code on the previous page** and learn the basics of detoxifying the body using Dr. Sebi's approved methods. After reading that, everything explained in the book will be easier to understand.

STEP 2: **Let me know how excited you are about having this book in your hands!**

SCAN THE QR CODE BELOW AND <u>LEAVE A QUICK REVIEW ON AMAZON</u> TO SHARE YOUR EXCITEMENT WITH THE FAMILY!

The best way to do it? **<u>Upload a brief video</u> with you talking about how you feel about it!**

Is it too much for you? Not a problem at all! **A review with a couple of photos of the book would still be very nice of you!**

<u>**NOTE:**</u> You don't have to feel obligated, but it would be highly appreciated!

Dedication to Dr. Sebi

Alfredo Bowman 11/26/1933 – 8/6/2016

Dr. Sebi was a resourceful knowledge bank on the power of natural alkaline plant herbs and foods in healing the body and reversing diseases. This transformed my life and made me passionate about spreading this knowledge to every part of the world to help as many people as I can live a healthier lifestyle.

Thank you, Dr. Sebi.

Rest in Peace.

Important Notice from the Author

Even if Dr. Sebi used to recommend different herbs and products for each ailment, the overall method is built on the same core concepts of his alkaline mucusless diet. For this reason, some info in this book will inevitably look similar to the ones in my other books.

Furthermore, each of my books is independent. Since everybody can read any of my titles as the first one on Dr. Sebi's diet, it's my duty to give all the tools needed to read them with complete understanding. In other words, every book is complete in explaining the core concepts of Dr. Sebi's diet because I don't want people to miss out on important information, even at the risk of being repetitive.

BOOK 1: DR. SEBI DIET

YOUR ESSENTIAL GUIDE TO REVERSING DIABETES AND HIGH BLOOD PRESSURE BY LIVING THE DR. SEBI LIFESTYLE. INCLUDES A 7-DAY DETOX PLAN TO CLEANSE YOUR LUNGS FROM MUCUS AND VIRUSES.

Chapter 1: About Dr. Sebi

Alfredo Bowman, whom most people know as Dr. Sebi, Is a well-known herbalist from Honduras. And according to what was on his website, he was self-educated, and he didn't have any formal physical training from anyone; he was not a medical doctor; therefore didn't hold a Ph.D.

He moved to the US to treat his many chronic disorders, including impotence, diabetes, asthma, and obesity.

On his website, it is stated that an herbalist in Mexico healed him, inspiring him to create his herbal mixtures that are generally known as dr Sebi's cell food today.

According to some of the health line's information about him, he initially claimed that his herbs could cure many chronic conditions like AIDS, lupus, and sickle cell anemia. In 1987, the authorities arrested him for practicing medicine without a license, but the jury acquitted him. A few years later, there was a lawsuit to stop making such claims by the State of New York.

And later, again, he was arrested for supposed money laundering in 2016. As he was jailed in Honduras, he there contracted pneumonia, and on the way to the hospital, he died.

Dr. Sebi's Teachings and Methods

Dr. Sebi proposed that the body is susceptible to contracting diseases when toxins and mucus accumulation increase.

He argued that people suffering from different diseases and those interested in preventing diseases should always eat an alkaline diet, bearing in mind that it becomes free from infections when the body removes the increased amount of acidic substances and mucus.

He also suggested that cleansing and detoxifying the body is an essential and significant tool necessary in dealing with any disease in the body.

Detoxification of the body helps eliminate mucus accumulated in the liver, lungs, and many other body organs and helps remove excess acidic substances, thereby freeing the body from disease-causing diseases.

Dr. Sebi also used herbs that are important in re-energizing and revitalizing the body. Our body's organs function correctly when there is an improvement in our health, indicating that the body is void of diseases.

Dr. Sebi's Classification of Food

Dr. Sebi classified food into six categories:

- Drugs
- Genetically modified foods
- Hybrid foods
- Dead foods
- Living foods

- Raw foods

He concluded that this list's first four food categories are a no-go area as they cause more body damage than good. These foods can cause a build-up of acids and mucus in the body. However, the last two categories of foods are the best types of food he classified as healthy because the nutritional contents are not lost in any way. For instance, thoroughly cooked, hybridized, and modified foods have lost the required amount of nutrients present in them. Hence, the reverse is the case instead of providing benefits for the body. However, raw foods, especially vegetables, fruits, and herbs, are excellent for building good health.

Basic info about Dr. Sebi's Diet

Dr. Sebi's diet is plant-based and electric. It also prevents various diseases (prevention) and boosts the immune system. When the body is immuno-compromised, it can accommodate any infection that sneaks in.

Dr. Sebi's diet is also beneficial for people who cherish living a healthy life by remaining clean and lean. But unfortunately, his diet was not created from heaven; they are common foods we ignore because of the love of modified, processed, refined, and hybridized foods.

Dr. Sebi's diet contains vegetables, fruits, grains, nuts, herbal teas, plant-based sweeteners, and seeds. Those who cherish animal products will not benefit from this diet as it does not encourage foods derived from animals.

According to Dr. Sebi, all infections grow well in an environment that makes them comfortable, such as acidic, mucus overloaded, and toxic.

When the body is in a limy condition, infections will find it difficult to thrive, and when it is in an acidic state, the reverse is the case. Hence, the acidic component in the body helps diseases multiply and thrive.

Likewise, he also declared that excess mucus' build-up in the body increases the infection's susceptibility. The mucus blocks the blood vessel and hinders the flow of blood smoothly.

He stated that the excess mucus must be removed to enjoy your health. The diseases are automatically removed when the mucus is removed either by detoxification or cleansing.

The diets of Dr. Sebi have been proven effective by those who genuinely love them. The diets re-energize and revitalize the body by returning it to its normal state.

The healing of many sufferers who suffer from hair loss and many other prevalent diseases didn't occur because of the medications they took but because of the self-healing that took place in the body due to Dr. Sebi's intake's alkaline diet.

Unknown Facts about Dr. Sebi

Dr. Sebi was a renowned herbal medicine practitioner, a biochemist, and a natural therapist. He is also known as Alfredo Darrington Bowman, who employed different herbs and foods to treat several diseases.

Dr. Sebi believed that things created by God are most important for human well-being, mostly plants.

He also believed that several electrical entities could be found easily in the environment, available for consumption and treating several ailments.

Dr. Sebi used these herbs, fruits, and vegetables to prevent and treat diseases. Dr. Sebi is the founder of the USHA Research Institute, which is regarded as the 'healing village.'

allowed many suffering from depressive illnesses to be free from their troubles by using herbs and alkaline foods.

d different illnesses such as cancer, asthma, impotence, eczema, epilepsy, diabetes, leukemia, HIV, fibroids, sickle-eart disease, hypertension, inflammation, lupus, and multiple sclerosis.

everal individuals have testified to their freedom from deadly diseases using Dr. Sebi's herbs and foods.

Benefits of His Treatments

Dr. Sebi's Diet offers a lot of benefits to dieters. While the foods recommended from this diet are known to reduce inflammation, there are other benefits that you can reap from following the Dr. Sebi Diet.

It Helps with Weight Loss

While this diet regimen is not designed for weight loss, it can help people lose weight. People who lose weight with this diet relies on the high fiber, and low-calorie foods encouraged to eat. Except for avocadoes, nuts, seeds, and oil, most foods encouraged by the Dr. Sebi Diet are low in calories. But even if you consume nuts and seeds, they are calorie-dense and rich in fiber and minerals.

Better Colon Health

Because this diet regimen encourages the consumption of large volumes of fruits and vegetables, it also benefits colon health. Foods rich in fiber can help promote healthy digestion; thus, people who follow the Dr. Sebi Diet do not suffer from constipation.

Appetite Control

Although many people think that this diet is very restrictive in terms of the number of calories a particular person takes in, studies indicate that this diet can help with appetite control. The high fiber in your food can provide a higher satiety level and make one feel full for much longer.

Better Gut Microbiomes

The stomach is the second brain. The enzymes and molecules released by the microbes in the gut affect not only your health but even your everyday mood. What you put inside your system also affects the microbes' molecules into the bloodstream. The type of food you consume can also affect the kind of microbes in your stomach. For instance, studies show that consuming greasy, fatty, and processed foods can decline good micro-organisms and promote harmful bacteria growth in the body.

Reduced Inflammation

While inflammation is one of the body's first lines of defense, indicating infection and diseases, chronic low-dose inflammation can also be harmful to the body. Chronic inflammation can result in diabetes, stroke, and even cancer. Thus, diets rich in fruits and vegetables are linked to reduced inflammation caused by oxidative stress. Studies that look into individuals consuming plant-based foods have a 31% lower incidence of developing heart diseases and cancer than those who consume animal products.

Dr. Sebi created this diet for anybody who wants to naturally prevent or cure any disease. It can also improve your overall health without using chemical medications.

Dr. Sebi's theory is that all diseases are caused by too much mucus building up in a specific body area. When you have too much mucus in your lungs, you get pneumonia. If you have too much mucus in your pancreas, it causes diabetes.

He believes that any disease won't exist in an alkaline environment but can happen if your body is too acidic.

Many people claim that his diet improved their health by using his compounds. The herbal approach to healing the body worked better than any medical approach ever did. You can find many of his thoughts about herbal therapy and Nutritional compounds on YouTube. They help promote and teach healthy living long after his death.

His diet does offer many health benefits. The main one is it can promote weight loss because it restricts processed foods, and you will be eating more plant-based, unprocessed meals. This diet consists of whole fruits and vegetables rich in plant compounds, minerals, vitamins, and fiber.

Diets that contain fruits and vegetables are related to oxidative stress and reduced inflammation, along with protecting you against most diseases.

Meatless diets have been linked to lower risks of heart disease and obesity. It also encourages foods that are high in fiber and low in calories. Regularly consuming fruits and vegetables can help protect your body against diseases and reduce inflammation.

Which Food Are Acidic?

Acidic products are found in a wide variety. Food, milk products, and beer are three common acid offenders. Such products can quickly increase the body's acid content and lead to poor health and a ready breeding ground for cancerous growth as a whole. Although an acid condition in the body delays cancerous development, it does not stop it generally. It is also considered a good probability that an alkaline pH-level body cannot cause cancer.

What about Protein?

Animal protein, dairy products, and other foods are very healthy to eat at sufficient portions from a strictly nutritional standpoint. Nevertheless, they increase the acidity of foods, which can affect the body's pH level. If consumed with caution when using more alkaline Ingredients, the pH balance should usually stay normal. Adjust this diet a bit more, and depending on the change, the risk of developing cancer is either increased or lower.

How Unhealthy Is A Diet With High Acidity?

A highly acidic diet is rich in animal protein and many other processed caloric items. Those foods can cause severe health problems without adequate portion control without considering their acid quality. Therefore, a high acid diet reduces the amount of oxygen entering the cells and allows internal acids, such as lactic acid, to build up in cells. That's usually why cancers develop if the cause is not certain external factors. Inhalation of asbestos is an example of an indirect cancer cause that has little to do with the acid content of food. However, all cancers seem to need a slightly acidic or balanced body.

Acid-based diets lead to waste materials and various free radicals that develop cancer within the body. The alkaline diet can purify free radicals and improve their oxygen content in cancer cells, killing them even as the increased blood flow and oxygen invigorate normal healthy tissues.

How Can I Test The Balance Of My Ph?

What are acidic foods? And how do I test my pH balance? The tools used for this purpose are called 'acid strips' or 'pH strips'. The individual's saliva is usually used as the body fluid is easy to reach and works well in pH balance testing. If the balance indicates a number below 7, the body is acidic. If it indicates a number above 7, the body is alkaline. For example, the blood in our veins is slightly alkaline with a pH of 7.4.

The influence of acidity is determined above all by erroneous dietary habits.

Mild Chronic Acidosis

That said, what is important to know is that what we are talking about is not acidosis itself but mild chronic acidosis. The critical problem is not exactly in the blood (which is also), but in our liquids, our extracellular matrix or the Basic System of Pischinger. Studies by Austrian Alfred Pischinger (1966) revealed the significance of the connective system for cellular function. Also known as connective tissue, mesenchyme, or extracellular matrix, SBP is responsible for life's most elementary essential functions: exchange of water, oxygen, electrolytes, acid-alkaline regulation, and everything related nonspecific defense systems. It is this "interior terrain" that slowly and chronically loses its "cleanliness" (alkalinity) and "gets dirty," creating mild chronic acidosis.

Acid Dietary Errors

All these problems and dietary errors make our digestion sick and cause or trigger what is surely the largest producer of acids in our system: a diseased colon. It is slowly irritated, inflamed, and hurt for months and years of receiving low-quality food like the ones mentioned above. Once these micro-wounds have caused the tissues, they will begin to let small particles and proteins pass without digesting into the bloodstream. This process is known as 'Intestinal Permeability Syndrome'. The immune system reacts violently to these unknown particles, causing "Allergic Reactions" when this occurs.

The mucoid plaque layers also stick to the tissue's interior and cause poor electrolytes' absorption (water and minerals). And this can be one reason for our mild chronic dehydration, dry skin, and a host of other health problems.

Eating Alkaline Foods

One of the things that we can do simply, cheaply and quickly is that our interior terrain is not too acidic to change our diet and lifestyle.

Our diet must consist of 60% alkaline foods and 40% acidic foods to be healthy. But to restore health, our diet must consist of 80% alkaline foods and 20% acidic foods. Unfortunately, the latter is the case for most populations in the countries that we believe to be "developed."

It should be evident that we are not trying to classify foods into "bad" and "good" categories. There are no bad foods in their natural form. Alkaline foods or acidic foods are only more useful or less useful, depending on the specific needs at any given time in a particular person.

Using alkaline foods or acidic foods to adjust your pH

This part is for those who want to "adjust" or balance their body's PH. The PH scale is 0 to 14, with the numbers below 7 being acidic (low in oxygen) and the numbers above 7 being alkaline. An acidic body is a magnet for the disease. What you eat and drink will have a decisive impact on the PH level in your body. Remember that balance is the key!

To function correctly, our bodies need to maintain many constants, including acidity. For example, if the blood's acidity, pH, comes out of the range 7.35 and 7.45, there is a risk of discomfort, even death. However, many health problems are linked to too high acidity without going that far. An often unbalanced diet and a sedentary lifestyle mean that many people are faced with chronic acidosis and its series of ailments.

Some Symptoms Encountered In Chronic Acidosis

- Fatigue
- dull
- brittle / split / scratched nails
- dry skin
- muscle or joint pain
- rheumatism
- osteoporosis
- chilliness
- cold extremities
- cramp
- spasms
- lack of energy
- difficulty recovering
- depressive tendency
- irritability
- nervousness
- emotionality
- dental problems
- kidney stones
- urinary or rectal burns
- inflammation of the mucous membranes
- lowered immunity
- allergies

How Acidosis Disrupts the Functioning Of the Body

By the loss of minerals (used to neutralize acids)
The various organs and tissues that provide buffer minerals do so by demineralizing. The bones are the first affected (calcium) and the nervous system (magnesium). Demineralization can prevent specific reactions from taking place, leading to an increase in acid charge, like enzymatic disturbances. Acidosis promotes osteoporosis by eliminating calcium from the bones, and neutralizing excess acidity.

By disrupting the proper functioning of enzymes
Thus the acidity can prevent the realization of physiological reactions and, in particular, the production of proteins and hormones. The intermediate stages of specific reactions go through the creation of acidic elements. Following an enzymatic problem, these products remain in the body, increasing acidity.

By affecting the immune system
By promoting the inflammation of the tissues by acids or deposits of crystals (the salts resulting from the buffer system by the basifying minerals), thus causing diseases in "it's" and in "oses." Inflammation of the tissues, in addition to the discomfort felt, weakens the tissues against infections.

The formation of deposits, blockage of joints, stones, and the formation of "crystals" during the neutralization of acids. Because an acid linked to a base gives a neutral salt and water, this neutral salt is not always easily eliminated and remains in the body.

How the Body Regulates Acidity

PH measures acidity on a scale of 0 (maximum acid) to 14 (maximum alkaline), passing through equilibrium 7 (neutral like water). The more acid an element, the more it contains H + ion.

In a healthy body, the blood's pH is between 7.35 and 7.45; that of the skin around 5.2; that of urine between 6.5 and 7.5. If the skin and urine pH can vary beyond their values, the blood should not go beyond its limits, at the risk of discomfort, even death.

Mucus and Diseases

Mucus is a liquid or a gel-like substance present in different lining surfaces of the body's organs and tissues. Mucus is excreted from different body organs such as the intestine, stomach, lungs, throat, eyes, cervical mucus, and mouth.

Mucus is a fundamental substance needed by the body to produce antibodies, provide a barrier against foreign bodies, lubricate the organs they are found in, and protect them.

Mucus protects the body's organs and possesses the ability to become hydrated. Hydration, in this sense, means the organs are always in liquid form and not dehydrated, which helps in the fight against bacterial, fungal, and viral invasion.

Mucus is a useful tool used by the body to filter any irritant, including allergens, dust, smoke, bacteria, fungi …and many more.

An active substance in the mucus makes it very useful in carrying out the above functions. The active substance is known as mucin.

Mucins are a family of molecular weight glycoproteins produced by the epithelial tissues in your body. Mucin is very important in producing gels, lubricating cells and tissues, and providing foreign materials barriers. This active substance in mucus is the primary functional substance that makes mucus very significant.

The volume of mucus produced by your body daily is about 1.5 liters. Most individuals are void of this because they believe mucus production is voluntary and refuses to pay keen attention to it.

The mucus consists of the following constituents:

- Water (95%).
- Protein (mucin).
- Inorganic salt.
- Ions.
- Antiseptics.
- Antibiotics.

The goblet cells are modified epithelial cells that secrete mucus directly from the surface of the mucous membrane of the major organs where mucus is located.

The primary importance of goblet cells is to secrete mucus known as Mucins, found in the goblet cells before being discharged into the organs. Goblet cells are spread between the enterocytes.

Mucus is found in different organs in the body. Let us look at the different functions in different organs.

The function of mucus in the stomach

Stomach mucus helps protect the gastrointestinal cells from any damage the gastric juices can cause.

Functions of mucus in the intestine

The mucus produced in the intestine helps protect the surface mucosal cells. In addition, the mucus in the intestine produces a gel that helps protect the mucosal surface from foreign bodies that attempt to alter digestion.

The function of the cervical mucus

The cervical mucus helps prevent any form of infection and aids the wetting and lubrication of the vaginal tract for easy sexual activities.

How hard or soft the mucus is, depends on the condition a woman is at a given time. For example, the mucus secreted during ovulation is very soft. It appears like a liquid gel, which helps sexual intercourse be easier. On the other hand, after the menstrual cycle, the mucus tends to become a bit thicker, thereby following the blockage of the migration of sperm.

Functions of Mucus in the Eyes

The mucus in the eyes is very thick and sticks to the eye's surface when relaxed.

The mucus in the sinuses is essential in providing tear film strength. It tolerates the aqueous layer to follow the cornea's epithelial cells.

When the surface tension is reduced between these two layers, it wets and stabilizes the thin

Pre-corneal tear film between blinks.

The mucus in the eyes also helps trap epithelial cells and removes excessive lipid contamination and bacteria.

These are then removed from the eye in the aqueous layer following the blinking of the eyes. The mucus layer becomes much thinner in blinking the eyes and spreads easily over the surface, providing lubrication.

The function of mucus in the mouth

The mucus in the mouth helps in the injection of food, and the swallowing process is very easy. However, the mucus present in the mouth is regarded as saliva. Many individuals do not know how vital the saliva in the mouth is.

Ultimately, the saliva's primary role in the mouth is to lubricate it and help in the digestion process via the enzyme present in the mouth to begin digestion.

What is the Role of Mucus in Protecting the Body?

The mucus in the body is essential, and they contribute immensely to protecting the body. For example, the mucus helps keep the body's internal organs lubricated and healthy, trapping foreign substances like bacteria, fungi, and viruses.

The mucus is then removed by coming out with the nose or mouth's help or swallowing into the stomach and is subsequently destroyed by digestive acids.

Micro-Organisms that Affect Healthy Mucus in the Body

Microorganisms are very important in the body. They almost dominate all the body, especially the mucus membrane, organs, and skin. Millions upon millions of micro-organisms in the body help fight against any organisms ready to cause harm.

They are significant because they help synthesize vitamins, facilitate an individual's immunity, and break down absorbable food nutrients into smaller forms.

These micro-organisms do not cause any problem in the body because they are found in their typical fauna. They undergo a symbiotic mutual relationship with humans.

A typical example of this beneficial micro-organism is lactobacillus bacteria, which help produce lactic acids to facilitate digestion.

However, some micro-organisms are hazardous to your body. These microorganisms' presence alone in your body is not harmful and cannot make you fall sick. Still, their growth and multiplication in the body can bring about different diseases, depending on the disease they cause.

Microorganisms can cause you to fall sick, grow and reproduce hastily in the body, especially when they find themselves in the mucus membrane. They deprive the mucus membrane of carrying out its normal activities.

As small as they appear, micro-organisms possess the ability to adapt to the environment they find themselves. The environment, especially the mucus membrane, is an excellent habitat for them.

The micro-organisms that affect the mucus membrane from performing their functions can cause disease and find their way to the body via the skin, mouth, nose, eyes, genitals, wounds… and many more.

Furthermore, when the micro-organisms become a disease in the body, they are easily transmitted via the mucus membranes. Some diseases that would be transmitted in this manner include; HIV, herpes simplex virus, flu, pneumonia, asthma…and many more.

There are different types of micro-organisms that affect the mucus membrane, such as:

- Bacteria.
- Protozoa.
- Viruses.
- Fungi.
- Helminthes.

The Effect of Excessive Mucus on the Body

The primary health problems associated with the respiratory system and other body organs are caused by over-secretion/overproduction of mucus in the mucus membrane.

The inability to remove mucus from the lungs and other body organs could result in serious health problems. An increasing amount of mucus could result in breathing and other infections that could be dangerous.

The mucus membrane produces excess mucus due to allergic reactions, too much spicy food, cold, flu…and many more.

Examples of infections associated with excess mucus in the body are discussed below:

Asthma

When you have asthma, the mucus lining the respiratory tract becomes a contract. This results in the over-production of mucus. Asthma is respiratory stress facilitated by the respiratory tract's exposure to external bodies such as airborne particles.

Bronchitis

Over-production of mucus by the goblet cells can result in bronchitis. Also, when your body cannot remove excess mucus, it results in cough and bronchitis. The over-production of mucus that leads to bronchitis occurs due to some form of lifestyle, including smoking a cigarette. It could also result from a viral infection, bacterial infection, or inflammation of the cell of mucin gene translation.

Pulmonary Edema

The lung is made up of several alveoli (elastic air sacs). The air sacs inhale oxygen and exhale carbon dioxide efficiently when you breathe. However, when the air sacs are accumulated with excess mucus instead of air, it hinders oxygen inhaling into the blood. The increased mucus production in the lung (respiratory system) could result in pulmonary edema. This increased level of mucus in the lung becomes accumulated, resulting in the inability to breathe. The accumulation of excess mucus makes it very difficult to sleep.

The accumulation of mucus could cause you cold and cough, bringing sputum stained with blood. There is also a condition that causes pulmonary edema, including heart problems. Hence, you have to understand your heart health to know the association between pulmonary edema and heart health.

Cystic Fibrosis

It is a disease that affects humans due to hereditary factors that result in problems in the lungs and digestive system.

This disease is characterized by the overproduction and coagulation of mucus in several body organs. The coagulation subsequently affects the airways of a sufferer having the disease or depressive illness.

Individuals who inherit this disease experience sticky and thick mucus, which is no longer lubricant. Hence, the airways, lungs, respiratory tracts, and pancreas become blocked or plugged up.

Furthermore, the cells that help produce and manufacture mucus become affected by this health problem.

When you have this kind of problem, you are expected to experience repeated lung infections, constant sinusitis, and wheezing.

Primary Ciliary Dyskinesia

Primary ciliary dyskinesia is a disorder inherited from the gene of one or both parents. This problem affects the cilia movement and damages the clearance of mucus. This disorder's symptoms are different among individuals, as some are affected by middle ear infections, chronic sinus, lung infections, hearing loss, excess mucus production, and coughing.

Chronic obstructive Pulmonary Disease

An increase in mucus production in the lung and mucus color changes are the major factors that make you vulnerable to chronic obstructive pulmonary disease. When the average daily limit production of mucus is changed or affected due to either cigarette smoking or when you have any prevailing illness, you could be exposed to chronic obstructive pulmonary disease.

Furthermore, you will get exposed to excess mucus production in the lungs when you have chronic bronchitis and chronic obstructive pulmonary disease symptoms. When your lung produces mucus more than recommended, you are expected to have a long-term (chronic) cough.

Chapter 2: Dr.Sebi Alkaline Diet

What if you heard of a reduction of weight plan to help you reduce weight and look younger? Will you try? Should you try it? Alkaline diets and behaviors have been around for more than 60 years. However, many people don't know about their normal, healthy, and tested weight-loss properties!

The alkaline diet is not a fad or a gimmick. It is a safe and quick way to experience higher fitness rates. This section will inform you what this diet program is, what makes it unique, and how it will result in life-changing outcomes for you, your tail, and your well-being.

Will you love today a lean and beautiful body? You are in the minority, if so. Unfortunately, more than 65% of Americans are overweight or obese. If you are overweight, you may suffer poor health conditions such as weakness, stiffness, swollen muscles, and other illnesses.

Worse still, you still have the impression that you still love the body you like and deserve. Maybe you were told you are growing older, but that's just not the truth. Don't give in to that myth. Don't fall into that myth. Many communities have strong, lean older adults who go to excellent health in their 1990s!

The reality is that the body is a computer of genius architecture. If you experience some adverse health effects, that is proof that the blood composition is too acidic. The signs are a call for assistance. That is, for one day, the body will not break down. Instead, your well-being is gradually eroding over time, finally slipping into 'disappointment.'

What's wrong with the way you're eating now?

The standard American Diet (S.A.D) relies on processed foods, fats, caffeine, meats, and animal goods. All of these products are incredibly acidic. Although we do not consume enough alkaline foods such as new fruits, vegetables, nuts, and legumes, diet experts appeal.

In brief, our S.A.D. Lifestyle upsets our species' normal acid-alkaline equilibrium. This illness induces malnutrition, higher rates of aches and pains, colds and flu, and disease inevitably develops.

We missed our path. We lost our way. It is where an alkaline diet will lead to improving our well-being.

I'm confident that you recognize the word pH relating to the acidity or alkalinity of something. Alkalinity on a scale is calculated. You should take a quick and economical home check to see your alkalinity and track your alkalinity periodically.

Scientific doctors and scientists have understood this lesser-established reality for at least 70 years... Your body requires a specific pH degree or delicate equilibrium of the acid-alkaline levels in the blood to ensure optimum well-being and longevity.

Perhaps you wonder, "Why do the pH balance and alkalinity mean to me?" I know these were my thoughts when I first learned of alkaline food.

Two definitions would demonstrate how acid and alkalinity are essential to the body.

We also realize that there is an acid in our throats. This acid is necessary in conjunction with enzymes to divide food into simple elements that can be ingested by the digestive tract. What if we have no fat in our belly? We can die of starvation in no time since the body can't use a whole slice of meat or whatever!

Can You Make Sense?

Various body parts need varying acidity or alkalinity amounts. The plasma, for example, needs a bit more alkaline than the stomach acids. What if you have so much acidic blood? It could nearly chew into the nerves and lungs, triggering major internal bleeding!

Although these explanations demonstrate that the body's various components or structures need specific pH values, we should not think about this. Our question is simple because it's that we're all mostly acidic.

It is the most critical thing to remember. Suppose the body becomes too acidic after a long time. In that case, it contributes to other diseases such as obesity, diabetes, lack of bone mass, high blood pressure, lung failure, and stroke. The list is infinite, as the organism eventually gives up the battle for life and falls into the state of survival for as long as possible.

What's the alkaline diet like, and what would you expect?

Like other adjustments in diet or lifestyle, a transition phase may occur. Yet if you're eating the cleanest food your body needs, you won't have to feel thirsty, unlike other diet strategies. Plus, once you're full, you can consume all you want. You won't have to count calories, either. And you can appreciate a lot of variety, so you're never going to be bored with cooking.

Find an alkaline diet as a kind of "juice fast" for the body. It's just not that serious. You consume rich and readily digestible foods that your body longs for. Once you supply all the cells in your body that it wants so badly, the appetite goes out. Yet dull vegetables don't have to fret, as there are plenty of tasty recipes on the internet and in books.

What would you find an alternate strategy, including an alkaline diet for other eating plans?

If correctly practiced, you should assume that the fat can dissolve more quickly than traditional plans. There are also accounts where individuals claim they drop more than two pounds a week. (And with most food plans, the weight will not be wise). In addition, when your skin becomes lighter, your vitality improves, looking younger.

Furthermore, the alkaline diet does two essential items to conventional diets.

It provides superior nourishment to your body's cells. It naturally helps to detoxify and cleanse the cells, too.

These factors illustrate why an alkaline diet operates both quickly and comfortably.

The Tips for Successfully Following the Alkaline Diet

Often, stretching for the additional mile, you get to the areas you had only dreamed about. Going well on an alkaline diet will be the battle that ultimately contributes to a balanced lifestyle. An alkaline diet assumes that certain products, such as berries, vegetables, roots, and legumes, leave an alkaline residue or ash behind in the body. The body is strengthened by rock's key ingredients, such as calcium, magnesium, titanium, zinc, and copper. Avoiding asthma, malnutrition, exhaustion, and even cancer is an alkaline diet. Conscious about doing something like that?

Below are ten strategies to adopt the alkaline diet effectively:

Drink Water

Water is probably our body's most important (after oxygen) resource. Hydration in the body is vital as the water content determines the body's chemistry. Drink between 8-10 glasses of water to keep the body well hydrated (filtered to cleaned).

Avoid Acidic Drinks like Tea, Coffee, Or Soda

Our body also attempts to regulate acid and alkaline content. There is no need to blink in carbonated drinks as the body refuses carbon dioxide as waste!

Breathe

Oxygen explains that our body works, and if you provide the body with adequate oxygen, it should perform better. Sit back and enjoy two to five minutes of slow breaths. Nothing is easier than you can perform Yoga.

Avoid Food with Preservatives and Food Colors

Our body has not been programmed to absorb such substances, and the body then absorbs them or retains them as fat, and they do not damage the liver. Chemicals create acids, such that the body neutralizes them either by generating cholesterols or blanching iron from the RBCs (leading to anemia) or by extracting calcium from bones (osteoporosis).

Avoid Artificial Sweeteners

These sweeteners, which tend to be high in low fat, are potentially detrimental to the body. Also, Saccharin, a primary ingredient in sweeteners, triggers cancer. Keep away from these things, therefore. Go for less healthy food, still a decent one.

Satiate Your Urges for Snack by Eating Vegetables

Whenever we are hungry, we tend to consume fast food. Instead, establish a tradition of consuming fresh vegetables or walnuts when you feel like eating something.

Eat the Right Mix of Food

The fats and proteins of carbohydrates need a specific atmosphere when digested. And don't eat it all at once. Evaluate the nutritional composition and balance it accurately to create the best combination of all the nutrients you consume.

Sleep Well, Remain Calm

Seek to escape the pain. Our mind regulates the digestive system, and only when in a relaxed, focused condition can you realize it functions properly. Relax, then, and remain safe

Chapter 3: Detoxing Your Body

Detoxification is the cleaning of unidentified body contaminants (toxins) and also the exclusion of body intoxicants (opioids, drugs, alcohol) until participation in something like a SUD (substance use disorders) or recovery program from addiction. They aren't the exact thing.

Uniform Alcoholism & intoxication Care Act (1971) suggested that better it was for those with an AUD (alcohol use disorders) to undergo medication instead of prosecution; detoxification became standard procedure for people with AUD (alcohol use disorder). They might "lead regular lives as citizens of the community" in that manner.

What does Detox Do?

For detox working, you should avoid utilizing or having a harmful substance that triggers your health issues, including lead-containing materials, fatty foods, or addictive things like alcohol or narcotics. Then the liver, digestive system, kidneys, lungs, and skin of your body remove the residual contaminants, taking the body back to its pre-toxin condition. The body typically needs time if it's healthy.

Some individuals claim that you will speed up the Process with an extreme diet, vigorously eliminating the toxins: supplements (natural), juicing foods, or proprietary tonics for best digestion.

Detox Full Body

In the common context, a cleanse or complete body detox is a way to purge "toxins" (chemicals and impurities and pollutants) to stay healthy and live happy and longer.

As long as you're healthy, drinking healthy fluids, sufficient water, and eating good food, this detox type is what your body is prepared to do without any support. It's a diet. Involves vegetables and Juicing fruits, taking away toxic things (coffee, sugar, tobacco, alcohol), and exercise.

If you eat vegetables and fruits instead of refined grains, beef, sugar, and wheat, you'll lose weight, get more stamina, and feel better, so you don't have to drink those juices. You should enjoy vegetables and fruit. Good for you is the food fiber. It is needless to juice food or purchase pricey juices containing dietary supplements.

Detoxing Misconceptions

Detox is a normal step in a balanced body and does not need attention. You will get fewer chemicals in your system once you avoid eating them, although there is no proof that diet programs quick up the method. If you have lesser toxins in the body, you will accumulate lesser toxins. Few popular misconceptions regarding detoxifying involve:

Using detox techniques would not accelerate the removal of contaminants from the system. All the so-called contaminants are not named. There is no proof of any contaminants exiting the body sooner due to detox.

Detox regimes do not help you shed weight. Yeah, once you avoid consuming sugars, fried products, and carbs, you are likely to lose fat; however, you are losing food, not pollutants. When you take diuretics and laxatives, you can lose weight throughout the near term, but you are often running to the toilet. You may end up becoming dehydrated dangerously.

Activated charcoal would not flush out liquor. It is utilized for purifying or aeration in manufacturing operations. Some also reported this to purify and avoid or ease cramps or even excessive drinking. Worse still, one contaminant that charcoal cannot flush off is liquor. It may inhibit the ingestion of many other compounds, but it may be the nutrients you require.

Chapter 4: Approved Food List

As a natural health and wellness specialist, Dr. Sebi created his specialized diets in his wealth of experience. His diets include fruits with seeds, agave syrup, wild rice, coconut oil, olive oil, and more. He further created his own fundamental six food groups: Dead, Raw, Live, Drugs, Hybrid, and Genetically Modified.

Dead Foods are foods that can stay for days without going bad. These are heavily processed, synthesized, and less nutritional; some examples are fruit snacks, flavored crackers, flavored beverages, and meal replacement bars. This food group is very common as they are fast, tasty, and convenient. Still, they contain chemicals, artificial colors and flavors, and unfamiliar ingredients. Such food consumption leads to diseases like diabetes, cancer, obesity, heart diseases, etc.

It has been detected that chemically processed and refined foods are significant players in body inflammation. When these dead foods accumulate in the body, it causes chronic inflammation, resulting in weight gain, increased blood pressure, arthritis, elevated blood sugar level, etc. Pains, aches, brain fog, hormonal imbalance, and poor sleep result from the body reacting to these dead foods.

Live Food

These are either natural or close to it; for example, fruits and vegetables, nuts and seeds. These foods have a contrasting fortune with the dead foods as they possess antioxidants that fight inflammation and phytochemicals. They help produce and activate enzymes that help produce hormones and chemical reactions in the body. These foods also boost your body's defense because they possess probiotics that promote healthy bacteria that act as the body's first response when fighting diseases.

Raw Food

As defined by the Natural Hygiene movement in the 1800s, Raw food is any food cooked below a temperature lower than 115 – 118 degrees Fahrenheit. Nutrients and enzymes are assumed to be preserved when cooked and keep food in its natural state. They are mostly vegetables, seeds, nuts, fresh fruits, and soaked legumes and grains.

Experts consider raw food diets as a natural diet for humans. They say raw foods would have been our food in the wild if we had not developed agriculture, created processed foods, and animal domestication. Some benefits of eating raw foods are improved sleep, energy, bowel movements, body fat loss, clear skin, a clear mind, etc.

Hybrids Food

These are foods formed from the combination of two different fruits or vegetables. The hybrid produce is referred to as hybrid foods; this rarely occurs in nature but is mostly engineered by men. Some hybrids are seedless apples, kiwis, seedless watermelon, seedless grapes, seedless citrus fruits, and seedless persimmons. There are no real health risks in the consumption of hybrid foods.

Genetically Modified Food

Foods made from organisms that have been genetically modified artificially are said to be GM foods. They are a significant health risk for consumers as good work has not been done to check GM foods' production. They are usually employed to help plant viability. Still, plans are ongoing to alter foods' nutrients to check allergenic potential.

Drugs

Some foods are grouped as drugs because they contain a high medicinal value, acting as a drug to the body. There are links between drugs and food; some food acts like drugs, while some drugs act as food. You should be aware of drugs considered food because they can be very harmful. Unlike food servings as drugs, such as green tea and coffee, they have far fewer health risks.

Approved Lists

Dr. Sebi created his diets from just live and raw food groups, virtually shutting out the rest of the food groups. He encourages dieters to consume more foods close to a raw vegan diet, such as vegetables and fruits that are naturally grown and whole grains. His thought line was that the live and raw foods were electric, and they combat the acidic food waste contained in the body. Dr. Sebi compiled his food list called 'Electric Food List', which he considered the best of his diets. This list continues to evolve and grow even after his demise.

It is always challenging for most people who eat out regularly to abide by Dr. Sebi's food diet. So it will be great to star

Vegetable Food list

Dr. Sebi strongly advocates that people consume non-genetically modified organism foods, including seedless vegetables and fruits, or those modified to contain more nutrients than the natural state. He has a long, diverse list of vegetables, providing more options to make amazing meals.

Approved vegetables are, for example:

- Amaranth
- Avocado
- Arame
- Bell Pepper
- Cherry and Plum Tomato
- Chayote
- Cucumber
- Dulse
- Dandelion Greens
- Garbanzo Beans
- Hijiki
- Izote Flower and Leaf
- Kale
- Lettuce, apart from Iceberg
- Mushroom, apart from Shitake
- Nori
- Nopales
- Onions
- Olives
- Okra
- Purslane Verdolaga
- Sea Vegetables
- Squash
- Tomatillo
- Turnip Greens
- Wakame
- Watercress
- Wild Arugula
- Zucchini

Fruit List

While Dr. Sebi proposes a wide range of vegetables, he restricts fruits. However, despite this restriction, fruits have diverse lists to choose from, including all berries apart from human-made cranberries.

Approved fruits are, for example:

- Apples
- Berries
- Bananas
- Cherries

- Currants
- Cantaloupe
- Dates
- Figs
- Grapes
- Limes
- Melons
- Mango
- Orange
- Plums
-
- Papayas
- Prunes
- Peaches
- Pears
- Prickly Pear
- Raisins
- Sour soups
- Soft Jelly Coconut
- Tamarind

Spices and Seasoning

- Achiote
- Bay Leaf
- Basil
- Cloves
- Cayenne
- Dill
- Habanero
- Oregano
- Onion Powder
- Pure Sea Salt
- Savory
- Sweet Basil
- Sage
- Thyme
- Tarragon

Alkaline Grain

- Amaranth
- Fonio
- Kamut
- Quinoa
- Rye
- Spelt

Alkaline Sweeteners and Sugars

- 100% Pure Agave Syrup from Cactus
- Date Sugar from Dried Dates

Nuts and Seeds

- Brazil Nuts
- Hemp Seeds
- Raw Sesame Seeds
- Walnuts

Oils

- Avocado Oil
- Coconut Oil
- Grapeseed Oil
- Hempseed Oil
- Olive Oil
- Sesame Oil

Guidelines

- Any food not listed above is not recommended.
- You should drink a gallon of water daily, preferably natural spring water.
- Take Dr. Sebi's product an hour before taking pharmaceutical drugs.
- Strict adherence to Dr. Sebi's nutritional guidelines guarantees the best result in disease reversal.
- No fish, no alcohol, no animal products, no hybrid foods, and no dairy.
- Consume only the above-approved grains.
- Many approved grains are sold in bread, pasta, cereal, or flour in health food stores.
- Dr. Sebi's products work for 14 days within the body, as it still releases therapeutic properties.
- Do not make use of microwaves, and it kills the food.
- No consumption of seedless or canned fruits.

10 Food You Should Never Eat and Why

Regardless of the diet, you're on, there are usually foods you should eat more of and those you should stay away from. Today, there are dozens of healthy as well as fad diets, and they all have their "followers." However, there are some foods everyone should avoid and avoid, like the plague. These foods are more than just unhealthy. Some contain so many artificial additives and synthetic chemicals; they are dangerous to eat.

Unfortunately, many of these foods are very popular, and we eat them all the time. Health food shops even offer some of them. When you go through this list, you'll understand why the so-called diseases of civilization are becoming a serious threat to global health.

Three things that most unhealthy foods have in common:

They are popular

Most of these foods are on our table every day. What's even worse, some of them are sold in health food shops as healthy alternatives to sugar, meat, or dairy.

They are aggressively marketed

The meat and dairy industries have powerful lobbies that successfully manipulate people into buying foods they shouldn't. In addition, aggressive marketing campaigns and misleading messages have resulted in consumers' inability to decide for themselves but do what they are told.

They are tasty, cheap, and convenient

What makes giving up these foods so difficult is that most of them are very tasty (because they are full of flavor additives), cheap (because they are mass-produced from the cheapest ingredients), and convenient (many of them are pre-packed and ready to use, requiring minimum preparation time). Unfortunately, the story of modern agriculture and the stressful, sedentary lifestyle we lead is long and complicated and beyond this book's scope. Suffice it to say that your diet should be much more than fuel that keeps you going.

A diet can be a source of healing or toxic foods.

It can improve or destroy your health. It can boost your mood and performance or contribute to premature aging and chronic disease.

So, whatever food you think is best for you, make sure it's free of the following foods:

1. Artificial sweeteners

Artificial sweeteners are found in many sugar-free products, ET chewing gums, baked goods, jams, etc. They are also what sugar replacements are based on, e.g., xylitol, erythritol, isomalt, lactitol, maltitol, mannitol, and sorbitol. Although these artificial sweeteners are marketed as natural, they are heavily processed and are often produced from GMO ingredients. Long-term use of artificial sweeteners can create an imbalance in your gut flora and contribute to the development of diabetes, gastrointestinal problems, weight gain, etc.

2. Soy protein

Most of the soy produced in the US (and some other countries) is genetically modified. GM soy is now farmed because it is resistant to glyphosate, commonly used in soy farming. A recent Norwegian study found that US-produced soy contains so much herbicide that it almost feels like eating weed killer. Glyphosate is linked to many life-threatening conditions, including several types of lymphoma cancer. So while fermented soy products, such as natto, tempeh, and miso soups, are perfectly safe to use, you must stay away from edamame, soy milk, and soy protein.

3. Farmed salmon (Atlantic salmon)

Most people eat salmon because it's high in omega-3 fatty acids. However, farmed salmon available today have considerably lower levels of these healthy fats than the salmon we could buy only five years ago. The most likely reason is that salmon is now fed much less nutritious food. Besides, dioxin levels are ten times higher in farmed salmon than wild salmon. This is bad news because this chemical is linked to cancer, organ damage, and immune system dysfunction.

On top of that, farmed salmon is regularly treated with banned pesticides. To make things even worse, it recently became legal to produce and sell genetically engineered salmon without labeling it as such.

4. Meat from large-scale farms

All animals raised this way are fed growth hormones, antibiotics, and food grown with chemical pesticides and fertilizers. A recent chicken meat and feathers analysis discovered banned antibiotics, allergy medications, painkillers, and arsenic.

5. Microwave popcorn

The microwavable bags are lined with perfluorochemicals that make the bags resistant to heat. Unfortunately, these chemicals are linked to cancer. Besides, the fake butter flavoring often used in popcorn production causes lung disease and inflammation in various organs.

6. Shrimp

Farmed shrimps contain a certain food additive used to improve shrimp's color. This additive has estrogen-like effects that can affect the sperm count in men and increase women's breast cancer risk. Besides, ponds, where shrimps are raised, are often treated with neurotoxic pesticides known to cause certain neurological problems, e.g., Attention-deficit symptoms, impaired memory, etc.

7. Fat-free and low-fat milk

When raw milk is pasteurized, it loses a lot of its nutrients. Long-life milk is particularly unhealthy because it first has to be dried at about 1000 degrees Centigrade, after which water is added. No enzymes or any other nutrients can survive these high temperatures.

People usually choose low-fat or fat-free dairy products because they don't want to gain weight. However, they don't realize that carbs or sugar are added when fat is removed. This is done so that milk would have flavor; otherwise, it would taste like water. So, fat-free and low-fat milk contains added sugar, which puts you at risk of developing diabetes or heart disease if you drink a lot of milk.

8. Seitan

We usually think of seitan as a healthy alternative to meat protein. However, it is simply wheat gluten. It means that even if you are not allergic to gluten. Still, you often eat seitan, you may develop gluten intolerance symptoms. Besides, seitan contains a lot of sodium, over 500 milligrams per 100 grams.

It gets even unhealthier if you add non-dairy liquid creamers based on corn syrup. Black coffee is the healthiest option because although these additives improve the taste of coffee, they also contribute to increased liver fat and gastrointestinal problems.

9. Canned green beans

For some reason, U.S.-grown canned green beans are some of the most toxic canned foods there are. This food is treated with some of the most dangerous pesticides. Eating just one serving a day puts you at risk of developing cancer and having other health problems. Besides, all cans are lined with materials that contain Bisphenol-A. It is a synthetic estrogen that can create fertility problems for men and women. Unless you can find fresh or frozen green beans, you must avoid this one of the foods at all costs.

10. Energy drinks

The reason they are so addictive is that they taste so good. That's because energy drinks are full of sugar and flavor additives. Long-term energy drinks are linked to inflammatory processes, heart disease, and neurological problems.

The list of unhealthy foods is much longer, but the bottom line is to try and stay away from all processed, instant, or foods that don't even look like food. Instead, stick to organically grown fruits and vegetables whenever possible.

Chapter 5: 7 Common yet Dangerous Disease You Can Treat

Asthma

Asthma is a long-term chronic inflammation due to environmental and genetic factors of excess mucus production. It's pretty hard to avoid, but it's easier to heal. Traditional medicine uses supplements, fatty acids, breathing exercises, and breathing strategies to ensure the lungs' proper functioning. Dr. Sebi encourages the use of fennel, anise, chamomile teas, and alkaline fruits and vegetables.

If you have asthma, your airways will still be inflamed. They get even more swollen, and the airways' muscles will relax when something causes the symptoms. That makes it difficult for air to pass in and out of the lungs, causing symptoms such as coughing, wheezing, shortness of breath, and chest tightness.

These symptoms are closely linked to physical activity for many people living with asthma. And, some otherwise healthy people may experience asthma symptoms only when they exercise. Exercise-induced bronchoconstriction (EIB) or exercise-induced asthma (EIA). Staying involved is an effective way to remain well, but asthma isn't meant to keep you on the sidelines. Instead, your doctor may establish a treatment plan to keep your symptoms under control before, during, and after physical activity.

People who have a family background of allergies or asthma are more likely to develop asthma. Many people with asthma, too, have allergies. This is called allergic asthma.

Occupational asthma is caused by inhaling chemicals, gases, dust, or other potentially dangerous substances while at work.

Childhood asthma affects millions of children and their families. However, most children who develop asthma do so before five.

There is no remedy for asthma, but if it is correctly diagnosed and a care plan is in effect, you will control the condition and improve your quality of life.

Cancer

Cancer is among one the leading causes of death around the world. Simple lifestyle changes, such as maintaining a balanced diet, could prevent up to fifty percent of all cancers from occurring. However, treating cancer and having the strength to cope with cancer can depend on the excellent quality of the food you consume. Foods themselves do not cause cancer, but they can lead to chronic health conditions leading to cancer growth.

You will suffer from an increased risk of developing cancer if your diet is low in nutrients and fiber and high in sugar and processed foods. High blood sugar levels can increase the risk of developing cancers of the colorectal system, breasts, and stomach. In addition, cell division is stimulated by higher insulin levels in the body, needed for cancer cells to divide and spread. And more elevated blood sugar and insulin levels in your body can lead to inflammation, leading to the growth of abnormal cells that may become cancerous.

What Is Cancer?

Cancer is an uncontrolled group of unusual cells that invades normal tissues in any part of the body. These irregular cells are called cancer cells, malignant cells, or tumor cells.

The three most common cancers among men, women, and children are as follows:

- **Males** → prostate, liver, and colorectal
- **Women** → breasts, lungs, and colorectal
- **Children** → leukemia, brain, and lymphoma

Hypertension

High blood pressure and hypertension are long-term health problems in which blood pressure gradually rises. It is a significant risk factor for strokes, heart disease, vision loss, and dementia. To be healed, we must keep away from meat and alcohol, drink not too much tea, and eat fruits and vegetables approved by Dr. Sebi. The vegetables to be consumed are olives, wild rice, cabbage, cucumber, bell peppers, kale, squash, valerian, and chickpeas. Dry fruit is the best choice for our diet.

Symptoms of high blood pressure

If your blood pressure is excessively high, there might be several signs to check for, including:

- Extreme headache
- Fatigation or confusion
- Vision problem
- Chest pain
- Nosebleed
- Pounding in your chest, neck, or ears
- Difficulty breathing
- Irregular heartbeat
- Blood in the urine
- Facial flushing
- Nervousness
- Sweating
- Dizziness
- Trouble sleeping
- Blood spots in eyes

Diabetes

Diabetes occurs when your blood glucose becomes too high. Blood glucose is what your body uses as energy and is created from whatever you eat. Insulin, a hormone that your pancreas makes, helps the glucose move into your cells to be used as energy. However, there are times when the body doesn't make enough insulin. Then there are times when the body doesn't use the insulin correctly. This causes the glucose to remain in your blood, which won't reach your cells.

The longer that this goes on, the excess glucose in the blood can create severe health problems. Luckily, there is a way to reverse diabetes. Modern medicine also can help manage diabetes if a person chooses not to make drastic dietary changes.

People can also be diagnosed with pre-diabetes. At this stage, it is easier to reverse things and prevent diabetes from developing at all. But that doesn't mean pre-diabetes is any less important than full-blown diabetes.

While type 1 and type 2 diabetes have different causes, two factors still work in both. First, a person inherits some predisposition to this particular disease, and then something in your environment triggers the onset. Genes by themselves are not enough. A good example of this is with identical twins. For identical twins, they have identical genes. Still, when one of them develops type 1 diabetes, the other one will only develop the disease, at most, half the time. If one of them Develops type 2 diabetes, the odds of the other one developing it is three in four.

CKD

Your kidneys are two organs about your fist's size located near the bottom of your rib cage. Each kidney will be on either side of the spine. In each kidney, there are millions of tiny things called nephrons. These nephrons filter the blood.

You need your kidneys to have a healthy structure. Your kidneys filter out all the impurities in the blood, excessive water, and waste products. All these toxins get stored in the bladder and then removed through the urine. Your kidneys regulate the potassium, salt, and pH levels in your body. They also produce hormones that can control red blood cell production and help regulate blood pressure. In addition, your kidneys create a type of vitamin D that can help your body absorb calcium better.

Kidney disease will attack these nephrons. The damage it causes might leave the kidneys unable to get rid of the waste. Millions of people in the United States are affected by kidney disease. That happens when the kidneys get damaged and can't function properly. This damage might be caused by different long-term chronic conditions, high blood pressure, and diabetes. In addition, kidney disease could cause other problems such as malnutrition, nerve damage, and weak bones.

HIV

Signs of HIV infection may differ in form and severity from person to person, and some people do not have symptoms for several years.

The steps below explain how HIV infection develops in the body if left untreated. Without HIV antiretroviral therapy, the virus replicates in the body and does more and more damage to the immune system.

However, you can keep the infection under control and prevent it from spreading with successful care. That is why it is essential to start care as soon as possible after positive tests.

Herpes

Herpes is a widespread viral infection that causes sores on your genitals and mouth. It can be irritating and painful, but it doesn't necessarily lead to severe health issues.

Herpes is a very common virus that stays alive in your body. A lot of people have genital herpes. But the chances are that a few people you meet are dealing with it.

Herpes is caused by two distinct but related viruses: HSV-1 and HSV-2.

Depending on the type a person gets infected with, it can potentially attack several different parts of the body, such as:

- Vulva
- Vagina
- Cervix
- Uterus
- Penis and scrotum (if you're a man)
- Butt area
- Inner thighs
- Lips
- Neck
- Throat
- And sometimes your eyes

Herpes spreads from skin to skin contact with infected areas, particularly during vaginal intercourse, oral sex, anal sex, and kissing. It causes itchy, painful blisters or sores that come and go. Unfortunately, many people don't notice the sores or make a mistake about anything else because they do not know they're infected. As a result, you can spread herpes even though you have no pain or symptoms.

There is no traditional cure for it, but medications will relieve your symptoms and reduce the risk of spreading the virus to other people. And the good news is that outbreaks typically become less common with time. Although herpes may sometimes be uncomfortable and painful, it's not harmful. People with herpes have relationships, have sex, and live a relatively safe life.

Chapter 6: How to Naturally Reverse Diabetes

Diabetes happens when your blood glucose turns out to be excessively high. Blood glucose is what your body utilizes as vitality and is made from whatever you eat. Insulin, which is a hormone that your pancreas makes, enables the glucose to move into your cells with the goal that it very well may be utilized as vitality. Unfortunately, there are times when the body doesn't make enough insulin. The body doesn't utilize insulin effectively. This makes the glucose stay in your blood, and it won't arrive at your cells.

The longer that this goes on, the excess glucose in the blood can create severe health problems. Luckily, there is a way to reverse diabetes. Modern medicine also can help manage diabetes if a person chooses not to make drastic dietary changes.

People can also be diagnosed with pre-diabetes. At this stage, it is easier to reverse things and prevent diabetes from developing at all. But that doesn't mean pre-diabetes is any less important than full-blown diabetes.

While type 1 and type 2 diabetes have different causes, two factors still work in both. A person in her first, as some predisposition Genes by themselves are not enough. A good example of this is with identical twins. For identical twins, they have identical genes. Still, when one of them develops type 1 diabetes, the other one will only develop the disease, at most, half the time. If one of them Develops type 2 diabetes, the odds of the other one developing it is three in four.

Types of Diabetes

There isn't just one type of diabetes that a person can be diagnosed with; there are three types:

- Type 1
- Type 2
- Gestational

Type 1 diabetes, previously known as juvenile diabetes, is an auto-immune disease normally found in childhood. In this case, your body doesn't make enough insulin. The immune system will also attack and destroy the pancreatic cells that create insulin. Most people with type 1 diabetes will have to take insulin every single day.

About 5% of people with diabetes have type 1 diabetes.

Potential symptoms of diabetes include:

- Weight loss without an apparent reason
- Fatigue and tiredness
- Unclear or blurred vision and problems with sight
- Frequent urination
- Increased thirst and hunger

Once diagnosed with type 1 diabetes, they enter the honeymoon phase. During this time, the cells responsible for secreting insulin could continue to make the hormone for a bit before stopping altogether. At this stage, they won't need as many insulin shots to keep their glucose levels.

People with type 1 diabetes face taking insulin for the rest of their lives. You will work with your doctor to figure out the best schedule for your insulin doses. There are now continuous blood sugar monitors and insulin pumps. This hybrid machine can act as an artificial pancreas and remove the need for remembering when to take insulin. They will still need to manually check their blood sugar levels to ensure things are still okay.

Diet as an infant may also play a role. Type 1 diabetes isn't as common in those who breastfed and started eating solid foods later. For most people, developing type 1 diabetes tends to take several years.

A man with type 1 diabetes has a 1 in 17 chance of having a child who develops it. For a woman with type 2 diabetes who gives birth before the age of 25, there is a 1 in 25 risks that your child will develop it. If you give birth after the age of 25, the odds go down to 1 in 100.

Type 2 diabetes is acquired during life because of poor dietary choices and genetics. It can be developed at any age and even as a child. However, it is more common for middle-aged and older adults to be diagnosed. It is known as the most common form of diabetes.

Common causes of developing Type 2 diabetes are:

- Leading a sedentary life
- Being older than 45
- Being of Asian-pacific islander, Latin American, Native American, or African American descent
- History of PCOS
- Give birth to a child that weighed more than nine pounds or has gestational diabetes
- History of high blood pressure
- Having an HDL cholesterol level that is less than 40 or 50 mg/dl
- Family history of diabetes
- Being overweight

The family lineage factor for type 2 diabetes is stronger than type 1 diabetes. Studies in twins have found that genetics plays a big role in developing type 2. Yet, the environment still plays a big role as well. Lifestyle tends to play a very big role as well. Obesity often runs in families, and families will often have similar exercise and eating habits.

Gestational diabetes only affects women during pregnancy. For the most part, diabetes will go away once the woman gives birth. However, the mother is also at a higher risk of developing type 2 diabetes later in life.

Pre-diabetes simply means having a higher blood sugar level than it should be but isn't high enough to be considered diabetes. It does place you at a greater risk of developing type 2 diabetes. They will suggest that the person start making healthy life changes to stop the progression. Eating healthier foods and losing weight will often prevent the development of diabetes.

How common?

In 2015, it was said that 30.3 million people in the United States had diabetes, which comes out to about 9.4% of the population. Of those, more than one in four didn't know they had the disease Race, physical inactivity, some certain health issues like high blood pressure can also affect your odds of developing diabetes. In addition, gestational diabetes and pre-diabetes also put you at a higher risk of developing type 2 diabetes.

Lifestyle Changes for Diabetes

At first, the doctor will tell a person with diabetes is to make some lifestyle changes to help support a healthy life and weight loss. Then, doctors may send you to a special nutritionist to help you manage the condition. Some of the most common changes diabetics are told to make include:

- When exercising, recognize the signs of low blood sugar, including profuse sweating, weakness, confusion, and dizziness.

- Take part in at least 30 minutes of exercise each day, five days a week. Some of the best exercises for people with diabetes include swimming, biking, aerobics, and walking.

- Abstaining from drinking alcohol or cutting back to one glass a day for women and two men.

- Staying away from high-sugar foods that only provide you with empty calories or calories won't provide you with any nutritional benefits, like sweets, fried foods, and sodas.

- Eating a high diet is healthful and fresh food, like whole grains, healthy fats, vegetables, and fruits.

- Lowering your BMI is also a great way to manage type 2 diabetes without medications. Making your weight loss slow and steady will help you retain the benefits.

Dr. Sebi's Diabetes Cure

Although there is a lot of good advice for people with diabetes that doctors will share, such as lifestyle changes, you could also end up being prescribed. And let's not get started on how scary it must be to learn how to give you insulin injections.

Dr. Sebi's diabetes cure is a super simple plan, and it doesn't cost that much. Very few people wanted to try his plan at first because it required fasting. Most would rather cut off their feet than not eat. However, Dr. Sebi could cure his diabetes with a 27 day fast.

Many other people have reported similar results as well. In addition, you can find many videos on YouTube, where people talk about having cured their diabetes with Dr. Sebi's plan.

Like with STD treatments, the goal is to rid the body of excess mucus. For people with diabetes, excess mucus is found in the pancreatic duct. Dr. Sebi's mother started fasting to help her diabetes, and after 57 days, she was cured.

During your fast, you should:

- drink water,
- have herbal teas

A great herbal tea to drink is a combination of burdock, black walnut leaf, red raspberry, and elderberry.

How to prepare it:

- Practice a tablespoon of each and mix them into one and a half liters of spring water.
- Carry this to a boil and let it steep for 15 minutes.
- Take this off the heat and mix in another half-litter of water.
- Strain out the herbs and place them to the side to use the next day.
- Store the tea in the fridge and drink as much as you want during the day.

When they overhear the word fast, many people assume that means they can't take anything by mouth. But that's not Dr. Sebi's fast. See, when Dr. Sebi fasted to cure his diabetes, he would take three green plus tablets each day and drink sea moss tea, spring water, and tamarind juice. You don't have to drink tamarind juice, though. Any juice that is on the approved list of foods is okay. It must be fresh juice, though. You don't want pre-made juice with a bunch of added sugars.

Once you have fasted for a while, and your body will tell you when you have had enough, you need to start the Dr. Sebi-approved diet plan. Along with that, you should also think about taking black seeds, mulberry leaves, and fig leaves. Research on black seeds has found that taking as little as two teaspoons of the powder each day can reverse diabetes.

Figleaves are the top alternative medicine for diabetes on the market today. Mulberry leaves are a common treatment for diabetes in the Middle East. These can be made into tea, and you can also mix in some black seeds.

Some other foods that you should consider adding to your diet are:

1. Ginseng
2. Okra
3. Ginger
4. Fenugreek
5. Red clover
6. Swiss chard
7. Avocado
8. Bitter melon

Chapter 7: How to Naturally Reverse High Blood Pressure

What is high blood pressure?

If the arteries' walls were clogged or packed with plagues, blood flow would become restricted as it pumps from the heart to the aorta. When the arteries create pressure in a situation like this, the blood pressure becomes higher than it should be, resulting in hypertension (high blood pressure).

Poor diet is the leading cause of high blood pressure in the United States as it has been reported that over 85 percent of reported high blood pressure cases are rooted in a poor diet. More than any other race in the United States, African Americans reported more high blood pressure cases. In addition, high blood pressure leads to other diseases such as kidney diseases, strokes, scarlet fever, large heart, typhoid fever, artery coronary diseases, and tonsillitis. These diseases are rampant among African Americans who have a hypertensive health history.

High blood pressure is caused when the blood flowing to the arteries is high due to consuming foods capable of clogging the arteries' wall. This act results in pressure through the arteries during blood flow distribution. First, blood is pumped by the heart to the aorta then the arteries. Peradventure, the arteries' walls become narrow and hardened due to excessive plague caused by poor eating habits, blood flow in the passageway of the arteries suppresses. Worthy of note is that as an individual gets older, the arteries get hardened bit by bit, and a bad diet will triple the possibility of high blood pressure.

Asides from clogged arteries, high blood pressure can also be caused by poor blood circulation, synthetic drugs, processed foods, and unhealthy behavior patterns.

These behavioral patterns include the following:

1. Bad diet
2. Tobacco intake
3. Stress
4. Excess coffee intake
5. Fried and processed foods
6. Over-eating
7. Aging

Symptoms of High Blood Pressure:

- Difficulty breathing
- Blurry vision
- Rapid pulses
- Constant headache

According to Dr. Sebi, high blood pressure symptoms can be likened to "navy seal snipers", as there are no signs of high blood pressure.

Dr. Sebi High blood pressure diet:

Every high blood pressure drug in the market imitates water. That's why it is important for you as an individual to drink a lot of clean water. To be effective, you will need to divide your weight by 2 and drink that much water daily. Why that much water? You may ask. Well, water thins the blood and makes passing through the arteries easy.

Taking five different types of fruits (vegetables included) a day will prevent the arteries from getting clogged due to excess plaque deposits. Fruits and vegetables containing many antioxidants protect the artery walls from plaque deposits. Such fruits include cabbage, tomatoes, oranges, seed grapes, and peaches.

Foods rich in potassium help reduce recurrent high blood pressure by expelling excess sodium from the body.

Fiber-containing fruits are also of high benefit to high blood pressure sufferers. It will lower blood pressure while simultaneously removing wastes from the artery walls.

Food-related high blood pressure knowledge is important. Not knowing what foods to eat and avoid is detrimental to blood pressure. No one wants to get high blood pressure from eating like everybody else.

Here are some tips about it:

- Avoid overeating even the healthiest of food.
- Avoid salty foods as much as possible as they transform into plaque in the artery walls. In essence, avoid sodas, baking soda, soy sauce, and meat tenderizers.
- Never eat canned foods.
- Eliminate dairy products such as sodium, cheese, and alcohol from your diet.
- Do not eat in the evening
- Avoid every other type of rice except wild and brown

Dr. Sebi High blood pressure medication natural herbs:

Dr. Sebi highly recommends these herbs like the one that helps open the blood vessels, open the arteries walls and eliminate plaques from the wall of arteries. They contain natural alkaline, are high in minerals, and have been medically proven effective as blood pressure medication.

Some of these herbs include:

1. Fennel
2. Oregano
3. Basil
4. Yellow dock
5. Cayenne

Chapter 8: Understanding Your Lungs Health and Diseases

Phlegm is nothing more than a jelly-like mucus produced by the mucous membranes. These fluids are also expelled from the body through the lungs, bronchioles, and diaphragm. This waste is disgusting and disgusting. Getting in contact with phlegm makes you want to vomit. Phlegm doesn't have a definite perspective; sometimes, it can be as clear as water; other times, it can be yellowish, green, dark, gray, light, or brown, depending on the type of food you eat. Some feel that the phlegm color expelled from your body indicates how healthy you are. Still, there is no substantial evidence to support this yet.

Phlegm can be compared to a chameleon that will take on the color of its surroundings. In this case, the color of the food consumed is considered. Mucus and phlegm are similar to inexperienced eyes. Still, they have their differences: one is more dangerous to human health than the other. You will soon find out how it happened.

Mucus is a gelatinous liquid secreted by the mucous membranes; the consistency is thick and slippery. This liquid contains abundant water and glycoproteins.

Difference between phlegm and mucus

Mucus and phlegm are not identical, although most people consider them one. Let me explain, our natural body produces mucus as a defense mechanism. For example, mucus captures bacteria so they do not enter the body. But eat too many unnatural foods that cause your body to produce excessive mucus. That will be a problem because your cells and organs will be starved of oxygen.

On the other hand, phlegm is very difficult to expel. The presence of phlegm in the body is an indication that there is a disease lurking somewhere. When phlegm is excreted, mucus accompanies it, just like bacteria. This is yet another reason why phlegm is more troublesome for our bodies.

Mucus disease

It is ideal to know the concept of disease, the environments in which it develops, and the causes. These are the keys to staying away from illnesses and ailments that your doctor will never tell you about. There will be no need for a healer when we know these things because getting sick will be rare. The disease is found in the body when you ingest a substance that does not live up to your body. This substance will conflict with our genetic structure, and this will end up making us sick and weakened. Almost everyone usually gets sick because of the excess mucus in the body. The cause of most diseases is the presence of excessive mucus in the body.

When mucus accumulates excessively in the body, the mucous membrane breaks, and the cells are covered with excess mucus. The mucous membrane serves to protect the body from invasion by aerobic bacteria.

When our diet consists of acidic foods, the mucous membrane breaks down, and the mucus already secreted enters the bloodstream. When this happens, the other groups of cells that belong to the organs are deprived of oxygen.

- When mucus reaches the nostrils → It is called Sinusitis;
- When it flows into the bronchial tube → It is called Bronchitis,
- When it enters the lungs →, It is called Pneumonia.
- When it enters the prostate → It is called Prostatitis
- When it enters a woman's uterus → It is called Endometriosis
- When it gets in your eyes → There will be a vision problem.

There you have it, six different diseases caused by mucus. There are many more of them.

When you have symptoms of one of these diseases, the underlying cause is the overproduction of mucus caused by an inadequate diet.

Phlegm, Mucus, and throat

Humans experience phlegm every time. When you cough with phlegm after eating, it results from consuming acidic foods. Now you understand that the overly acidic food you eat is the cause of your phlegm cough. If you start producing a lot of phlegm through coughing after eating a certain type of food, you need to stay away from that food. The production of excess phlegm due to consuming a certain food type indicates unhealthy food. Excessive secretion of phlegm will deprive your body of oxygen and other parts of your internal organs.

Acidic foods do not complete the biological structure of the human body. The body's reaction is to make more mucus each time you eat acidic foods. The excess mucus in the lengths will spread to the throat. This situation will lead you to cough up phlegm after every meal you eat. A temporary solution to this condition is to gargle with salt water, but what is needed is a diet change to prevent the body from producing excess mucus. If you refuse to change your diet to one that eliminates excess phlegm production, there will be more to cough up each time you eat acidic foods. Every organ in the body that houses this excessive mucus will experience one disease or another.

To help your body create a balance in mucus and phlegm production, herbs such as:

1. Wild cherry bark
2. Echinacea
3. Slippery elm bark
4. Chickweed
5. Ginkgo biloba
6. Burdock
7. And lobelia

It should be considered an essential part of your diet.

Dieting tips for mucus relief

Avoid eating the following to help your body get rid of excessive phlegm and mucus:

1. **White flour and white sugar** → they are highly processed acidic foods
2. **Eggs** → it is difficult for the body to digest a fetus, which is what eggs are.
3. **Sugar** → It is one of the main causes of severe diseases, such as Diabetes and High Blood Pressure.
4. **Bread** → processed, dairy, and acidic ingredients like white flour, eggs, white sugar, or GMO grains.
5. **Dairies** → due to thick phlegm and excess mucus that dairy produces in the body.

Also, stop smoking and remove tobacco from your home. Phlegm and mucus should not be played with, as leaving them unattended can lead to conditions such as pneumonia, lung congestion, acute bronchitis, chronic bronchitis, and bronchiectasis.

Chapter 9: Everything You Need to Cleanse Your Lungs

Mucus is an aqueous secretion produced by the cells of the mucous glands. It serves as a covering for the mucous membranes. Mucus is mainly composed of water, which is the mucin secretion.

It is an important element of the epithelial lining fluid, the airway surface liquid, the respiratory tract's lining. Mucus helps to protect the lungs during breathing by trapping foreign particles and infectious agents like dust, allergens, virus, bacteria, etc.

The human body always produces more mucus to protect and prevent airway tissues from drying out. Thus, there is a continuous production of mucus in the respiratory system.

When foreign objects get trapped by the mucus, the mucus becomes thick and changes color most of the time. This thick mucus usually coughed out as sputum is known as phlegm.

Mucus also plays an important role in the digestive system. The layer formed by the mucus in the small intestine and colon helps to protect the intestinal epithelial cells from bacterial infections. It also serves as a lubricant for the movement of foods through the esophagus.

Interestingly, mucus is the body's natural lubricant in females, which helps during sexual intercourse. It also helps to fight against infection in the reproductive system.

Mucus and Body Health

There is a continuous process of mucus production in the body, which protects the body systems from infections and provides the necessary lubrication.

Thus, the presence of mucus in our bodies is important. When mucus traps foreign and infectious bodies, it becomes phlegm. Phlegm and excess mucus in the body are not healthy. As the body produces up to a liter of mucus every day, it is vital to get rid of it to keep it healthy.

Accumulation of mucus in the body is the major cause of illnesses, as claimed by Dr. Sebi. So, excess mucus can be a red flag for the unhealthy state of the body.

Causes of Mucus Buildup in the Body

Its production triggers snails and other animals that secrete mucus. However, the major triggers in human beings are dryness and inflammation of the body.

Some factors that may lead to dryness, inflammation, and other mucus secretion triggers are:

- Dry air
- Smoking
- Allergies
- Infections
- Acid reflux
- Asthma
- Low water/liquid consumption
- Medications

These factors and more contribute to excess buildup of mucus in the body. The body naturally produces it to ensure that foreign objects (toxic or infectious) don't interact with the body cells. The more we have these foreign bodies, the more the body produces mucus.

When these objects get trapped by the mucus, they become thick and build phlegm.

Moreover, our body must stay lubricated for the swift movement of particles and cells in the body. Thus, the body's dryness makes the body produce more mucus, which is the liquid the body can produce naturally.

Mucus Natural Cleanse - The Dr. Sebi Way

If you are on the Dr. Sebi Diet, below are simple steps to clear out and prevent excess mucus and maintain the diet recommendations.

Hydration

Enough liquid in the body, especially warm liquid, can help drain the sinuses and thin the mucus. Thus, drinking high amounts of water can help clear out mucus from the body.

Dr. Sebi recommends a high intake of water. Also, most fruits and vegetables recommended by Dr. Sebi's diet have high water content. These foods help to keep the body hydrated and prevent excess mucus production.

Moreover, some drinks like coffee and alcohol can cause dehydration in the body. Therefore, anyone on the Dr. Sebi diet must stay away from alcohol; it helps to avoid dehydration.

Action:

Take a lot of water, smoothies, and juice made with Dr. Sebi-approved foods.

Expectorant:

An expectorant is known to help in clearing mucus. Expectorant loosens and thins mucus, making it easy to cough it out of the system.

Some herbs in the Dr. Sebi diet can serve as expectorants. However, the Red Clover's major and most used herb in the Dr. Sebi approved herbs.

Red Clover is a super healthy herb that aids circulation in the body. It is a natural blood purifier and also serves as an expectorant. It is widely used by women in treating menopause-related conditions like hot flashes and lumbar spine protection.

So taking red clover can help loosen and clear mucus from the body.

Action:

In 8 oz of hot water, steep 1 - 2 teaspoons of the dried flower, allow up to 30 minutes. Then drink at least 2 and not more than 3 cups per day.

Or sip 1ml of the fluid extract with hot water three times daily.

Essential Oils:

Some essential oils have been proposed to effectively treat lung disease-related symptoms. For example, people use essential oils to treat and prevent chest colds and sinusitis. These essential oils can be obtained from Dr. Sebi-approved products like eucalyptus, oregano, and thyme.

Eucalyptus has been widely used to treat coughs and reduce mucus production for many years. It helps to loosen the mucus so it can be easily coughed out. Thus, it relieves nagging coughs.

Action:

Make your homemade vapor rub by adding 12 drops of eucalyptus oil to ¼ cup of coconut oil.

Alternatively, add 1 drop of eucalyptus oil to 1 teaspoon of water.

First, test the mixture to know whether it is safe for use. Then apply it directly to your skin, especially your throat and chest. That makes the scents easily reach the nose and mouth.

Note: These recommendations are for adults only.

Additional tips

- Eating many high-fiber foods may help treat respiratory issues linked to phlegm. So there are loads of fiber-rich foods in Dr. Sebi's diet.
- Capsaicin in cayenne may help to thin and clear out sinuses temporarily. This gets the mucus to move easily.
- Drinks and foods containing ginger can help clear excess mucus and treat cough.
- Gargling with warm salt water may not only kill germs. In addition, it can help to remove mucus that accumulates on the back of our throat.

The methods we have discussed truly help cleanse the mucus from the body. But the result might not be as fast as we want it.

However, we can catalyze the process and make it faster. So, yes, we can cleanse mucus as soon as we desire, depending on the program we follow. But before you follow any program, consult your health professional. Remember, developers of any health program only give you what works for them.

They do not know your health condition. So, they use the health condition they know as a standard or reference. So, do your due diligence and consult your doctor first.

To boost the mucus cleansing process, below are listed simple steps I found to be very effective on myself:

- Every morning, do 5-10 minutes of breathing exercise upon arising.
- Immediately after, drink 16 ounces of prune juice.
- Drink grape juice throughout the day, especially after lunch.
- Eat your dinner before 7 pm every day. About 15 minutes later, drink 3-4 tablespoons of onion water. Grate the onion and soak in the water around noon to stay in the water for about 7-8 hours before use.
- Finally, do another 5 minutes of breathing exercise before you sleep.

Righteously follow this simple program for at least 7 days for results to be noticeable

Note: Mucus is not a harmful substance in our bodies. It is a vital element in the system, as discussed in its roles in the body. So, having it does not mean illness.

We are much concerned about having excess or accumulation of this liquid in our body systems. Accumulation is not good for the body and may lead to various diseases.

But before you take any action regarding mucus, or any health-related issue in your body, consult your doctor first.

Chapter 10: Tips for a Good Kickstart and a Longer Life

To properly switch to Dr. Sebi's diet plans, it will be best to make small changes at the beginning of your overall eating habits. Gradually, these small changes will prepare you mentally and emotionally.

Emotional and Mental Preparation

Eating is an essential part of our lives. It is important to provide everyday energy and nutrition requirements for our bodies. The types of foods and substances we eat every day become our habits, and these habits can last for our life if we do not try to mind them.

Usually, these habits can be extremely hard to change or stop. Moreover, our friends, family, and colleagues' influence makes it hard to change our daily habits. For example, you can't deny a piece of cake and other junk foods if it is a birthday party at your own home.

Therefore, before you rush to start with Dr. Sebi's diet, you should make a plan about changing your diet habits. A start without a proper plan and understanding may fail due to a lack of preparation. It will be best to discuss and reveal your plans to all the people you interact with within your regular life.

Drink More Water

Water is essential for our bodies. It is well known that around 75% of our body is water and can't survive even for three days without water.

Drinking more water cleanses our bodies and maintains our healthy brain and body functions. Among Dr. Sebi's products, Bromide plus Powder has natural herbs like Bladderwrack that induce laxative effects and promote urination to remove toxins. Drinking more water will replenish this lost water and will keep you hydrated.

It is recommended to drink up to one gallon of spring water every day. Spring water is recommended because it is alkaline. It is different from tap water, high in chloride and other contaminants.

Add Whole Foods to Your Diet

You should add more whole foods to your existing diet. The basic idea is to consume whole foods to replace packaged foods full of additives. Cutting off these additives from your diet will help you later in your plans.

Also, note that refined sugar is extremely addictive, causing food cravings.

Switch slow

You should start with the foods you already eat as a part of your diet. It doesn't matter if you are taking a vegan diet, but make sure that you are not using processed meals. It will be best to cook your food, that means homemade food is recommended. For example, if you are taking fish in your meals, it is okay to just reduces the frequency at the beginning without cutting it cold turkey. Eventually, you want to switch to a full alkaline electric diet in around 30 days.

After you leave the processed food completely and homemade food becomes your daily habit, you are on the right path to regain your health. Your next steps will bring you totally towards the right diet.

You should research new recipes with the same ingredients and learn them to remain monotonous. For example, you can cook a single vegetable in many different ways to change its taste and feel without losing the nutritional qualities.

Read Ingredient Labels

It won't be easy for some people to quit processed food at once. But before you consume such foods, be sure to check the food ingredient labels. This will help you stay alert about what you are eating or drinking.

In the beginning, as you are not eating a strict diet, checking the labels will make you nutrition-conscious, and it will help you change your habits as you progress.

Later, when you switch to a proper strict diet plan, you will still be conscious about your nutrition if you go astray from it.

Snacks

Snacks are very addictive. It becomes your compulsive habit, and you eat and eat without watching the nutrition status. Many people like to have snacks now and then, but instead of eating chips, why not try a mixture of walnuts, raisins, and other dried fruits? These dry fruits will replace processed snacks and will provide you the right nutrition.

Chapter 11: Alkaline Herbs and Spices

Detoxification or cleansing depends on the types of fasting you desire. Trust me; it will do better if you consume some cleansing herbs during your fasting period. However, suppose you decide to do the water fasting for a week, then throughout that week. In that case, you should consume only water and the cleansing herbs in a tea, and nothing else should be consumed.

Herbs that you should use as part of the detox process are:

Cascara sagrada

Most people only know a shrub plant as a "dietary supplement" sold in pharmacies as a counter drug. However, in 2002, the FDA declared that it doesn't meet the standards to be sold over counter drugs (OTC) or prescription drugs. Before then, the dietary supplement or the bark of Cascara Sagrada was used as a purgative for constipation. One sweet thing about this shrub is that it is a bitter, less extract that can also be used as a flavoring agent.

Rhubarb Root

It is the root and underground stem (that is, rhizome) of the Rhubarb plant. The traditional Chinese people have used this plant's root to treat digestive tract disorders, including stomach pain, constipation, menstrual cramps (dysmenorrhea), diarrhea, and swelling of the pancreas. This plant's stems are also used as a flavoring agent and mostly used to make pie and serve as great recipes. Because of the chemicals that Rhubarb root contains, such as fiber, research has it that it a potent laxative has the potency to reduce swelling, treat cold sores and improves the tone and health of the digestive tract, clean heavy metal and harmful bacteria, improve the general movement of the intestines and also, reduce cholesterol levels.

Prodigiosa

It is a flowering plant/shrub from the daisy family and is native to Mexico and California. The Mexican has used these plant/shrubs as a tea to treat diarrhea, diabetes, and stomach pain. Research carried on Prodigiosa shows that the plant is an antioxidant. It contains chemical compounds that help stimulate the pancreatic gland to be secret and reduce or lower blood sugar levels, aid the digestion of fat in the gallbladder, and improve the stomach digestive system's health.

Burdock root

It is the root of a plant called Burdock that can be found worldwide. Virtually everything about Burdock is important. The root is used as food and medicine, while its leaf and seed are used for medicinal purposes. Many people believe that consuming Burdock helps increase urine flow, eradicate germs, purify the blood, prevent and treat cancer, joint pain, cold, diabetes, anorexia, fever, bladder infections, syphilis, stomach and intestinal complaints. However, this plant does not stop there as it also helps treat and prevent skin diseases such as; acne and psoriasis. Burdock also helps in boosting sex drive (libido), lowering high blood pressure, and cleansing the liver and lymphatic system.

Dandelion

It is a flowering plant, also known as "Taraxacum officinale," native to Europe. However, it is commonly found in the mild climates of the northern hemisphere. These flowering plants have been in use for centuries before now to treat swelling (inflammation) of the pancreas, cancer, tonsils (tonsillitis), acne, bladder or urethra, digestive, and liver disorders. Because of the vitamin (A, B, C, E, and K), mineral (iron, potassium, magnesium, and calcium) and other compounds (Polyphenols,

Chicoric and Chlorogenic acid) that Dandelion contains, research has it that it has the potency to detoxify gallbladder, kidney and purifies the blood. It also dissolves kidney stones, treats and prevent diabetes and relief liver and urinary disorder. It also contains chemicals that may increase urine production, preventing the urinary tract and preventing crystals from forming in the urine.

Elderberry

It is also known as European elderberry, black elder, or Sambucus nigra. It is a flowering plant that belongs to the family of Adoxaceae and the native to Europe. These flowering plants are common in Europe and many other parts of the world. This plant can grow as long as 9 meters. That is 30feet tall and has many clusters (white or cream-colored flowers) known as elderflowers. The elderberry leaves have been used to treat pain, inflammation, swelling, stimulate urine production, and induce sweat. The bark is not left behind as it was also used as a laxative, diuretic, and to induce vomiting.

Guaco

It is a climbing plant known as "Guace" or "Ventolin". This climbing plant is rich in various minerals and compounds. It is from the family of Asteraceae and the species of cordifolia. Its leaf is very medicinal and nutritional.

Mullein

It is a flavorful beverage plant that is also known as 'Aaron's rod, Candlewick, American mullein, Adam's flannel, Denseflower mullein, Candleflower, European or orange mullein etc. this flavorful beverage plant has been used for centuries before now for the treatment of diverse sicknesses, which include; asthma, tuberculosis, pneumonia, chills flu, gastrointestinal bleeding, colds, chronic coughs and others.

Natural Herbal Teas

According to Dr. Sebi, it is important to maintain a "consistent use of natural botanical remedies' and doing so will cleanse and detoxify the body.

While using herbs and natural remedies is an important step on your journey to greater health, you must also make the correct adjustments to your eating habits by following the recommended food list.

We have seen that plant-based nutrition is fundamental for a healthy diet. But when we talk about plants, we can't consider only fruits and vegetables; there is also an incredible variety of herbs with a powerful alkaline effect. We need to understand how important they could be for our health: they have a real healing effect that prevents many diseases.

Herbal medicine is a very ancient practice. It consists of a series of healing techniques based on plants. The official modern medicine is also aware of many plants' extraordinary properties. Therefore, it uses them for many common drugs.

We can naturally assume most of their macronutrients simply through infusions, so we can't neglect them in our alkaline diet.

Chamomile

Many people use it to relax or sleep. Still, very few people know its important alkaline effect: when you're stressed or worried, your body increases acid production, so chamomile tea, thanks to its relaxing effect, helps your body balance its pH value. Moreover, chamomile fights arachidonic acid, resulting in an important anti-inflammatory effect.

Alfalfa

Also called Lucerne, it is a less-known herb with an incredibly high level of nutrients. Its name means "Father of All Foods"; it contains many vitamins, minerals, protein, and essential amino acids. Beyond its alkalizing effect, it allows you to reset your metabolism and stay away from different common diseases.

More in details, it can:

- Lower the cholesterol level
- Increase immune system functionality
- Clean the blood
- Support digestion

- Alleviate allergies
- Relieve all forms of arthritis
- Relieve headaches and migraines

You should drink alfalfa tea daily, mixing it with another flavored tea if you prefer, since alfalfa is very mild in flavor. Or you could take this herb in capsule form. Whatever you decide, remember that this herb should never be missing; it is one of the biggest secrets for an incredibly healthy life!

Dandelion

It is another alkaline herb that you can eat as tea or a salad. It is an effective aid against kidney stones; it promotes weight loss and contains potent Antioxidants. Dandelion is very rich in vitamin C and folic acid, which are susceptible to heat: for this reason, I suggest you consume this herb as a fresh vegetable, preparing delicious salads with other vegetables. Dandelion is, of course, very cheap. You can easily collect it in the fields or cultivate it in your garden, so you should seriously consider adding this herb to your daily healthy diet.

Red Clover

A particular and almost unknown medicinal herb tea is based on red clover. It contains flavones, natural phytoestrogens with high antioxidant effects, cancer prevention, indigestion, asthma, and bronchitis. Red clover is particularly suitable for women because it promotes female reproductive health, reducing breast cancer risk.

Many herbs are undervalued: usually, people think that their only purpose is to add flavor to our dishes, but they add much more than that.

For example, I think of:

- Parsley
- Basil
- Cilantro
- Oregano
- Sage
- Thyme

Nobody knows that parsley contains more vitamin C than oranges! It also has a very high percentage of vitamin K and a lot of iron.

Basil releases high eugenol quantities into our body, a powerful anti-inflammatory, while oregano is one of the best sources of free-radical fighters.

Among the other alkaline herbs, we can use to prepare excellent infusions, we can mention lime, sarsaparilla, verbena, sage, and laurel.

Laurel is a valid ally against respiratory diseases like flu, bronchitis, cough, and pharyngitis. Moreover, it has positive effects on treating vascular problems and arteriosclerosis. You should also consider buying the essential oil, which has antibacterial and antitussive properties (I suggest taking 4 drops of this essential oil 3 times a day).

Chapter 12: Dr.Sebi Supplements

Besides eating the foods listed in Dr. Sebi's nutritional guide, I recommend buying his proprietary supplements. Dr.Sebi guaranteed they would aid in cleansing your body and nourishing your cells.

The recommended package is the all-inclusive option, consisting of all 20 available supplements. This is the best option because it quickly cleans and restores the body.

Alternatively, you can purchase individual supplements based on your health goals. Each has its unique benefits. For more details, let's take a look at some of the supplements and what they offer:

- **Sea Moss/Seaweed →** This nutritious plant has rich calcium, magnesium, iron, and ninety-two other essential minerals. It also contains many vitamins and is quite versatile in ingesting them. Sea moss can be incorporated in baking, blended into smoothies, used as an ingredient for gravies, ice creams, and fashioned into desserts. It is well known for its healing aspects and ability to promote a balanced restoration of the mucous membrane, thus improving your overall health. The ailments it can help treat include skin conditions.

- **Uterine Wash and Oil →** It is used to clean and restore your vaginal canal's natural state. Pour boiling water (8 0z) over one tablespoon of the herb, wait for it to cool, and use it to douche.

- **Viento** – This is an energizer and cleanser. It will revitalize your body and increase the oxygen levels in your brain and blood. It is rich in iron, which forms hemoglobin in red blood cells. The supplement also works on your kidneys and the lymphatic, respiratory, and central nervous systems. Also, it combats addiction to a substance, such as drugs. Take a daily dosage of four capsules.

- **Tooth Powder** – This unique herb combination helps cleanse your teeth. It also nourishes gums and retards gum disease and tooth decay. After wetting the brush, add about 1/8 of the powder, then brush.

- **Testo** – By nourishing your endocrine system, this supplement aids in balancing your hormones. As a result, it increases virility and betters sexual responsiveness. Additionally, Testo encourages a healthy flow of blood to male genitalia.

- **Green Food Plus** – This formula contains several minerals. It consists of herbs rich in chlorophyll for the whole body. Apart from promoting nourishment and good health, this supplement also helps the heart, the central nervous system, and the brain. Take four capsules daily.

- **Banju** – Conditions of the central nervous system—such as irritability, stress, insomnia, and irritability—can be addressed with this supplement. It was made for kids with ADD and ADHD but is also effective in mature people. The dosage is two tablespoons twice a day.

- **Iron Plus** offers iron-rich nourishment to the brain, blood, and central nervous system. It was developed to purify and provide strength to your entire body. This supplement also prevents inflammation. The dosage is two tablespoons per day.

- **Hair Food Oil** – It provides nourishment to the scalp and hair. For best results, apply daily.

- **Hair Follicle Fortifier** – Its role is cleansing and strengthening hair follicles to promote new hair growth.

- **Bio Ferro Capsules** – They purify and nourish your blood and contain herbs rich in iron phosphate and several other minerals that nourish and strengthen your entire system.

It is worth noting that these supplements do not guide all the nutrients and quantities. Therefore, it makes it difficult to know if, by taking them, you will meet your daily nutritional requirements. Contact your doctor to discuss this further.

Conclusion

Dr. Sebi's diet is planned to prevent and cure several diseases, but it is also planned for people who love to live healthy by remaining lean and clean.

His diet comprises alkaline grains, vegetables, fruits, nuts, tea, seeds, natural alkaline sweeteners, etc... At the same time, all animal products are not included.

Dr. Sebi argued that all diseases thrive in an acidic environment and cannot survive when the body is alkaline. That means that when the body is acidic, it contains an increased amount of toxic substances that promote diseases.

He argued that mucus accumulation in the body is one of the major factors predisposing you to disease. He concluded that you are getting rid of any disease you are suffering from when you remove the excess mucus in the body.

The diet of Dr. Sebi has been proven effective by dieters who truly use them. The diets re-energize and revitalize the body by returning it to its normal state.

Dr. Sebi's foods and herbs are used to cure asthma, diabetes, obesity (over-weight), erectile dysfunction, hypertension, Lupus, Leukemia…and many more.

"The healing of many sufferers who have asthma and many other prevalent diseases didn't occur because of the medications they take but because of the self-healing in the body due to an alkaline diet", as Dr. Sebi stated.

He learned that the body is contracting diseases with excess toxic substances and mucus accumulation.

He stated that people suffering from depressive illness or who want to prevent diseases should always eat an alkaline diet. When the body removes the increased amount of acidic substances and mucus, it becomes free from infections.

Dr. Sebi argues that the body's cleansing and detoxification is an essential and significant tool essential in dealing with infectious illnesses.

Detoxification assists the body in eliminating excess mucus accumulated in the liver, lungs… and many other body organs; it also helps in the removal of excess acidic substances, thereby making the body free from problems and sicknesses caused by acidity like ulcers, inflammation, internal heat, gastrointestinal disorder, heartburn, intestinal perforation, self-cellular digestion, nervous disorder, chronic fatigue, infertility, hormonal depletion, nervousness, dizziness… and many others.

The great herbalist also used herbs to re-energize and revitalize the body of the major nutrients required for proper functions.

Your body's organs function properly when there is an improvement in your health, indicating that your body is void of infectious diseases.

BOOK 2: <u>DR. SEBI TREATMENTS</u>

HOW TO GET RID OF THE 11 MOST COMMON YET LIFE-CHANGING CHRONIC DISEASES NATURALLY USING DR. SEBI'S OFFICIAL TREATMENTS | CURE FOR ACNE, ASTHMA, HYPERTENSION, AND PCOS INCLUDED.

Chapter 1: Dr. Sebi and His Philosophy

The man behind the Dr. Sebi Diet is Alfredo Bowman. He is a Honduran self-proclaimed herbalist and healer who uses food to improve health. Although he is already deceased, he has many followers in the 21st century. He has claimed to cure many diseases using herbs and a strict vegan diet because of his holistic approach. He has set up a treatment center in his home country before moving to New York City. He has continued his practice and extended his clienteles from Michael Jackson, John Travolta, Eddie Murphy, and Steven Sea gal, to name a few.

Although he calls himself Dr. Sebi, he does not hold any medical nor Ph.D. degree. Moreover, the diet has claimed to cure different conditions such as sickle-cell anemia, lupus, leukemia, and HIV-AIDS. That led to many issues, particularly that he practiced medicine without a license. While he was charged for practicing without a license, he was acquitted in the early 1990s due to a lack of evidence. After that, however, he was instructed to stop claiming that his diet could treat HIV-AIDS. Nevertheless, while controversies surround his name, there are so many benefits of his alkaline vegan diet that it is still popular even to this date.

Dr. Sebi believed that acidity and mucus could cause different types of diseases. For instance, mucus build-up in the lungs can lead to pneumonia. He noted that eating certain food types and avoiding others like the plague can help detoxify the body. It can also bring the body to an alkaline state, reducing the risk of developing many diseases. The cells can be rejuvenated and easily eliminate toxins by turning the blood alkaline. Moreover, he argues that diseases cannot exist in an alkaline environment. His principle of making the body more alkaline is what other plant-based diets are banking on.

This diet relies on eating a list of approved foods and certain supplements. For the body to heal itself, Dr. Sebi noted that this diet should be followed consistently for the rest of your life.

The Dr. Sebi Diet is plant-based, but there are some differences, unlike other plant-based diets.

Here is a compiled list of what differentiates the Dr. Sebi Diet from a plant-based diet:

- **No processed foods**: Tofu, veggie burgers, textured vegetable protein, canned fruits, canned vegetables, oil, soy sauce, and other condiments are considered processed. The Dr. Sebi Diet encourages dieters to consume unadulterated food. Some plant-based diets still allow processed foods as long as they are made from plant-based ingredients.
- **No wheat products allowed:** Under this diet regimen, you are not allowed to consume wheat and wheat products such as bread, biscuits, and others as they are not naturally growing grains. Naturally growing grains include amaranth seeds, wild rice, and triticale, to name a few.
- **The need to adhere to the food list:** In general, plant-based diets are not so restrictive for the food that dieters can eat (unless you are specifically following a strict plant-based regimen such as the plant-based keto diet). However, the Dr. Sebi Diet requires dieters only to eat foods listed in the nutritional guide.
- **Drink one (1) gallon of water daily:** Water is the most hydrating liquid on the planet. The Dr. Sebi Diet requires dieters to consume 1 gallon of water daily or more. Moreover, tea and coffee should be avoided as these drinks are highly acidic.
- **Taking in Dr. Sebei's supplements:** If you take any medications for a particular health condition, this diet regimen will require you to consume proprietary supplements an hour before taking your medication.

Chapter 2: Dr. Sebi Teaching and Methods

Dr. Sebi proposed that the body is at the state of becoming susceptible to contracting diseases when the level of toxins and mucus accumulation increases.

He argued that people suffering from different diseases and those interested in preventing diseases should always eat an alkaline diet, bearing in mind that it becomes free from infections when the body removes the increased amount of acidic substances and mucus.

He also suggested that cleansing and detoxifying the body is an essential and significant tool necessary in dealing with any disease in the body.

Detoxification of the body helps eliminate mucus accumulated in the liver, lungs, and many other body organs and helps remove excess acidic substances, thereby freeing the body from disease-causing diseases.

Dr. Sebi also used herbs that are important in re-energizing and revitalizing the body. The body's organs function properly when there is an improvement in your health, which indicates that your body is void of diseases.

Dr. Sebi classified food into six categories:

- Drugs
- Genetically modified foods
- Hybrid foods
- Dead foods
- Living foods
- Raw foods

He concluded that the first four food categories in this list are no-go areas as they cause more body damage than good. These foods can cause a build-up of acids and mucus in the body. However, the last two categories of foods are the best types of food he classified as healthy because the nutritional contents are not lost in any way. For instance, thoroughly cooked, hybridized, and modified foods have lost the required amount of nutrients present in them. Hence, the reverse is the case instead of providing benefits for the body. However, raw foods, especially vegetables, fruits, and herbs, are excellent for building good health.

Dr. Sebi's plant-based and electric diet is based on the 'African bio-mineral that helps dieters fight diseases. The diet also prevents various diseases (prevention) and boosts the immune system. When the body is immuno-compromised, it can accommodate any infection that sneaks in.

Dr. Sebi's diet is also beneficial for people who cherish living a healthy life by remaining clean and lean. But unfortunately, his diet was not created from heaven; we ignore common foods because of the love of modified, processed, refined, and hybridized foods.

Dr. Sebi's diet contains vegetables, fruits, grains, nuts, herbal teas, plant-based sweeteners, and seeds. Those who cherish animal products will not benefit from this diet as it does not encourage foods made from animals.

According to Dr. Sebi, all infections grow well in the environment that makes them comfortable such as acidic, mucus overload, and toxic environs.

When the body is in a limy condition, infections will find it so difficult to thrive, and when it is in an acidic state, the reverse is the case. Hence, the acidic component in the body helps diseases multiply and thrive.

Likewise, he also declared that the build-up of excess mucus in the body increases the susceptibility to an infection as the mucus blocks up the blood vessel and easily hinders blood flow.

He stated that the excess mucus must be removed to enjoy your health. The diseases are automatically removed when the mucus is removed either by detoxification or cleansing.

The healing of many sufferers who suffer from hair loss and many other prevalent diseases didn't occur because of the medications they took but because of the self-healing that took place in the body due to Dr. Sebi's alkaline diet.

Dr. Sebi's Nutritional Food Lists

Vegetables

- Izote flower and leaf
- Kale
- Mushrooms except for Shitake
- Bell Pepper
- Chayote
- Cherry and Plum Tomato
- Dulse
- Garbanzo Beans
- Arame
- Wild Arugula
- Avocado
- Cucumber
- Dandelion Greens

- Amaranth
- Watercress
- Tomatillo
- Turnip Greens
- Wakame
- Lettuce
- Olives
- Purslane Verdolaga
- Squash Okra
- Hijiki
- Nopales
- Nori
- Zucchini
- Onions

Fruit Diets

- Peaches
- Orange
- Soft Jelly Coconuts
- Cantaloupe
- Prickly Pear
- Cherries
- Prunes
- Bananas
- Dates
- Figs
- Plums

- Grapes
- Apples
- Pears
- Limes
- Mango
- Berries
- Raisins
- Papayas
- Melons
- Currants

Alkaline Grains Diets

- Kamut
- Tef
- Wild Rice
- Spelt

- Fonio
- Amaranth
- Quinoa
- Rye

Alkaline Sugar Items

- Date Sugar
- Agave Syrup from cactus (100% Pure)

Herbs Item

- Dill
- Onion powder
- Basil
- Pure sea salt

- Oregano
- and Cayenne

Spices and Seasoning Diets

- Dill
- Achiote
- Habanero
- Savory
- Basil
- Thyme
- Pure Sea Salt
- Bay Leaf

- Cayenne
- Sweet Basil
- Cloves
- Onion Powder
- Sage
- Oregano
- Powdered Granulated Seaweed
- Tarragon.

Dr. Sebi Diet for Weight Loss

While it is not designed for weight loss, this diet can ultimately help you shed some extra pounds. It discourages the consumption of ultra-processed foods and other western diets high in fat and sugar.

People who stick to plant-based diets, for the most part, have lower body weight and fewer cases of congenital medical conditions.

Moreover, most foods eaten with this program have a low-caloric content, aside from the oils, avocados, nuts, and seeds. Although this diet may help you lose weight, it does not guarantee that you will maintain your new weight once you resume your previous eating patterns. Studies have shown that most people gain weight once they stop following the Sebi diet. Perhaps reiterate that the diet is intended to be followed for life.

The absence of calorie valuation with each recipe and supplement makes it challenging to gauge weight loss sustainability on a diet.

Meanwhile, you will eat many veggies and fruits; it offers you numerous health benefits. For example, diets rich in veggies and fruits have contributed to less oxidative stress and concentrated inflammation. In addition, they can help defend you from many different diseases.

One of Doctor Sebi's most significant benefits is its promotion of the consumption of fruits and vegetables.

These two food categories have high:

- Fiber content
- Antioxidants
- Many essential minerals and vitamins

The diet contains many plant compounds that have been known to combat inflammation and improve immunity against a myriad of illnesses.

Studies done by scientists and other experts have shown that people who consume fruits and vegetables in high amounts every day have reduced risk and fewer cardiovascular diseases and cancer incidents.

This diet is rich in fibers, especially from whole grains and vegetables. Fibers are beneficial because they help deal with constipation and ease bowel movements.

Limiting ultra-processed foods improves the quality of the diet in the overall scheme of things.

Chapter 3: Benefits of Dr. Sebi Treatments

Dr. Sebi's Diet offers a lot of benefits to the dieters. While the foods recommended from this diet are known to reduce inflammation, there are other benefits that you can reap from following the Dr. Sebi Diet.

It May Helps with Weight Loss

While this diet regimen is not designed for weight loss, it can help people lose weight. Studies show that people who consume a whole plant-based diet experience significant weight loss. People who lose weight with this diet relies on the high fiber, and low-calorie foods encouraged to eat. Except for avocadoes, nuts, seeds, and oil, most foods encouraged by the Dr. Sebi Diet are low in calories. But even if you consume nuts and seeds, they are calorie-dense and rich in fiber and minerals.

Better Colon Health

Because this diet regimen encourages the consumption of large volumes of fruits and vegetables, it also benefits colon health. Foods rich in fiber can help promote healthy digestion; thus, people who follow the Dr. Sebi Diet do not suffer from constipation.

Appetite Control

Although many people think that this diet is very restrictive in terms of the number of calories a particular person takes in, studies indicate that this diet can help with appetite control. The high fiber in your food can provide a high satiety level and make one feel full for much longer.

Better Gut Microbiome

The stomach is the second brain. The enzymes and molecules released by the microbes in the gut affect not only your health but even your everyday mood. What you put inside your system also affects the microbes' molecules into the bloodstream. The type of food you consume can also affect the kind of microbes in your stomach. For instance, studies show that consuming greasy, fatty, and processed foods can decline good microorganisms and promote bad bacteria growth in the body.

Reduced Inflammation

While inflammation is one of the body's first lines of defense, indicating infection and diseases, chronic low-dose inflammation can also be bad for the body. Chronic inflammation can result in diabetes, stroke, and even cancer. Thus, diets rich in fruits and vegetables are linked to reduced inflammation caused by oxidative stress. Studies that look into individuals consuming plant-based foods have a 31% lower incidence of developing heart diseases and cancer than those who consume animal products.

He created this diet for anybody who wants to naturally prevent or cure any disease. It can also improve your overall health without using chemical medications.

Dr. Sebi's theory is that all diseases are caused by too much mucus building up in a specific body area. When you have too much mucus in your lungs, you get pneumonia. If you have too much mucus in your pancreas, it causes diabetes.

He believes that any disease won't exist in an alkaline environment but can happen if your body is too acidic.

Many people claim that his diet improved their health by using his compounds. The herbal approach to healing the body worked better than any medical approach ever. Many of his thoughts about herbal therapy and nutritional compounds on YouTube help promote and teach healthy living long after his death.

His diet does offer many health benefits. The main one is it can promote weight loss because it restricts processed foods, and you will be eating more plant-based, unprocessed meals. This diet is full of whole fruits and vegetables of plant compounds, minerals, vitamins, and fiber.

Diets that contain fruits and vegetables are related to oxidative stress and reduced inflammation, along with protecting you against most diseases.

Meatless diets have been linked to lower risks of heart disease and obesity. It also encourages foods that are high in fiber and low in calories. Regularly consuming fruits and vegetables can help protect your body against diseases and reduce inflammation.

If you can switch from your normal diet that is full of fast foods, saturated fats, refined sugars, and grains to Dr. Sebi's diet could help you lose some weight—increasing your intake of grains, vegetables, and fruits while getting rid of pork and beef can decrease your risk of elevated cholesterol, high blood pressure, Type 2 diabetes, heart disease, and cancer. In addition, most people eat way too much sodium, which can drastically reduce this amount. Lowering sodium intake can lower your blood pressure, which reduces your risk of heart disease and stroke.

In one study, people who ate seven servings of fruits and vegetables each day had between 25 and 31 % lower heart disease chance and cancer.

Most Americans don't eat enough produce. During 2017 it was reported that between 9.3 and 12.2 percent met all their recommended daily intake of fruits and vegetables.

Dr. Sebi's diet encourages eating healthy fats like plant oils, seeds, nuts, and whole grain-rich fiber. These foods have a lower risk of developing heart disease.

Any diet limiting processed foods can help you have a better diet quality.

Chapter 4: Asthma

Asthma is a long-term chronic inflammation due to environmental and genetic factors of excess mucus production. It's pretty hard to avoid, but it's easier to heal. Traditional medicine uses supplements, fatty acids, breathing exercises, and breathing strategies to ensure the lungs' proper functioning. Dr. Sebi encourages the use of fennel, anise, chamomile teas, and alkaline fruits and vegetables.

If you have asthma, your airways will still be inflamed. They get even more swollen, and the airways' muscles will relax when something causes the symptoms. That makes it difficult for air to pass in and out of the lungs, causing symptoms such as coughing, wheezing, shortness of breath, and chest tightness.

These symptoms are closely linked to physical activity for many people living with asthma. And, some otherwise healthy people may experience asthma symptoms only when they exercise. Exercise-induced bronchoconstriction (EIB) or exercise-induced asthma (EIA). Staying involved is an effective way to remain well, but asthma isn't meant to keep you on the sidelines. Instead, your doctor may establish a treatment plan to keep your symptoms under control before, during, and after physical activity.

People who have a family background of allergies or asthma are more likely to develop asthma. Many people with asthma, too, have allergies. In this case, it is called allergic asthma.

Occupational asthma is caused by inhaling chemicals, gases, dust, or other potentially dangerous substances while at work.

Childhood asthma affects millions of children and their families. In reality, most children who develop asthma do so before the age of five.

There is no remedy for asthma, but if it is correctly diagnosed and a care plan is in effect, you will control the condition and improve your quality of life.

Symptoms

The symptoms of this disease differ from person to person. You may have infrequent asthma attacks, symptoms only at some times — such as during exercise — or symptoms all the time.

Signs of asthma include:

- Breath shortness
- Chest of tightness or pain
- Wheezing while exhaling is a typical sign of asthma in children
- Trouble sleeping due to coughing, shortness of breath, or wheezing
- Coughing or wheezing episodes are caused by a respiratory infection, such as cold or flu.

Signs that your asthma is getting worse include:

- Symptoms of asthma are more severe and bothersome
- Trouble breathing, as calculated by the system used to check how well the lungs are functioning (peak flow meter)
- When there is the need to use a quick-relief inhaler, more often than not
-

Causes

It's not clear why some people get asthma, and others don't. Still, it's possibly due to a combination of environmental and hereditary (genetic) factors.

Some Asthma Triggers are:

- Exposure to various irritants and substances that cause allergies (allergens) can trigger asthma symptoms and symptoms. Asthma causes vary from person to person and can include:
- Airborne allergens such as pollen, dust mites, mold spores, pet dander, or cockroach waste particles
- Respiratory diseases, such as common colds
- Physical movements
- Cold air
- Air contaminants and irritants, such as smoke;
- Some medications, including beta-blockers, aspirin, and nonsteroidal anti-inflammatory medicines, such as ibuprofen (Advil, Motrin IB, others) and sodium naproxen (Aleve)
- High emotion and tension
- Sulfites and preservatives have been applied to many foods and drinks, including seafood, dried fruit, cooked potatoes, beer, and wine.
- Gastroesophageal reflux disease (GERD) is a disorder in which stomach acids migrate to your mouth.

Risk factors

A variety of factors are thought to increase the risk of developing asthma. They shall include:

- Getting a blood relative with asthma, whether a parent or sibling
- Getting another allergic disorder, such as atopic dermatitis, which causes red, itchy skin or hay fever, causes runny nose, cough, and itchy eyes.
- To be overweight
- To be a smoker
- Exposure to second-hand smoke
- Exposure to traffic gases or other sources of emissions
- Exposure to occupational causes such as chemicals used in agriculture, hairdressing, and manufacturing

Complications:
- It may interfere with sleep, work, and other activities;
- Sick days at work or school during asthma flare-ups
- A persistent narrowing of the tubes that bring air to and from your lungs (bronchial tubes) affects how well you can breathe.
- Emergency department visits and hospitalization for severe asthma attacks
- Side effects of long-term use of some drugs used to control extreme asthma

The proper treatment makes a big difference in preventing short-term and long-term asthma complications.

Chapter 5: Diabetes

Having Diabetes indicates that your blood sugar level, often called blood glucose, is too high. A hormone named insulin is usually used to help convert food into energy. When a person has diabetes, his body either does not create insulin or cannot properly use insulin. It may cause severe health complications, kidney failure, heart disease, and blindness if diabetes is not managed.

By maintaining blood sugar within a reasonable range, eating healthy, and becoming physically active, diabetes may be treated.

You have got to improve your style of dieting. Sometimes diabetes is like a lifestyle condition, usually known and managed by modifying it. If you're eating the wrong way, your body is more likely to be in an acidic state because, according to Dr. Sebi, the source of all sickness is mucus. Mucus would be abundant where illness is present.

Through his methodology, Dr. Sebi helped millions of people. Unfortunately, his death did nothing to alter this; he left behind therapeutic healing methods for diabetes.

You will benefit from his philosophy about what he truly felt about this dangerous illness to remove

A common misconception is that diabetes has just a form. Still, there isn't just one type of diabetes a person can be diagnosed with.

There are three known types of diabetes:

- Type 1
- Type 2
- Gestational

Type 1 diabetes can't be avoided and is normally found in childhood and is often referred to as juvenile diabetes. It is a type of auto-immune disease. In this case, your body doesn't make enough insulin. The immune system will also attack and destroy the pancreatic cells that create insulin. Most people with type 1 diabetes will have to take insulin every single day.

About five percent of people with diabetes have type 1 diabetes. Type 1 diabetes is considered incurable, but there are a lot of management tools out there.

Some of the most common symptoms of type 1 diabetes are:

- Weight loss without an apparent reason
- Fatigue and tiredness
- Unclear or blurred vision and problems with sight
- Frequent urination
- Increased thirst and hunger

Once diagnosed with type 1 diabetes, they enter the honeymoon phase. During this time, the cells responsible for secreting insulin could continue to make the hormone for a bit before stopping altogether. At this stage, they won't need as many insulin shots to keep their glucose levels.

That often causes the sufferer to think they are getting better. However, even if things seem good, they need to ensure they are still closely monitoring their numbers.

People with type 1 diabetes that go unmanaged can face dangerous complications, including:

- Diabetic retinopathy – Too much glucose can weaken the retina walls, which is the part of the eye that detects color and light. As this progresses, small blood vessels behind the eye could bulge and rupture, creating vision problems.

- Diabetic neuropathy – Too much glucose can reduce your circulation and damage the nerves in the feet and hands, causing pain, tingling, and burning sensations.

- Kidney disease – Since the kidneys filter glucose out of the blood, having to do this too much can cause kidney failure.

Some other issues people could face are depression, gum disease, and cardiovascular disease. Diabetic ketoacidosis is a complication when the body is not given the right amount of insulin. It places the body under great stress. This causes very high levels of blood sugar. At this point, the body has started to break down fat and not sugar and produces ketones. These ketones can become harmful if too many are produced, which causes acidosis. It is a medical emergency, and it will require hospitalization.

People with type 1 diabetes face taking insulin for the rest of their lives. You will work with your doctor to figure out the best schedule for your insulin doses. There are now continuous blood sugar monitors and insulin pumps. This hybrid machine can act as an artificial pancreas and remove the need for remembering when to take insulin. However, they will still need to check their blood sugar levels manually to ensure things are still okay.

Most of the time, for a person to develop type 1 diabetes, people will have to inherit a risk factor from both of their parents. It is believed that these factors tend to be higher in Caucasians because there is a higher rate of type 1 diabetes among Caucasians.

Since most people at risk don't develop diabetes, researchers want to determine the environmental triggers. One trigger could be cold weather. Type 1 diabetes tends to show up more often during the winter months than summer and tends to be more prevalent in colder climates. They also believe that viruses could be another trigger.

Diet as an infant may also play a role. Type 1 diabetes isn't as common in those who breastfed and started eating solid foods later. For most people, developing type 1 diabetes tends to take several years.

A man with type 1 diabetes has a 1 in 17 chance of having a child who develops it. For a woman with type 2 diabetes who gives birth before the age of 25, there is a 1 in 25 risks that your child will develop it. If you give birth after the age of 25, the odds go down to 1 in 100.

A child's risk becomes doubled if you ended up developing diabetes before you were 11. If you and your partner have type 1 diabetes, the risk becomes 1 in 10 and 1 in 4. Some tests can be given to determine your child's risk of developing type 1 diabetes.

Type 2 diabetes is acquired during life because of poor dietary choices and genetics. It is most often caused by depleting your insulin resources when the body cannot make or use insulin correctly. It can be developed at any age and even as a child. However, it is more common for middle-aged and older adults to be diagnosed. It is the most common form of diabetes.

There are many risk factors for developing type 2 diabetes.

They can include:

- Living a sedentary life
- Being older than 45
- Being of Asian-Pacific Islander, Latin American, Native American, or African American descent

- A History of PCOS
- Give birth to a child that weighed more than nine pounds or has gestational diabetes
- History of high blood pressure
- Having an HDL cholesterol level that is less than 40 or 50 mg/dL
- Family history of diabetes
- Being overweight

The family lineage factor for type 2 diabetes is stronger than type 1 diabetes. Studies in twins have found that genetics plays a big role in developing type 2. Yet, the environment still plays a big role as well. Lifestyle tends to play a very big role as well. Obesity often runs in families, and families will often have similar exercise and eating habits.

Gestational diabetes only affects women during pregnancy. For the most part, diabetes will go away once the woman gives birth. Still, it puts the baby at a higher risk of developing diabetes. The mother is also at a higher risk of developing type 2 diabetes later in life.

There are also less common types of diabetes, such as monogenic diabetes inherited and diabetes-related to cystic fibrosis. As mentioned earlier, people can be diagnosed with pre-diabetes. Doctors diagnose people with pre-diabetes when blood sugar reaches a range of 100 to 125 mg/dL. Normal blood sugar levels are normally 70 to 99 mg/dL. A person who has diabetes will have a blood sugar high than 126 mg/dL when fasted.

Pre-diabetes simply means having a higher blood sugar level than it should be but isn't high enough to be considered diabetes. However, it does place you at a greater risk of developing type 2 diabetes. If a doctor finds that a person has pre-diabetes, they will suggest making healthy life changes to stop the progression. For example, eating healthier foods and losing weight will often prevent the development of diabetes.

While there is a lot of good advice for people with diabetes that doctors will share, such as lifestyle changes, there is also a lot of medication that you could prescribe. And let's not get started on how scary it must be to learn how to give yourself insulin injections.

Dr. Sebi's diabetes cure is a super simple plan, and it doesn't cost that much. Very few people wanted to try his plan at first because it required fasting. Most would rather cut off their feet than not eat. Dr. Sebi was able to cure his diabetes with a 27 day fast.

Many other people have reported similar results as well. You can find many videos on YouTube where people talk about curing their diabetes with Dr. Sebi's plan. Like with STD treatments, the goal is to rid the body of excess mucus. For people with diabetes, excess mucus is found in the pancreatic duct. Dr. Sebi's mother started fasting to help her diabetes,

During your fast, you should drink water, and you can also have herbal tea. A great herbal tea to drink is a combination of burdock, black walnut leaf, red raspberry, and elderberry. Use a tablespoon of each herb and mix them into one and a half liters of spring water. Bring this to a boil and let it steep for 15 minutes. Take this off the heat and mix in another half-liter of water. Strain out the herbs and place them to the side to use the next day. Store the tea in the fridge and drink as much as you want during the day.

When they hear the word fast, many people assume that they can't take anything by mouth. But that's not Dr. Sebi's fast. See, when Dr. Sebi fasted to cure his diabetes, he would take three green plus tablets each day and drink sea moss tea, spring water, and tamarind juice. You don't have to drink tamarind juice, though. Any juice that is on the approved list of foods is okay. It must be fresh juice, though. You don't want pre-made juice with a bunch of added sugars.

Once you have fasted for a while, and your body will tell you when you have had enough, you need to start the Dr. Sebi-approved diet plan. Along with that, you should also think about taking black seeds, mulberry leaves, and fig leaves. Research on black seeds has found that taking as little as two teaspoons of the powder each day can reverse diabetes.

Figleaves are the top alternative medicine for diabetes on the market today. Mulberry leaves are a common treatment for diabetes in the Middle East. These can be made into tea, and you can also mix in some black seeds.

Some other foods you should consider adding to your diet are ginseng, okra, ginger, fenugreek, red clover, Swiss chard, avocado, and bitter melon.

Chapter 6: HIV

The same strategies to prevent any other STD are the same strategies you should use to decrease your risk of contracting HIV. In addition, there are some medications that people can take to keep them from contracting HIV. Still, these are normally only given to patients at a higher risk of contracting it.

Dr. Sebi offers an alternative to modern medicine when treating HIV. He believes that cleaning the mucus build-up in the lymphatic system and blood can help HIV.

Dr. Sebi didn't create something specifically to treat HIV/AIDS or any specific disease. Instead, he came up with compounds meant to cleanse the body and provide important nutrition. However, when you focus on cleansing your body of major illnesses, the interest will turn to compounds found in his therapeutic packages.

We are all dealing with the fatigue and cellular stress because we constantly exhaust our oxygen supply. And we are constantly trying to find any means to remain hydrated to deal with our suffocation through animal products, medical chemicals, starch, and sugar.

We need our mucous membrane to maintain health because it helps to protect the cells. If this mucus is broken down, it becomes pus and will expose your cells, causing disease.

When we are fasting, it will cause our bodies to form more oxygen. Then we start to provide our bodies with rich foods in potassium phosphate and iron fluorine, which helps to flush out toxins, tumors, and mucus from our internal walls. We need to cleanse ourselves because our liver, intestines, and pancreas are power players for the best circulation. It will help to treat HIV/AIDS.

The only thing that will cause your body to start harming your mucous membranes is acid. This erosion in the body will create greater oxygen deprivation. You must consume natural greens and fruits when you eat. Any grains you eat should not be human-made, and all oils you use can retain nutrition once it is processed. Springwater will also help you to maintain your mineral content.

Dr. Sebi has come up with more than 40 herbs to flush your body of inflammation as well as nourish it. While many people will travel to Usha Village in Honduras to be cured of HIV/AIDs, you don't have to travel that far. All you need to do is stick to the nutritional guide and consume only alkaline foods.

The lymphatic system, skin, and blood make up the immunological system. You must adhere to a strict diet to clear these areas of mucus. If you don't, it will take a lot longer to heal.

To help boost your healing, you should consume only green leafy plants such as:

- Nori
- Hijiki
- Arame
- Dulce
- Wakame
- Burdock plants
- Lams quarters
- Purslane
- Nopales
- Dandelion greens
- Lettuce

You can also eat mushrooms, spices, and peppers on the approved foods list. When you start to follow this diet, you must make sure you drink a gallon of water every day and do some light exercise. Having a gallon jug prepared for the day is a good idea at the start of the day, and you can count any water used in teas. You should drink red clover tea instead of chamomile.

The first thing you need to do is address your iron deficiency because your immune system requires plenty. You need to take a bottle a day of either Bio Ferro or Iron Plus for ten days. After that, you only have to take two to three spoonfuls once you begin your therapeutic package. You can also consume a cup of bromide tea at noon and in the evening each day.

After the initial first ten days, you should start taking a mixture of different supplements. Some people will take all of them, while others only choose a few. Again, they are on Dr. Sebi's website

The following products are the ones you should look at:

- **Electra Cell** – breaks down calcification, strengthens your immune system, and clears out mucus build-up.
- **Cell Cleanser** – Gets rid of mucus, acids, and toxins on the intracellular level and will improve your bowel movements.
- **CC4** – Gets rid of mucus, acids, and toxins on a deeper intracellular level and helps provide you with mineral nourishment.
- **Chelation** – Helps to cleanse you on an intracellular level and improves your bowel movements. It also helps your digestive tract.
- **DBT** –Helps to nourish and cleanse your pancreas.
- **ECAL** – Removes fluid and toxins from your cells' mitochondria. It is high in carbonates, phosphates, bromides, and iodides.
- **Fucus** – This is a natural diuretic. It will flush out stagnant fluids dead cells and promotes healthy skin. It contains phosphates, calcium, magnesium, and other important minerals.
- **Lino** – Get rid of calcification in the body. It has many important minerals, which are important for the body and help break up and dissolve calcification.
- **Lupulo** – Calms the nervous system, relieves pain, and breaks up inflammation.

If you follow Dr. Sebi's diet and start taking his supplements, you can improve HIV/AIDs. That being said, it is still a good idea to continue to go to your doctor for monitoring. It is okay to take medications that your doctor prescribes while doing this. As you will read in the nutritional guide, the important thing is to take your supplements an hour before taking medications. It allows the supplements to help your body heal from any ill effects the medications could cause.

Lastly, you may have noticed that Dr. Sebi's treatments for herpes and HIV are very similar. While there are slight differences, most treatments will follow along the same lines. That means if you start following the treatment for one disease, you will be helping to prevent other diseases.

Chapter 7: Hair Loss

Hair loss is a problem that affects both men and women frequently, accumulating over the years. Hair loss is most common in men as they experience complete baldness. However, women also experience hair loss through thinning, weakness, breakage, and falling off.

The following are Dr. Sebi's recommended herbs for hair growth and hair abnormalities treatment:

- **Marshmallow root:** It is rich in proteins and vitamins. It helps treat hair problems such as eczema, psoriasis, and dry scalp. It does this with mucilage, a gel-like substance that becomes slippery when wet. It also helps in softening hair and helps in improving healthy hair growth. This herb could also be responsible for calming dry hair.
- **Nettle** helps alleviate hair loss through the scalp's stimulation, improves blood circulation, and protects against further damage and the hair's breakage.
- **Licorice**: It helps in moisturizing the scalp and hydrating the hair. This herb also prevents and fights many common hair problems such as dandruff, scabs, and itching. This herb can also help fight baldness and improve hair growth.
- **Dandelion:** This herb is rich in vitamin A, magnesium, iron, potassium, phosphorus, calcium, choline…and more. These nutrients effectively improve hair growth by treating the scalp and follicles.
- **Watercress**: it is rich in Vitamin A, biotin, and potassium. That makes it an excellent herb for treating hair loss, helps active hair growth, nourishes the hair shaft, and supports new hair growth.
- **Flaxseed** is rich in fatty acids essential for your hair and antioxidants that remove free radicals. As a result, it nourishes the hair, strengthens
- **Coconut oil:** it helps in facilitating hair growth. Coconut oil protects the hair scalp and gives you smooth, shiny, and soft hair. This oil is also essential in preventing and fighting
- **Sage:** it contains antiseptic and astringent components that help in promoting longer, fuller, thicker, and shiny hair.

Preparation of the Herbs

- Rinse, dry, and grind the following herbs together:
- Dandelion
- Saw palmetto
- Sage
- Nettle
- Marshmallow
- Licorice
- Watercress
- Flaxseed.

- Collect half tsp. of each herb and add into two cups of water.
- Boil for about five minutes.
- Drain and drink two times daily.

Note:

- You can collect half tsp. of each herb and boil with three cups of water.
- Steep and use it to wash your hair once a day.

Or:

- Collect two tbsp. of undiluted coconut oil and two tbs. of olive oil.
- Add two tbsp of powdered thyme and curry herbs.
- Mix thoroughly and apply to your hair.
- You can add the mixture to your hair cream and apply it thoroughly.

Chapter 8: Hypertension

High blood pressure is initiated when the blood flowing to the arteries is high due to consuming foods capable of clogging the arteries' wall. An act that results in pressure through the arteries during blood flow distribution. Blood is pumped by the heart to the aorta then the arteries. Peradventure, the arteries' walls become narrow and hardened due to excessive plague caused by poor eating habits, blood flow in the passageway of the arteries suppresses. Worthy of note is that as an individual gets older, the arteries get hardened bit by bit, and a bad diet will triple the possibility of high blood pressure.

Some of the numerous causes of high blood pressure are:

- Bad diet
- Tobacco intake
- Stress
- Excess coffee intake

- Fried and processed foods
- Over-eating
- Aging

Natural Remedies for Hypertension

Every high blood pressure drug in the market imitates water. To be operative, you will need to divide your weight by two and drink that much water daily. Why that much water? You may ask. Well, water thins the blood and makes passing through the arteries easy.

Taking five different types of fruits (vegetables included) a day will prevent the arteries from getting clogged due to excess plaque deposits. Vegetables and fruits that contain a high percentage of antioxidants protect the artery walls from plaque deposits. Such fruits include peaches, oranges, cabbage, seeded grapes, and tomatoes.

Foods rich in potassium help reduce recurrent hypertension by expelling excess sodium from the body. Fiber-containing fruits are also of high benefit to high blood pressure sufferers. They will lower blood pressure while simultaneously removing wastes from the artery walls.

High blood pressure after eating:
Knowledge of food-related high blood pressure is important as knowing what foods to eat and avoid is detrimental to the blood pressure level. No one wants to get high blood pressure from eating like everybody else.

Here are some things to avoid:

- Avoid overeating even the healthiest of food.
- Avoid salty foods as much as possible as they transform into plaque in the artery walls. In essence, avoid baking soda, sodas, soy sauce, and meat tenderizers.
- Never eat canned foods.
- Eliminate dairy products such as sodium, cheese, and alcohol after your diet.
- Avoid every other type of rice except wild and brown

The herbs listed below are recommended by Dr. Sebi. They support opening the blood vessels, exposing the arteries' walls, and eliminating plaques from the wall of arteries. These herbs are alkaline high in iron and other minerals. They are not hearsays; they have been medically proved to be effective as blood pressure medication.

Some of these herbs include:

- Fennel
- Oregano
- Basil
- Yellow dock
- Cayenne

About Hypertension

If the arteries' walls were clogged or packed with plagues, blood flow would become restricted as it pumps from the heart to the aorta. When the arteries create pressure in a situation like this, the blood pressure becomes higher than it should be, resulting in hypertension (high blood pressure).

Poor diet is the leading cause of high blood pressure in the United States as it has been reported that over 85 percent of reported high blood pressure cases are rooted in a poor diet. More than any other race in the United States, African Americans reported more high blood pressure cases. In addition, high blood pressure leads to other diseases such as kidney diseases, strokes, scarlet fever, large heart, typhoid fever, artery coronary diseases, and tonsillitis. These diseases are rampant among African Americans who have a hypertensive health history.

To be certain of your blood pressure, you will need a blood pressure gauge for accuracy. This gauge is often called a sphygmomanometer. It records two basic types of information: the first is systolic, which the higher reading is, while the second is diastolic, which the lower reading is.

Consequently, the diastolic high blood pressure is less problematic than the systolic high blood pressure readings. The systolic shows the blood pressure built as pumped through the passageways in the aorta's arteries. The blood pressure is high when your systolic reading is high due to the clogged artery walls, limiting blood flow. A regular systolic hypertension reading is usually among 120 – 150 millimeters. On the other hand, a high understanding is 140/190; the sign of a systolic hypertension reading is over 180/115.

Symptoms of High Blood Pressure:

According to Dr. Sebi, high blood pressure symptoms can be likened to "navy seal snipers", as there are no signs of high blood pressure.

The few noticeable pointers of high blood pressure have always been:

- Difficulty breathing
- Blurry vision
- Rapid pulses
- Constant headache

My mother, when alive, had high blood pressure. She once told me that her blood pressure symptoms are dizziness and that her pulse gets fast often.

Chapter 9: Lupus

Having lupus isn't a joking matter. This disease is even worse because healthcare professionals work with lupus patients. Some doctors want to kill your immune system with chemotherapy or begin giving you shots of concentrated starch, which is worse than alcohol. They might as well just put lupus in the same boat as AIDS. The main reason it hasn't been considered AIDS is that it doesn't shatter the immune system. The truth is that for people who have lupus, their immune system is so screwed up that you would be better off not having one. This is why I said it might as well be AIDS.

What has Dr. Sebi taught us about lupus?

Your central nervous system has been compromised because there is a yeast infection that no one has addressed right. As a result, the mucous membranes are continually attacked and turned into pus. Mucus contributes to the cells being deprived of oxygen. Because the cells are exposed, and our bodies are stressed to function correctly, our central nervous system needs some serious help.

The lives of our cells and nerves responsible for sending signals through our bodies have been challenged and diminished as more cells get compromised, contributing to more mucus forming in other parts of our bodies. Our bodies are still smart enough to know that they need to be cleansed since mucus stops the cells from doing their job correctly. Mucus will soon keep your organs from doing what they are supposed to do. That causes your pain receptors to go on overload to tell you that something is wrong with the body. Your brain and body want you to quit eating specific foods, and you should know what you need to leave eating. When it seems like your organs don't want to work right, they start acting like an enemy rather than a friend. Can you guess what your immune system is saying about all this? What do you think your immune system is going to do? It is going to start attacking everything in sight. Now your organs are being attacked. They can't fix themselves anymore, and you can't even get a good night's sleep.

Our bodies need to protect and repair the central nervous system because it protects our immune system. They do things simultaneously as long as our bodies are producing dopamine naturally. Our body can instinctively and immediately defend itself by sending out phagocyte cells to protect and defend it. It already has these cells placed throughout our bodies. Phagocyte cells called neutrophils are what begin attacking your organs. This causes organs to die and turn into pus or mucus. We have more of these cells in our bodies than any other kind of phagocytes. These stationary cells, called macrophages, will begin eating right where they are. They only follow orders, and they don't know right and wrong. Pain receptors start going off. But they aren't finished yet. Our central nervous system has some tough guys in the blood. They are called our "natural killer cells." These cells patrol the lymphatic and blood systems, just trying to find abnormal cells. They will kill off healthy cells faster than they can erode.

You Now Have a Compromised Central Nervous System

Your body is confused, and your immune system sets off a fever so that your metabolism gets faster, trying to repair everything quickly. Unfortunately, this fever begins attracting histamines to areas that have been damaged to help call the phagocytes. Now, your body feels as if it has the flu. The immune system uses the fever to heal; it also calls the bones to help trigger leukocytosis. This is when the bone marrow begins producing more neutrophils to help fight. While all this is happening, guess who was supposed to be making sure that everything is being done correctly and that the right enemies have been found: your lymphatic system.

Your lymphatic and immune systems are the same. It is supposed to clean up the dirty cells and make them all clean and new. If it fails to do this, your blood pressure is going to drop, your lungs will fill with fluid, your ankles are going to start swelling, and your body wants to give up and die.

How to Handle Lupus?

You get rid of lupus the same way you get rid of AIDS, cancer, and tumors. You use the bio-mineral balance along with intra-cellular chelation. These require you to eat a rigorous diet. Intra-cellular chelation means that you will clean your cells; every single cell makes up your central nervous system and organs. You won't just be washing your organs but every cell that makes the organ. Why do you need to do this? If you have cancer present in your body, it tells you that it has a high acid level. We have to nourish every part of our bodies at the same time. The disease requires us to nourish our bodies back to health. We need to give them a bio-mineral balance. Along with the intra-cellular chelation, that will bring our bodies back to the way they were before.

So, what are we going to do?

- We give our bodies' electric cell nutrition
- We get rid of the mucus
- We stay away from foods that create mucus, hybrid grains, synthetic sugars, and starches
- We fast

Support and Coping

If you have lupus, you will probably have many painful feelings about your disease, from extreme frustration to fear. There are challenges to living with lupus that can increase mental health problems like low self-esteem, stress, anxiety, or depression. To help you cope, you can try:

Connecting with Others

You can try talking to others who have lupus. Through message boards, community centers, and support groups, you can find people. Other lupus people could give you amazing support since they face the same frustrations and obstacles you face.

Time for Yourself

You can cope with the stress by taking time for yourself. Use this time to write in a journal, listen to music, meditate, or read. Find an activity that will renew and calm you.

Get Support

Find support from your family and friends. Talk about your lupus with family and friends and explain how they could help you when you have flares. Lupus is a frustrating disease for a loved one since they can't feel or see it, and you might not look like you are sick.

Educate Yourself

Write down all the questions you have about lupus when they come to mind so you can ask your doctor. You can ask your nurse or doctor for reputable sources for more information. The more you know about your disease, the more confident you feel about your treatments.

Your Appointment

Since lupus symptoms mimic other health conditions, you might need to have some patience while waiting on your diagnosis. Your doctor has to rule out other illnesses before they diagnose lupus. You might need to see many specialists like a neurologist, hematologist, or nephrologist. It all depends on what symptoms you are experiencing.

Things You Can Do

Before you go to your appointment, write down answers to these questions:

- What supplements and medications do you regularly take?
- Have your siblings or parents been diagnosed with an autoimmune disease or lupus?
- Do you have any symptoms?
- When did the symptoms start? Do they go away and come back?
- Write down some questions for your doctor like:
- Do I need to see a specialist?
- Are there any restrictions I need to adhere to while waiting for a diagnosis?
- What type of test are you recommending?
- What other tests will I need if these don't point to a specific cause?
- What are the causes of my condition or symptoms?
- I am thinking about getting pregnant. What do I need to do? Are there certain medicines that I can't use if I am pregnant?
- Never hesitate to ask any question that might pop into your mind while you are at your doctor's office or something; they bring you what you don't understand.
- What to Expect from the Doctor?
- Your doctor is going to ask you a lot of questions. It would be best if you were ready to answer them. Your doctor could ask:
- Are you pregnant? Do you have plans on having a child?
- Do you have any other medical problems?
- Do your symptoms limit your ability to function at home, work, or school? How much do they define you?
- Are you having problems concentrating or with your memory?
- Do your fingers get uncomfortable, numb, or pale when you are in the cold?
- Do you get rashes when you are out in the sun?

Chapter 10: PCOS Treatment

Polycystic ovary syndrome (**PCOS**) is a hormonal disorder that affects women within their reproductive age range. That is from 15 to 44 years. Research shows that 2.2 and 26.7 percent of women within the range of 15-44 years of age have PCOS, and about 70% of the women don't even know they are suffering from PCOS.

What Are The Causes Of PCOS?

Today, most doctors believe that PCOS is caused by the excess of male hormone (androgen). Things like insulin resistance, genetics, and inflammation cause women to produce more androgen hormones, usually linked to PCOS.

Insulin resistance

Let's look at the number of women suffering from PCOS. Approximately 70% have issues with their cells trying to use insulin properly. So, if their cells cannot use insulin, the body will demand more insulin. As the pancreas keeps producing more insulin, the ovaries will be forced to produce more male hormones, leading to obesity or type 2 diabetes.

Genes

Research shows that PCOS can be transferred from one mother to the other.

Inflammation

When you don't watch your weight, you might suffer from inflammation, and research shows that excess inflammation can lead to excess production of androgen hormone by women. However, Dr. Sebi state that there is only one disease, compromising the mucous membrane. Wherever the mucous is compromised, determine the sickness that will manifest. When it is in the ovaries, it is called PCOS.

What Are The Symptoms Of PCOS?

Some women might be lucky to experience some symptoms around their first period. In contrast, others may only get to know after gaining a lot of weight and others when they find it difficult to get pregnant.

However, the symptoms that one will experience when suffering from PCOS include:

- **Irregular or unusual periods:** if you have PCOS, one of the symptoms is that you might only experience eight periods in a year because of the in-between delay periods.
- **Heavy bleeding:** because of the uterine lining that will build up for a longer period without experiencing a period, when it comes, it will be heavier than a normal period.
- **Hair growth:** The women will show masculine features like hair growth on their bodies and faces because of the excess male hormone. Research has that more than 70% of women suffering from PCOS experience or have hair on their face and body.
- **Break out like acne:** The male hormones allow men's skin to be oilier than usual, which will lead to breakouts on the face, chest etc.
- **Weight gain or obesity:** research shows that more than 80% of women with PCOS have excess body weight (obese).
- **Hair loss:** some women with PCOS experience that their scalp's hair will become thinner and fall out.
- **Sometimes Headaches:** hormonal change can lead to headaches in some women.

How Do I Know If I Have PCOS?

If you experience any two out of these three symptoms, you should go and see your doctor or lab technician for an ultrasound scan.

The three symptoms are:

- High level of androgen hormone.
- Experiencing heavy menstrual flow or irregular menstrual cycles.
- If there are cysts in your ovaries

Meeting with your doctor or lab technician, you will be asked some questions like:

- Do you have symptoms like acne on your face?
- Are you experiencing a fat gain?
- Are you experiencing hair growth on your face and body?
- Have you missed your periods, and you're not pregnant?
- Have you been trying to get pregnant for more than 12 months without any good news?
- Do you have diabetes symptoms like excessive thirst or hunger, possibly blurred vision, or unexplained weight loss?

Once you are experiencing any other symptoms, the lab technicians will recommend an ultrasound scan for confirmation.

What Are The Complications Of Suffering From PCOS?

There are some severe complications that one can suffer from if she is suffering from PCOS.

For example:

- Suppose you have a higher-than-normal level of androgen hormone as a woman. In that case, there is a tendency that your fertility will be affected. To be pregnant, you have to ovulate. Women suffering from PCOS do not ovulate regularly. Women who do not ovulate regularly often have issues releasing enough eggs for fertilization. PCOS is the major cause of infertility in women.

- Metabolic syndrome: research has it that more than 80% of women that are suffering from PCOS are suffering from an obese or overweight issue, which is one of the major causes of; high blood sugar level, high blood pressure, low HDL and high LDL that increase the risk of heart disease, diabetes, and stroke.

- Women overweight or suffering from obesity always suffer repeated pauses in breathing during the night, interrupting their sleep. Women with PCOS have the chance to suffer from sleep apnea 5-10 times higher than normal women suffering from obesity without PCOS.

- Women who do not ovulate (shedding uterine lining) regularly because they are suffering from PCOS will build up the lining, which will increase the chances of endometrial cancer.

- Unwanted hair growths from women and hormonal changes can negatively affect women's emotions.

What Can I Do To Treat And Prevent PCOS?

According to the late Dr. Sebi, there have never been two diseases in this world. The only one disease is the compromising of the mucous membrane, which is caused by our dieting plan and the only way to get rid of PCOS is by eliminating mucus from the entire body and eating the alkaline diet, which will help the body to reverse it to its original alkaline state where sickness cannot withstand.

Chapter 11: STD Treatments

STDs, which stands for sexually transmitted diseases, are still fairly prevalent even though there are well-known ways to prevent them. Numerous diseases fall into STDs and are spread by sexual intercourse but can spread through other ways. The most common STDs are trichomoniasis, syphilis, some types of hepatitis, gonorrhea, genital warts, genital herpes, Chlamydia, and HIV.

At one time, STDs were referred to as venereal diseases. They are some of the most common contagious infections. About 65 million Americans have been diagnosed with an incurable STD. Every year, 20 million new cases occur, and about half of these are in people aged 15 to 24. All of these can have long-term implications.

These are serious illnesses that need to be treated. Some are considered incurable and can be deadly, such as HIV. Learning more about these diseases can teach you how to protect yourself.

STDs can be spread through oral, vaginal, and anal sex. Trichomoniasis can be contracted through contact with a moist or damp object, like toilet seats, wet clothing, or towels. However, it is mostly spread through sexual contact.

People who are at a higher risk of STDs include:

- Those who have more than one sexual partner.
- Those who trade sex for drugs or money.
- Those who share needles for drug use.
- Those who don't use condoms during sex.
- Those who have sex with a person who has had several partners.

Herpes and HIV are the two STDs chronic conditions that modern medicine can cure but only manage. Hepatitis B can sometimes become chronic. Unfortunately, you sometimes don't find out that you have an STD until it has damaged your reproductive organs, heart, vision, or other organs. STDs can also weaken the immune system, which leaves you vulnerable to contracting other diseases. Chlamydia and gonorrhea can cause pelvic inflammatory disease, leaving women unable to conceive. It is also able to kill you. If an STD is passed onto a newborn, the baby could face permanent damage, or it could kill them.

Causes of STDs

In modern medicine, STDs are caused by all types of infection.

- Syphilis, gonorrhea, and Chlamydia are bacteria
- Hepatitis B, genital warts, genital herpes, and HIV are all viral
- Parasites cause trichomoniasis

The STD germs live within vaginal secretions, blood semen, and, in some cases, saliva. The majority of the organisms will be spread through oral, anal, or vaginal sex. Still, some, like genital warts and genital herpes, can be spread simply through skin-to-skin contact. Hepatitis B can also be spread through sharing personal items, like razors or toothbrushes.

Prevention

The most obvious step in healing for STDs is not to get one in the first place. The first tip people give in preventing STDs is not having sex or avoiding sex with people who have genital discharge, rash, sores, or other symptoms. The only time you should have unprotected sex is if you and your partner are only having sex with one another, and you have both tests negative for STDs in the last six months. Otherwise, you need to make sure you:

Use condoms whenever you have sex. If you need a lubricant, make sure that it is water-based. Condoms should be used for the entire act of sex. Remember that condoms aren't 100% effective in preventing pregnancy or disease. However, they are very effective if you use them the right way.

Other useful tips I can give you are:

- Avoid sharing underclothing or towels.
- Bathe after and before sex.
- If you are okay with vaccination, you can get many STDs, specifically Hep B and HPV.
- Make sure you are tested for HIV.
- If you abuse alcohol or drugs, please seek help. It is more common for people under the influence to have unsafe sex.
- Lastly, abstaining from sex completely is the only 100% effective way to prevent STDs.

There was a belief that using a condom with nonoxynol-9 would prevent STDs by killing the organisms that caused them. However, a new study has found that this can irritate the woman's cervix and vagina and increase her risk of an STD. Therefore, it is recommended that you avoid condoms with nonoxynol-9.

Chapter 12: Herbal Medicine

Herbal medicine is "the expertise, techniques, and procedures centered on the philosophies, values, and interactions indigenous to various societies, utilized in the health preservation and health prevention, evaluation, enhancement or cure of the mental and physical disorder." Traditional medicine has several distinct structures. The theory and each activity are regulated by the environment, different conditions, and geographical location of the area where it is evolved. Generally, regardless of the underlying ailment or illness, the patient suffers, the emphasis is on the person's general health. Therefore, the usage of the herb is a central aspect of many conventional medicine programs.

Traditional Chinese medicine (TCM) has been a significant representation of how classical and acquired information is implemented through a systematic approach to present-day medical care has been traditional Chinese medicine (TCM). TCM has over 3000 years of history. The book 'The Devine Farmer's Classic of Herbalism' was composed in China around 2000 years back. It is the world's oldest documented herbal text. However, the historical and methodically gathered herbal knowledge has evolved into numerous herbal pharmacopeias. In addition, there are several monographs on herbs individually.

Treatment and diagnosis, represented in light of the combination of Yin - yang, are centered on a balanced perception of the disease and its effects. Yin portrays femininity, earth, and ice, while the sky, masculinity, and heat are depicted by yang.

Yin and yang's acts impact the relationships of the five elements that make up the world:

- Wood
- Water
- Metal
- Earth
- Fire

TCM practitioners strive to regulate the degrees of Yang and yin across 12 meridians that carry and guide energies (Qi) via a body. TCM is a rising procedure worldwide, and it is used both to improve well-being and avoid and prevent disease. TCM contains several activities, but traditional remedies and natural elements are crucial.

In some regions of the planet, health treatment has been revolutionized over the last 100 years by the invention and industrial manufacturing of chemically manufactured medicines. However, in developed countries, significant parts of the community also depend on conventional practitioners and natural remedies for primary treatment. Up to 90 percent of the people in Africa and 70 percent in India rely on traditional medication to treat their medical needs. In China, conventional medicine contributes to around 40 percent of all healthcare provided. More than ninety percent of public hospitals have traditional medicine units. However, the usage of herbal remedies is not restricted to emerging nations. The general interest in herbal remedies has significantly expanded in developed countries during the past two decades, with ethnobotanicals' increasing use.

The most popular motives for utilizing natural medications are that they are more accessible, more generally correlates to the patient's lifestyle, allays fears regarding the harmful consequences of artificial (synthetic) drugs, fulfills a need for more customized healthcare, facilitates a more comprehensive community approach to health records. In addition, herbal medications' main application promotes human health and therapy of chronic diseases and prevents life-threatening disorders. However, natural remedies grow as current therapy is inadequate in clinical management, such as advanced tumors and modern contagious diseases. In comparison, natural drugs are commonly accepted, not poisonous, and are safe healthy.

Whether a person needs it, herbal medicine offers an essential health care commodity, whether individuals have financial or physical exposure to allopathic medication, and is a growing worldwide market.

Herbs are currently used to cure chronic and severe illnesses and different disorders and issues, such as heart disease, prostate disorders, obesity, asthma, anxiety, and improve immunity. Traditional natural remedies played a leading key role in the technique for controlling and curing SARS (severe acute respiratory syndrome) in China in 2003. A conventional herbal medication, the African flower, has been used in Africa for ages to manage HIV-related symptoms. Natural medicines are still trendy in Europe. In most developed countries, France and Germany, leading overall purchases by European countries, herbal extracts or teas, and essential oils may be found in pharmacies selling prescription medications.

Herbs and seeds, including whole herbs, teas, syrups, lavender oil, ointments, salves, rubbers, tablets, and capsules comprising a powdered type dry extract of a raw herb form, may be manufactured and may be taken in numerous ways and styles. Plant and herb extracts differ and include vinegar (extracts of acetic acid), alcoholic extracts, hot water extracts (tisanes), long boiling extracts, generally bark and roots (decoctions), and cold plant infusions. There is little specification, and an herbal product's ingredients differ significantly across batches and manufacturers.

Plant species are abundant with a diversity of substances. Most are secondary plant metabolites containing aromatic compounds, mostly phenols or phenols supplemented with oxygen, like tannins. Many of those substances are antioxidants.

Herbal Treatment For Aging

In several developing nations, life expectancy rose, in the early 1950s, from about 41 years to about 80. Consequently, the proportion of the aged among our communities (sixty-five years and over) is growing. The greying of our societies carries a growing burden of illness and dependence correlated with chronic aging. Aging is linked with a gradual deterioration in neurological activity and an enhanced risk of death, coronary disease, hypertension, diabetes mellitus, dementia, osteoporosis, etc. Factors in lifestyle such as exercise or diet play a significant role in assessing the length and quality of healthy life and even treating infectious diseases. There is no apparent reason for aging, though multiple aging hypotheses have been proposed over the years. Genetic influences are undeniably significant, but the most widely supported theory of aging's metabolic explanations is the oxidative stress hypothesis (Beckman and Ames 1998; Harman 1992). This hypothesis postulates that aging is triggered by the accumulation of permanent damage, i.e., oxidative stress generated by oxidation arising from the association between reactive oxygen species and cell DNA, protein, and lipid components. And as it is observed that the aging mechanism itself is unlinked to oxidative stress, widely frequent chronic age-related illnesses have indeed raised oxidative stress. In herbs, antioxidants can contribute to at least some of their renowned therapeutic effects.

Natural-Derived Analgesic Agents

Different natural ingredients have been used to cure pain problems since the first documented reports, about 7000 years ago. Examples of those genuine items are opium poppy (Papaver soniferum) and willow tree bark (Salix spp.). It was not until the nineteenth century that particular molecules were extracted and believed to obtain the desired results from these chemicals. The identified origins of such compounds were studied in detail. More analgesic compounds have been removed from natural materials during the last few decades, resulting in new molecular groups and action mechanisms. In drug research attempts, plants or other natural remedies mentioned in historical ethnopharmacological and ethnobotanical literature have been of more recent importance. Such records and studies classify better herbal ingredients traditionally used in pain treatment. The simple knowledge of the intricate pain transmitting processes in the nervous system has been a significant factor in finding new compounds to relieve pain. Nociceptive synthesis includes various types of receptors, enzymes, and signaling pathways. Identifying novel groups of compounds through natural sources can contribute to a greater understanding of the pharmacological mechanisms underlying them. With the ability to identify new substances with favorable pharmacological characteristics (i.e., no health risks, no addictive capacity), natural products also carry tremendous promise for the future of drug development, especially in the treatment of pain conditions and possibly opioid addictions.

Anti-Inflammatory Action of Natural Products

Many inflammatory disorders are being widespread in the world's aging population. Unfortunately, the anti-inflammatory medications used clinically suffer from the downside of adverse effects and rising medication costs (in biologic drugs). Alternatively, these drugs are natural remedies and natural ingredients that offer great hope in discovering and producing biologically active lead compounds into medicines to treat inflammatory diseases. Herbal drugs and phytopharmaceuticals have prevented inflammation and other diseases since ancient times. The metabolites listed belong to various chemicals, such as steroids, alkaloids, polyphenolics, and terpenoids, which play a vital role in their anti-inflammatory properties.

Plants Induced Antifungal Agents

A modern continuum of human fungal infection is growing because of intensified cancer, AIDS, and impaired immune system patients. The increased usage of antifungal agents has also developed tolerance to existing medications. New groups of antifungal substances to treat fungal infections continue to be identified. Plants are a rich source of many biologically active secondary metabolites, such as tannins, terpenoids, saponins, flavonoids, alkaloids, and other substances, reported to have antifungal properties in vitro. Research into natural products and substances extracted from natural resources has also increased in recent years, owing to their significance in discovering medicines. In plants of considerable value to humans, several compounds have been identified with antifungal action against various fungus strains. These molecules may be used as a guide to creating better molecules.

Chapter 13: Fasting to Prevent all Diseases

The main contributors to self-sustainability, disease recovery, and quality of life are nutritional status. Obesity can result from overeating, dietary errors, or other various metabolic, genetic, and behavioral defects, causing both insulin resistance and dysfunction of pancreatic beta-cells and is therefore considered the foundation of diabetes type 2.

To promote weight loss, intermittent fasting, wherein people fast on sequential or alternating days, was being reported to prevent diabetes type 2 and boost cardiovascular risk. Substantial evidence indicates that the imposition of fasting periods on laboratory animals enhances survival, promotes health, and decreases illness, including multiple morbidities with neurological cancer disorders and circadian rhythm disorders. Fasting is being used in religion. Fasting is usually carried out for three weeks. During Ramadan, all Muslims worldwide fast during the daytime of this month, the 9th month of the Muslim calendar, which is considered one of Islam's five critical pillars.

These fasting periods can reduce inflammation, amplify pro-inflammatory immune cells and cytokines, boost circulating lipids and glucose levels, and decrease blood pressure. Besides, experiments on humans and animals have indicated that fuel selection is changed, metabolism efficiency increases, and oxidative stress decreases.

Animal models indicate that some cardiac benefits are caused by random fastings, such as raising heart rate and blood pressure, circulating triglycerides and cholesterol, and reducing intima-media carotid thickness. Besides, it enhances myocardial ischemia survival by anti-apoptotic, pro-angiogenic, and anti-remodeling impact.

Intermittent fasting also tends to be cardioprotective, offering resistance to ischemic injury, to laboratory animals, in a way likely associated with a rise in adipokine adiponectin levels. Adiponectin is a distinctive adipokine that tends to have positive effects and has circulation levels associated negatively with the body's composition. Intermittent fasting, however, attenuates visceral fat levels and multiple specific adipokines, like IL-6, IGF-1, TNF-alpha, and leptin.

Although Ramadan fasting is compulsory for all the Muslims who value the religious atmosphere throughout the month of Ramadan, the Qur'an disallows from fasting those who are sick, traveling, expectant mothers, mothers during feeding, or females during their menstrual phase. In particular, fasting can be dangerous with diabetes as it could raise the incidence of postprandial hyperglycemia, dehydration, hypoglycemia, and thrombosis, both with and without diabetic ketoacidosis.

Fasting promotes blood sugar control

Intermittent fasting enhances blood sugar-lowering insulin hormone sensitivity and defends against fatty liver disease. In addition, researchers have now revealed that mice often display lower fat cells in the pancreas on a fasting schedule. In their recent study, the researchers demonstrated printed in a journal the pathway through which fat cells in the pancreas would lead to diabetes type 2.

The fatty liver was extensively studied as a recognized and commonly occurring condition. However, little is understood about the accumulation of fats in the pancreas caused by the extra weight and its impact on diabetes type 2. Work has shown a high concentration of pancreatic fat cells in obese mice vulnerable to diabetes. Despite the extra weight, mice immune to diabetes because of their genetic sequence had barely any pancreatic fats but had excess fat in the liver. The accumulation of fats external to the fat tissue, such as in the liver, bones, or even muscles, has a detrimental impact on these structures and the body.

Pancreatic fat is decreased by intermittent fasting

The team of experts split the diabetes-prone overweight animals into two categories: the first group was permitted to consume ad libitum — as much as they wished. The second group endured a random fasting routine: one day, the animals received an unlimited meal and were not fed the next day. The researchers noticed differences in the last five weeks. They concluded that the fat cells are accumulated in group 1 animals. Meanwhile, there are rarely any fat deposits in group 2 animals.

Hypersecretion of insulin by pancreatic adipocytes

Researchers extracted precursor cells of adipocytes from the mice pancreas to determine how fat cells could inhibit the pancreas' functioning, enabling them to develop into matured fat cells. If the grown fat cells were ultimately cultivated along with the pancreas islets of Langerhans, insulin was gradually secreted by the beta cells of the 'islets.' The rise in the production of insulin results in the quick depletion of Langerhans islets of the diabetic animals and after a while it terminates functioning entirely. In this way, the accumulation of fats in the pancreas results in the occurrence of diabetes type 2

Fasting Intermittently

In some clock cycles, intermittent fasting involves not eating. However, unsweetened tea, water, and black coffee are permitted around the clock. Depending on the process, fasting lasts between 16 to 24 hours or, instead, on two days within a week. An average of 500- 600 calories is consumed. The most known type of intermittent fasting seems to be the 16:8 method that includes eating only during a week

Langerhans Islets

Langerhans' islets — also referred to as islet cells or islets of Langerhans — are islet-like deposits in hormone-producing cells in the pancreas. There are about one million islets of Langerhans in a healthy person. Each islet has a diameter of 0.2-0.5 millimeters. The β – cells produce insulin from the blood sugar-lowering hormone and pay about 65 - 80 percent of the islet cells. When the blood sugar level rises in the body, these cells secrete insulin in the blood to normalize it again.

Fasting enhances heart health

Fasting can enhance heart health to refine blood pressure, cholesterol levels, and triglycerides.

Heart disease is recognized internationally as the leading cause of death, responsible for approximated 31.5% of deaths internationally. Among the most important ways to reduce the risk of heart disease is to mix up the diet and lifestyle. Some studies have found that it can be incredibly helpful for heart health to integrate fasting into your routine.

Research showed that intermittent fasting for eight weeks decreases "poor" LDL cholesterol levels by 25% and reduces blood triglycerides by 32 %.

Another analysis of 110 overweight individuals demonstrated that, under medical supervision, fasting for three weeks substantially lower blood pressure and blood triglyceride levels, total 'bad' LDL cholesterol, and total cholesterol.

Furthermore, in one study of 4,629 individuals, fasting was associated with a reduced risk of coronary artery disorder and a slightly reduced risk of diabetes, a risk factor for heart disease.

Fasting boosts brain function

New research shows that fasting can improve brain function by raising protein levels that encourage neuron growth.

The results suggest the treatment and prevention of age-related neurodegenerative diseases such as Alzheimer's disease correlated with diabetes type.   Researchers examined brain neurochemistry and brain activity of mice placed on intermittent fasting and normal eating.

Many studies are conducted on neurodegenerative diseases underlying molecular and cellular processes. They have also thoroughly studied how fasting can increase the amount of energy in neurons and enable the brain to resist disease.

Earlier work indicates that fasting is a brain challenge that activates chemicals that encourage greater neuron efficiency and development. It can also have this effect by performing rigorous exercise.

One unique chemical shift potentially gives more energy to neurons and improves links to other neurons. Researchers noticed that fasting mice displayed a 50% rise in a chemical in the brain called BDNF (brain-derived neurotrophic factor), triggered by a surge in beta-hydroxybutyrate in the ketone body as fasting burns fat.

It is known that BDNF facilitates the development of new stem cell neurons, greater neuronal Conn exons, and strengthens the synapses. In addition, previous literature indicates that a drop in BNDF levels is a characteristic of Alzheimer's.

The fasted mice and the rise in BDNF showed increased alertness and activation in brain regions involved in learning and memory.

The cognitive advantages of fasting may originate from a rise in the number of nerve cell mitochondria due to increased levels of BDNF. Neurodegeneration has historically been associated with a deficiency or dysfunction of brain mitochondria.

Increasing the number of mitochondria in neurons will improve their ability to shape and sustain synapses and, therefore, likely increase learning and memory capacity.

Fasting can delay aging and increase longevity

The anti-aging molecule caused by fasting preserves young blood vessels.

New studies have shown that fasting activates a molecule, slowing our arteries' aging. The results might help avoid chronic age-related diseases like heart disease, cancer, and Alzheimer's.

Researchers have discovered a new function for a molecule created during fasting: it can sustain our young and supple vascular system.

In a new analysis, researchers have restored aging symptoms such as wrinkles and hair loss in mice. Even more magnificently, another group of scientists has succeeded in rejuvenating aging human cells.

Fasting or reducing the intake of calories may generate a molecule that slows vascular aging.

How a ketonic molecule holds youthful cells?
Vascular aging is an essential part of aging. When people get older, the arteries that serve various organs are the most susceptible and the most resistant to damage from aging, so it is crucial to know vascular aging. t Therefore, the researchers agreed to concentrate on vascular aging and the events that happen with cell aging and how to avoid them.

The researchers explicitly observed the link between vascular aging and the restriction of calories. They used atherosclerosis mouse models, researched their aortas post-mortem, and conducted a series of experiments on cell culture. In the mice, they also caused malnutrition and performed similar experiments.

They saw that the hungry mice created the beta-hydroxybutyrate molecule, as predicted. Interestingly, however, vascular aging was also stopped by that compound.

Beta-hydroxybutyrate is a ketonic molecule formed by the liver and used when glucose is not available as an energy source. During fasting or famine, on low-carb diets, or after extended exercise, the body releases ketones.

The analysis also showed that beta-hydroxybutyrate encourages the cells that line the blood vessels inside to divide and multiply. An indicator of cellular youth is cellular division.

The beta-hydroxybutyrate molecule can slow vascular aging. That provides a chemical connation between the restriction of calories and the effect of anti-aging. This compound may delay vascular aging by endothelial cells that line the lymphatic vessels' inner surface and blood vessels. One type of cell aging, called senescence, can be prevented.

A target for drugs to avoid aging chronic illness:

The study also showed that the compound causes yet another chain of events that holds the DNA of such endothelial cells undamaged and young.

More precisely, when beta-hydroxybutyrate binds with heterogeneous nuclear ribonucleoprotein A1, an RNA-binding protein, it enhances the function of an Oct4 (Octamer-binding transcriptional factor), which is a stem cell transcription factor

BOOK 3: <u>DR SEBI'S CURE FOR HERPES</u>

DISCOVER THE PROVEN 3-STEP METHOD THAT ALLOWED 7000+ PEOPLE TO GET RID FOREVER OF COLD SORES AND GENITAL HERPES WITH NO MEDICATION

Chapter 1: Herpes Simplex Virus

What's Herpes?

It is indeed a virus that might stay inactive or allow the body to undergo the flare-up. Two major strains are known.

While the herpes virus group has eight variants, including the Epstein-Barr virus, we will concentrate on the two most prevalent HSV types.

HSV-1, or oral herpes, is a type of herpes spread by saliva. Many persons with oral herpes were possibly compromised during infancy or adulthood by exchanging a straw, cup, eating utensils, toothbrush, gum, or kissing.

The most prevalent sexual disease is HSV-2, also identified as genital herpes. As per the C.D.C, the incidents involving genital herpes within the U.S. are above 1 in 6 people aged 14-49. In women, it is often around twice as high as in males.

Herpes infection is drawn-out contamination brought about by the herpes simplex virus (HSV). The genital district, the oral locale, the skin, and the butt-centric area are the body areas influenced by this infection.

This ailment is known for an extremely prolonged period. It normally assaults people causing a few ailments; some are mellow, and some are perilous.

Genital herpes is one of the most widely recognized herpes simplex infections. The genital herpes infection is an explicitly transmitted disease that affects genital, and butt-centric rankles. There might be bruises that additionally influence the mouth and face.

A few instances of the rehashed appearance of genital herpes are brought about by H.V.S. 2. A large portion of this disease is spread from victims who don't realize they have it, and more often than not, the side effects are asymptomatic in a victim.

People can contract this contamination through a sexual relationship with a victim infected with HSV. Additionally, you can get contaminated by your sex accomplice, who doesn't encounter any indications of this disease whatsoever.

More so, the subsequent kind can be brought about by oral-butt-centric contact or butt-centric contact with a victim. HSV 2 is the most predominant herpes infection disease, yet HSV 1 happens less ordinarily.

HSV-1

The primary way that the HSV-1 virus spreads is through an outbreak from an affected person. In America alone, it is estimated that 67% of people under the age of 49 are infected with the HSV-1 herpes virus. But most of these people may not experience an outbreak throughout their lifetime.

The Ways You Can Contact the Herpes Simplex Virus

The ways you can contact HSV-1 includes:

- Kissing someone infected.
- Using the same eating utensils that an already affected person uses.
- Using the same lipstick or lip balm with an affected person.
- Engaging in oral sex with an infected person.

HSV-2

The primary way to contact HSV-2 is through sexual contact with an already affected person. According to the American Academy of Dermatology (A.A.D.), 20 to 25% of active sexually infected with the HSV-2 herpes virus.

This one is not that common as type one as only 15.5% of people from the age of 14—49 are suffering from this type of herpes in the U.S.A.

It is 100% impossible for you to get infected with genital herpes through a toilet seat.

You can also get infected through oral sex.

Different Manifestation of the Herpes Virus

Cold Sore

We'll expose many herpes myths in this book, but here's one of the most prevalent; the idea that a "cold sore" is NOT herpes. Unfortunately, many people believe this because of how the virus is marketed.

Knowledge about herpes is mostly the result of marketing firms tinkering with public perception.

However, not all mouth sorer is related to the herpes virus... A dermatologist can identify a herpes sore versus a different type of mouth ulcer.

Herpes Zoster

Herpes zoster is the clinical manifestation of the reactivation of the Varicella Zoster virus (VZV), the primary infection of chickenpox, an exanthemata disease affecting mainly children and characterized by maculae, bumps, blisters (vesicles), and crusts. The viral D.N.A. finds shelter in the posterior sensory ganglia or the cranial pars. Different factors comprising stress, immune depression, lymphomas, or immunosuppressive drugs may trigger this genetic material's activation and progress towards the epidermis. This triggering effect can take place at any time. However, it prevails in older people who have a depressed immune system. It is not season-related.

The VZV belongs to the Herpes virus family and comprises a double-chain D.N.A. genome with a lipoprotein layer that helps the virus adhere and get into.

It gains access through the airway and replicates in the rachidian nerves' ganglia, resulting in the first viridian.

Chickenpox

The virus gains access through the respiratory epithelium. It replicates in the lymph nodes, spreading through the blood and resulting in chickenpox. Symptoms do not take more than 15 days. The virus remains inside the posterior lymph nodes.

It starts as a hyperesthetic, painful, prodigious area preceded by fever, cephalea, asthenia, and local discomfort. Then, small blisters appear erythematous, the well-delimited place that adopts a radicular distribution. These blisters, which completely cover the area, tend to meet and group into one. Finally, scorching, neritic pain is characteristic and can persist for months (post-herpetic neuralgia).

Pyogenic impetiginization is frequent at the skin level and mucopurulent conjunctivitis in the ophthalmic region. It can mainly be seen in older people. It can be continuous or parodist. There is also paralysis, esp. in the face and the lumbosacral region and paresis. Despite its low incidence, encephalitis can also be a complication, presenting with fever, meningeal signs, disturbance of consciousness, hallucinations, and delirium.

What Are the Causes of Herpes?

There are some primary causes of herpes, which I am going to talk about below:

Oral sex

Oral sex is good, and I do not deny it, but it is wise for us to know who and how healthy our partner's mouth is. If the mouth of the person giving you a leader has cold sores around their mouth, there is a tendency that you might get infected with herpes.

Unprotected sex

Having unprotected sex with someone suffering from herpes transmits the virus.

Sharing sex toys with someone infected with the herpes virus transmits the virus rapidly and very fast.

Transmitted through birth

Another craziest thing about this virus is that it can be transmitted from the mother to her newborn baby through birth delivery if the mother's genital herpes have sores while giving birth.

Please note that sharing towels, chairs, kitchen utensils, or toilet seats with someone with herpes cannot get you infected because the viruses need a moist environment to be transmitted. That is why it can be transmitted through the eyes, anus, vagina, mouth, and wounds.

The Symptoms of the Herpes Virus Include

The main symptoms of the herpes virus are something that everyone needs to recognize to be careful because a lot of people with the herpes virus show no symptoms or visible signs such as:

Urine and Discharge Problems for Women

Stinging is a familiar sensation when pee comes into contact with an open injury. Ladies experience more difficulty with pee ignoring the wounds than men due to the shape and position of the urethra. Ladies may likewise observe a release adjustment when the herpes infection is dynamic. The release might be thick rather than white, watery, and normally unscented, with a yellow tinge and a sharp smell. This is an indication of disease in the cervix.

Blisters inside the Urethra

The urethra is the cylinder that interfaces the urinary bladder to the private parts. In the two people with herpes type-2, difficult bruises can frame this cylinder's inward coating. While peeing, an individual may feel a consuming or extremely sharp steel sensation when pee disregards these bruises. Not at all like genital or mouth bruises, the specialist may need to lead tests to affirm a herpes disease when the urethra is influenced.

Fatigue

Individuals with a herpes infection contamination may see general sentiments of tiredness, shortcoming, and an absence of vitality. Weakness may likewise discover its way into the muscles, leaving them feeling agonizing or substantial. This side effect can likewise cause brevity of breath, weight reduction, uneasiness, and gloom and leave individuals feeling like they have to nap as often as possible during the day.

Spinal pains

The herpes type-2 infection can influence the lumbar and sacral nerve roots, prompting nerve and nerve endings. As a result, individuals with herpes viral contamination Are regularly intermittent and can be very awkward and excruciating.

Flu-Like Symptoms

Influenza-like side effects that can create alongside herpes contamination include a fever with cools, an irritated throat, diligent hack, and a runny or stuffy nose. A few people may encounter sickness and retching or runs. The safe framework kicks vigorously to battle the contamination. Yet, the herpes infection leaves many people feeling exhausted until it can finish its work.

Headaches

Headaches and the herpes infection go connected at the hip when a flare-up happens. Indications of headaches incorporate general head torment, which can move from a moderate, dull yearn to an extreme, throbbing agony behind the eyes. Different side effects incorporate peevishness and affectability to sound and light. This cerebral pain may cause summed up muscle throbs, inconvenience dozing or focusing, obscured vision, nausea, and craving loss.

Swollen Lymph Nodes

Lymph hubs are little bean-formed organs all through the body. The lymphatic framework goes about as a seepage or sifting activity, conveying lymph liquid, supplements, and waste material through the tissues and the circulation system. Generally found in the neck, the crotch, and under the arms, these hubs expand and become delicate during disease or damage. When somebody has genital herpes, the organs around the genital territory will expand and might be sore.

Blisters on the Genitals

When genital rankles happen, the herpes type-2 infection (HSV 2) is as often as possible suspected as a reason. It will initially begin with a comparative inclination to the mouth wounds, yet with greater power because of the zone's affectability.

Around 12 to 24 hours before noticeable rankles, the skin will be bothersome and excruciating and might be red, crude, and broken. At that point, a rankle will show up burst open to turn into an ulcer before scabbing over to mend. The herpes episodes can repeatedly happen; however, the manifestations of bunched rankles will here and there become less extreme than the underlying disease. The infection is infectious both during an episode and when there are no manifestations or wounds.

Mouth blisters

As often as possible, mouth blisters on the mouth brought about by the herpes type-1 infection (HSV-1) are a typical event. After they initially create individuals powerless to them contract the bruises repeatedly. Most normally found around the lips, the herpes infection can cause rankles in the mouth and throat.
The mouth blisters start as little red fixes that transform into a rankle or a bunch of rankles that blast and leave a crude, sobbing region in the long run blast. This territory normally recuperates and scabs over without assistance. Yet, over-the-counter creams can help alleviate and fix the skin.

Itching or Tingling Around Genitals or Anus

The main indication of the herpes infection flare-up is tingling and bothering around the influenced zone. The tainted individual may feel a shivering or tingling sensation around the private parts of the butt or some other delicate tissue territory like the mouth or nose. This is an indication that will create in this limited territory. The skin will get red, irritated, and may break a bit. It will feel crude and sore, and contact is prompted against as this can move germs and microorganisms.

What Triggers Herpes?

Through skin-to-skin touch with anyone who got the infection, herpes can quickly be transmitted. You will get it, typically through anal, oral, & vaginal intercourse, anytime your mouth or genitals meet their mouth and genitals.

If there's a path for herpes to get through, such as a wound, rash, burn, or other infections, other skin areas may get contaminated. To get herpes, you may not have to have intercourse. Herpes may also be spread in non-sexual contexts, such as whether you are pecked on the lips by a parent with a cold sore. While they were children, most individuals having oral herpes developed it. While vaginal childbirth, a mother may transfer herpes to the newborn, but that's very uncommon.

Suppose you tap herpes sore and touch your genitals, eyes, or mouth without washing your hands first. In that case, you will transmit herpes to any other areas of your body. This way, you will even move herpes onto somebody else.

Herpes is more common when the sores are exposed and moist. The infection is quickly transmitted by fluid through herpes blisters. Although there have been no sores, herpes may still "shed" & get passed on to someone, and the skin appears perfectly fine.

Most people receive herpes through someone who has no sores at all. It will remain in the body for a long time without showing some signs, but it is impossible to tell for certain how and where you caught it. That's why it's a pretty sly virus that so many individuals have herpes.

You can't catch herpes by hugging, shaking hands, sneezing, coughing, or using toilet seats because the infection dies rapidly outside of the body.

The individual must refrain from oral, anal, or vaginal sex with someone affected with HSV-2 to avoid contractions with genital herpes. To do this, you should refrain from sex entirely or just have sex in a legally monogamous partnership in which neither spouse exhibits genital herpes.

The use of contraceptives might even minimize the risk of genital herpes. Still, lesions could be present in places not covered by condoms, and no lesions need to be visible for the disease to spread. Some strategies to avoid or minimize the transmission of the infection can involve taking medicine each day to avoid an epidemic, or after an epidemic, avoiding participating in anal, oral, or vaginal intercourse.

The factors that can trigger an outbreak of the herpes virus include:

1. Prolonged stress or stressful activities

2. Excessive heat or sunburn

3. Fever

4. Menstruation

Manifestations of Herpes Virus

There are three manners by which herpes infection show:

1. **It happens through the change of existing infections**

 In general, R.N.A. infections will have an uncommonly high pace of change since mistakes in recreating their R.N.A. genomes are not rectified by editing. Some transformation changes their current infections into new hereditary assortments that can cause illness, even resistance to the infection.

2. **Distribution of herpes infection from a little secluded human populace**

For example, aids went un-named and unnoticed for a considerable time before it started to spread the world over. Accordingly, mechanical and social elements, including reasonable worldwide travel, blood transfusions, extramarital perversion, and the maltreatment of intravenous medications, permitted a formerly uncommon human illness to turn into a worldwide one.

3.   The spread of existing infections from different creatures

Researchers evaluated that seventy-five percent of new human infections start along these lines. Creatures hold and transmit a specific infection; however, they are commonly unaffected by it are said to go about as a characteristic supply for that infection (Campbell Reece, 2008).

The Risk of Contracting the Herpes Virus

Everyone can contract the herpes virus, but certain factors expose some people to the risk of contracting the herpes virus.

Some of such risk factors include:

1.   Having a weak immune system

2.   Having oral and unprotected sex with affected partners

3.   Having a previously untreated sexually transmitted disease

4.   Having multiple sexual partners at a young age

5.   More risk as a woman

Who's at risk of getting diseases of herpes simplex?

Anyone, irrespective of age, may be contaminated by HSV. But, almost exclusively, the probability is dependent on susceptibility to the virus.

Individuals are increasingly at risk in sexual transmission instances because they have intercourse not covered by contraceptives or other protective techniques.

Some HSV-2 risk factors include: • Having several sex partners • Physical intercourse at an earlier age • Female being • Getting another virus spread via sex • Possession of a compromised immune system When a pregnant lady has a genital herpes infection at the period of delivery, the infant will be subjected to both forms of HSV and will be at risk of severe complications.

What is the future regarding herpes simplex in the long term?

For the remainder of their life, individuals who get contaminated from HSV may have the infection. The infection can continue in an infected individual's nerve cells, although it doesn't show symptoms.

Frequent outbreaks can occur in certain persons. After they have become bitten, some can only undergo one infection, and afterward, the virus might be inactive.

Over time, it is suspected that occurrence -becomes less frequent when the body continues to produce antibodies. Therefore, there are normally no risks if a typically stable individual is afflicted with infection.

Preventing the transmission of diseases with herpes simplex

While there is no treatment for herpes, you should take precautions to discourage or avoid the spread of HSV to some other person from transmitting the virus.

If you have an HSV-1 epidemic, try taking a few protective steps: • Try preventing overt physical interaction with many other persons.

• Don't exchange certain things such as towels, cups, clothes, silverware, lip balm, or makeup, which can transmit the virus.

• In an occurrence, do not partake in sexual contact, kissing, or some such form of sexual interaction.

• To avoid contact with lesions, clean your hands well & use medicine using cotton swabs.

Individuals with HSV-2 can prevent some form of sexual contact with other persons. A contraceptive must be used through sex if the individual is not having signs but has also been confirmed to have the virus. However, the infection may also be transmitted from exposed skin to a mate, including contraceptive use.

To keep the pathogen from harming their newborn infants, people who are expecting & contaminated might just have to use medication.

Chapter 2: Genital Herpes

Anyone sexually active can be infected with herpes. Herpes is a sexually transmitted disease caused by the herpes simplex virus. One can live with the virus without any symptoms, and that's the major reason it's easily spread through sexual intercourse. You can have the virus and spread it to your partner without knowing.

Generally, there are two types of viruses responsible for herpes infection. These viruses are; type 1 herpes simplex virus (HSV-1) and type 2 herpes simplex virus (HSV-2).

It's important to know that herpes doesn't only attack the genitals. Its infection can be oral. Oral herpes is mostly caused by herpes simplex virus type 1, which has a fever, blisters, cold sore, etc. However, there may be no virus symptoms until its outbreak in some cases. It can be transmitted through saliva or oral sex.

Genital Herpes

Genital herpes is very common in the United States, and one in every six persons has the virus. This is so because it can easily be spread through sex. And one can easily be infected once one comes in contact with the virus. Therefore, using protection during sex does not guarantee that the virus will not be transmitted.

If your skin touches your partner's infected area, whether genital or oral, you can be easily infected. The infected person's saliva alone is enough to spread the disease with oral infection. In addition, general secretions of someone infected with genital herpes can spread the disease.

So, herpes is a disease that can be spread, even without explicit sex. If you have oral sex with someone infected with oral herpes, you can get infected easily.

Though herpes can be spread easily through contact, the virus doesn't survive easily outside the body. Therefore, you cannot contract the disease from objects like toilet seats, swimming pools, soap, towels, etc.

The best way to avoid herpes and other sexually transmitted diseases (S.T.D.s) is to avoid sex. However, if you are in a relationship, do your best to stick with your partner. Discuss with your couple if you notice any signs or symptoms of herpes. It's better to avoid sex if you have S.T.D.

Genital herpes is one of the most common sexually transmitted diseases in America; a clear understanding of this condition allows us to take appropriate measures to prevent it or even treat it if we have already acquired the disease.

Genital herpes is caused by the herpes simplex virus, which is estimated to be present in the body of one in five adults in the United States. Many people have no symptoms; therefore, they have no idea that they are infected with the virus.

After acquiring the disease, many victims have had recurrent genital ulcers for years. Genital infection can be managed with proper self-care and medication.

People with genital herpes are generally encouraged to discuss with their sexual partner, use condoms while having sex, and practice other preventive measures to prevent transmission to others. Genital herpes is transmittable even when there are no visible signs of ulcers and blisters.

Genital herpes is an infection that occurs near or on the genitalia. The type 2 herpes virus usually causes it. On the flip side, type 1 herpes infection is becoming more and more popular in recent years due to increased oral sex practice.

Contrary to popular belief, skin contact is the only way to spread genital herpes. It can't be gotten through the sharing of towels, toilet seats, or swimming pools.

A significant outbreak is usually more severe than the subsequent ones. When the initial attack is over, it becomes inactive and does not cause symptoms again. This period is known as the dormant infection; the herpes virus can pop up again at any point after this. It then becomes reactive and once again causes sores.

Once a victim has contracted herpes, it is there for life (which isn't true). The person may experience repeated recurrences or outbreaks. Every single person has a unique recurrent pattern while experiencing episodes.

The frequency, severity, and duration of outbreaks can significantly be reduced with herbal treatments and mixtures.

What's the distinction between oral herpes & genital herpes?

Many people are uncertain about what to name these diseases. There are two distinct forms of herpes viruses, HSV-1 & HSV-2, on multiple body sections. But it's pretty easy actually: It's labeled genital herpes anytime you either have HSV-1 or two on or near your vulva, vagina, butt, cervix, scrotum, penis, anus, inner thighs).

It's labeled oral herpes anytime you have HSV-1 or 2 in or near your mouth, lips & throat. In addition, fever blisters or Cold sores are often called oral herpes.

HSV-1 tends to cause oral herpes, & genital herpes is typically induced by HSV-2, with each strain choosing to reside in its favorite location. But with all forms of herpes, infecting a region is entirely probable. For starters, when somebody having a cold sore over their lips offers you oral sex, you might develop HSV-1 over your genitals. And when you provide oral sex to someone having HSV-2 over their genitals, you will develop HSV-2 on the mouth.

Herpes and H.I.V.

Herpes sore on the skin, vagina, mouth, or rectum can provide a pathway for H.I.V. to easily enter the body. Moreover, genital herpes increase CD4 cells count in the lining of the genitals. CD4 cells are what H.I.V. usually targets to gain entry into the body.

When H.I.V. and Herpes are present in a person, they can easily spread the viruses during sexual intercourse.

Chapter 3: Herpes and Relationships

Telling Your Partner About HSV

So, now you're in the awkward position of having to explain to your significant other about being infected with genital herpes. Mainstream advice says: "tell your partner right away, always use condoms and take antiviral medication to lessen your partner's chance of contracting the disease."

What this common advice does not mention is the fact most people are terrified of HSV, and it's not uncommon, at all, for boyfriends and girlfriends to leave their partners over such a matter. So it is not an easy subject to bring up!

Also, there's no mention of the severe side-effects of antiviral, and some doctors suggest taking them for the rest of your life to keep your partner from becoming infected!

While yes, obviously you need to tell your partner right away, I suggest approaching the topic from a slightly different frame of mind:

1. Explain You Have Hsv-2 Not "Genital Herpes"

Hysteria and taboos sometimes surround words and concepts more than anything else. Call the virus what it is. One of the reasons genital herpes is a bit of a misnomer is because sometimes HSV-2 isn't even located on the genitals, so if you're diagnosed with it, consult with your doctor to see if it's even latent on your nether region or not.

2. Explain the Virus Is Dormant and Prove It with a Medical Test

Prove your low viral count and the static nature of the illness by having a urine test.

Explain the truth that catching HSV-2 is not a big deal, unlike what media/society/commercials say. Furthermore, provide some of the pamphlets provided by the herpes virus association.

Explain That You Take Natural Anti-Virals and You Lead a Lifestyle to Minimize Chances of Spreading It

Don't take dangerous antiviral pharmaceuticals if you're not having reoccurring outbreaks and you don't need it. But reassure your partner that you're taking all the necessary precautions to prevent infecting anybody else.

Ask Them If They've Ever Had a Cold Sore Before

If so, they are infected with HSV-1, a far more dangerous form of herpes. Explain that 30-40% of the adult population also has HSV-2, growing.

Should I Tell My Partner About It?

It is a moral question, for which the answer is obviously "yes", but I can perfectly understand why many people debate the idea. Given the extreme social taboo of the virus, we've almost reached a point where people have no choice but to hide the fact they're infected, and I don't blame them. Again, I don't condone it, but I perfectly understand why people feel this way.

It comes down to you; you can either be honest about your illness and risk having your partner leave you or be a liar and hide it. But, of course, if it becomes apparent later that you're infected (or if they catch it from you), you'll risk having your partner leave you, and you'll be called a liar.

However, the big problem with revealing to a partner about herpes infection is that it's not realistic at the beginning of a relationship to wear the disease around your neck as a badge of dishonor. If you're single, and you meet the future love of your life. You guys are tearing each other's clothes off in the heat of passion. Do you think this is a good time to say, "wait, baby, I'm infected with genital herpes!"

Seriously, you'll never date again. Until the social taboo of HSV-2 is lifted, this will remain a big issue for everybody infected (which is currently 60+ million Americans).

For this reason, if you opt not to disclose herpes, make sure your viral count is as low as it can go, and wear a condom for added protection. The odds of a new partner contracting herpes, in this case, is very small.

If you're having any kind of outbreak whatsoever, you have to refrain from sex. Furthermore, if you're entering a relationship or a reoccurring series of physical encounters, reread the above steps for explaining your infection properly so as not to harm your relationship.

Dealing with the Herpes Stigma

The reason herpes is "the world's most annoying virus" is not so much because of the outbreaks as it is the social stigma associated with having it.

Herpes is considered a social taboo. It's used as an insult against people and used by people who probably have HSV-2 without realizing it to denigrate others.

Which is a shame considering it's one of the most benign illnesses. HSV-1 does have some dangerous health ramifications, but HSV-2 (genital herpes) does not—unless you have an autoimmune disorder like H.I.V.

So why would anybody make something seem worse than it is? The answer is profit.

Because it's such a common illness, by scaring or shaming the people who catch it, it's possible to up the sales of Valtrex or whatever the latest pharmaceutical is. That's tens of millions of potential customers.

That is why many doctors indirectly exaggerate HSV in the media or commercials. You'll never hear them say, "if you're one of the 2-4% who develops chronic HSV symptoms..." As far as they're concerned, everybody infected needs immediate pharmaceutical treatment.

Chapter 4: Dr. Sebi Thoughts on Herpes

An alkaline-rich diet rich in essential nutrients will help rid your body of the herpes virus. It can be achieved by creating an environment that can't support the growth of diseases causing substances.

The cells in your body require oxygen to perform to their optimum capacity. Still, the chemicals and substances found in some medicines and foods rob your cells of the much-needed oxygen to thrive.

Curing the herpes virus requires adequate cleansing of your body, and Dr. Sebi's plant-based alkaline diet does just that.

It is essential to know that curing herpes depends on your food and what you feed your body.

You should avoid eating sweets and starchy foods. Instead, eat foods that are bitter instead of sweet.

Eat more healthy vegetables such as zucchini, mushrooms, squash, cactus leaf or cactus plant flowers, and sea vegetables. Plant-based iron, such as dandelion, burdock, and yellow dock, is also helpful.

Dr. Sebi also emphasizes fasting because fasting helps you eat less and heal fast. Another good reason Dr. Sebi's diet can cure herpes is that it eliminates mucus in your body. That is because once your mucus membrane is compromised, your immune system becomes weak, and you become to disease.

Your mucus membrane needs to remain healthy for you to be healthy because it is your mucus membrane in charge of protecting your body's cells.

The plant-based diets and herbs that are the main constituents of Dr. Sebi's alkaline cell foods are very effective for curing herpes.

Dr. Sebi cured herpes by detoxifying the body and effectively nourishing the body.

You presumably know at this point what Dr. Sebi herpes fix is. Truly, Dr. Sebi's solution for herpes is continuously arriving at each side of the world. The purpose of it picking up prevalence so brisk isn't many dollars spent on commercials. Nor is it well known because some big-name is embracing it. Instead, it dazzles the hearts of herpes patients in such a case that its adequacy.

Basic because the recuperating standards of this incredible cultivator are successful, the present reality is discussing him. Everybody today knows him as a man who helped millions conquer the illnesses wherein allopathy helped less. Notwithstanding, later on, it was understood that Dr. Sebi's standards were extraordinary in all the wellbeing inconveniences. Today, we won't just discuss what Dr. Sebi's herpes fix is about, yet we will reveal to you why Dr. Sebi's herpes fix is the best alternative you ought to go for.

Dr. Sebi was a famous herbalist who mended numerous patients when allopathic specialists couldn't assist. He identified the enchantment that herbs conveyed and, utilizing that supernatural made numerous lives excellent and sickness-free. Similar standards of mending, when applied to herpes, gave sudden and incomprehensible outcomes. What the allopathic specialists couldn't reply to, what the researchers couldn't stop, can be fixed with the assistance of Dr. Sebi's remedy for herpes.

Nothing was taking a shot at mouth blisters and different manifestations of herpes. Yet, this botanist had at the top of the priority list some marvel herbs that can give another opportunity for herpes patients to live.

Even though it is likewise critical to perceive how it is done, at the same time, before that, let us see why Dr. Sebi's method is the best accessible option for you.

1. *It is the best because it works in herpes:* This is the best treatment far from the effectiveness. There is very little effective herpes treatment around the globe. There are antiviral drugs that are expensive but ineffective. They only give you a fake feeling of wellness when, in fact, nothing is working as it should in your body. Despite the intake of antiviral drugs by some herpes patients, the herpes simplex virus still thrives without limitation. It is a lot of sacrifices to choose antiviral drugs over traditional medicines as the former only pamper the symptoms of herpes with many underlying side effects. Some other herbs are safe but do not produce the same effect as Dr. Sebi's cure. It makes Dr. Sebi's treatment the only perfect solution for every herpes patient, as nothing comes close to its healing prowess.

2. *It is the best option because it is safe:* Dr. Sebi's cure is all-natural. All the ingredients contained therein are devoid of any synthetic material. Herbs have been in existence since the time the very first man was made, and the reason they are still preferred over conventional medicine is that they have zero side effects. Since Dr. Sebi's cure is entirely made up of herbs, you do not have to worry about your present and future health. These herbs work like magic, not only in curing you of herpes but also in improving your health every day. Those who have used Dr. Sebi's herpes cure in the past have backed up the claim that these herbs indeed improved their health as they felt more energetic after starting the course. This makes Dr. Sebi's herpes cure the only alternative you should consider.

3. *It is the best because it is cost-effective, too:* With antiviral drugs, you need a prescription. Dr. Sebi's herpes cure is different, as you do not need a prescription when you purchase. This alternative medicine is much less than the money that goes into consultation. Health is essential, but the money spent on antiviral drugs is excessive, not guaranteeing their effectiveness. On the other hand, Dr. Sebi's herpes cure is available in nature. You do not need to pay a consultation fee, and zero marketing cost is involved. You only pay for what you get. Since it is effective and gets the job done, you are not throwing away your hard-earned cash.

4. *It is the best because scientists certify it:* various medical and scientific research has verified Dr. Sebi's claim to cure herpes with herbs. In addition, some studies established more facts about the herbs' antiviral properties used in the herpes cure. Natural antiviral properties can rid the body of the herpes virus without any side effects. In addition to the antiviral properties found in these herbs, they have also been found to be immune-modulatory. That means they directly boost the body's disease-fighting mechanism. A more muscular immune system means that the herpes simplex virus's replication can be put under control for every herpes patient to live a herpes-free life. All the research about Dr. Sebi's herpes cure proves it is the best solution for herpes.

5. *It is the best because it gives you herpes free life:* The efficacy of Dr. Sebi's herpes cure is the sole reason it is considered the best herpes treatment worldwide. No other treatment has been verified to cure herpes, only this one. Therefore, you need to trust Dr. Sebi's methods to live a herpes free life.

The highlighted points are why Dr. Sebi's herpes cure is the best one around. So if you think it is time to end the pain herpes is putting you through, you should give this cure a try.

In the wake of taking a gander at the fixings, it is by all accounts all the more encouraging solution for herpes, isn't that so? Indeed, it can murder the herpes simplex infection. Everything is expected to help herpes patients carry on with a herpes-free life. You may be on antiviral medications at present and can remain on the equivalent in the future too. Only for a couple of days, give this supernatural item a possibility, and you will never need to glance back at some other herpes treatment.

Herpes fix is a typical point encompassed with such a significant number of inquiries and no reliable answer. If you have herpes, your brain might be loaded with questions identified with herpes treatment. Herpes is a disease spreading worldwide; many individuals are influenced by herpes, yet nobody thinks about it regarding herpes fix. The ongoing revelation of herpes treatment is Dr. Sebi's herpes fix.

This isn't just a name; however, the most anticipated comprehensive solution for herpes can cause your fantasy about getting the chance to be free of herpes to work out as expected. Dr. Sebi is the author of the Dr. Sebi inquiry about the foundation, which professes to fix illnesses like malignancy, A.I.D.S., lupus, diabetes, fibroids tumor joint inflammation, sickle cell sickliness, and now herpes as well.

These illnesses, including herpes, are a large difficulty for a human to deal with. Now it is an ideal opportunity to get an answer for every one of them. The sicknesses like herpes need more mindfulness and information because you deal with the successive episodes of herpes and control the transmission up partly with these. You ought to know about the infection; you can discover your responses to the herpes treatment at exactly that point.

The following steps were what Dr. Sebi used to cure herpes:

Put an end to consuming acid foods. Ensure your body is not fed with acidic foods.

Clean your body of acids and toxins and start eating alkaline diets and herbs that increase your cells' oxygen level.

Feeding your body with the needed nutrients can repair, rebuild, and completely strengthen your body at the cellular level.

Practice fasting. Take herbs and water only during fasting. You can add green juice if fasting becomes too difficult for you.

Eat vegetables and fruits immediately after fasting.

Endeavor to eat foods from Dr. Sebi's nutritional guide after your body has been cured of herpes. Detoxification is at the heart of ridding the body of the herpes virus-there is no other way that will bring the necessary results."

Ways to cure herpes

Herpes and Alkaline diets

For the healing of herpes, an alkaline diet is needed. Dr. Sebi emphasized the significance of this and how important it is to eliminate 'blood and starch,' as he calls it, referencing animal flesh-like all sorts of animals, seafood, and starchy foods. However, it is essential to move beyond this when it applies to herpes recovery since even some things on Dr. Sebi's food list or dietary guide can be avoided. And why? Only that some of the ingredients are soothing better than others. Dr. Sebi stated that his collection comprises 'least harmful' foods; nevertheless, you want food as alkaline as possible and refreshing as possible. For this cause, fasting was believed to be such an essential factor in Dr. Sebi's recovery – it helped the body break from the ingestion of mucus-forming foods and acids; cleaning will begin, and the oxygen amount to the cells may improve.

An alkaline diet is essential for the whole process of herpes cure. On numerous occasions, Dr. Sebi stressed the vitality of avoiding "blood and flesh," that is, animal flesh, meats, fish, and starchy foods. However, when it comes to healing herpes, you need to go over and beyond by avoiding some of the foods on Dr. Sebi's list.

That is simply because some foods have more healing factors than others. Dr. Sebi has always referred to his food list as "least detrimental" as the diet is alkaline and cleanses the body. That is the sole reason why fasting boosts this healing method's effectiveness, as it allows the body to break acid consumption and begin the cleansing process.

During this time, alkaline herbs should be consumed in a high quantity. It helps cleanse and nourish the body and strengthen the immune system.

During this time, eat alkaline herbs to detox, rejuvenate, recharge the body, and improve immunity.

What exactly do you have to do?

1. Stop foods that are fried.

2. Delete all acid-forming items from the diet.

3. Take just the water and herbs for fasting (if you can't incorporate green juices).

4. Instantly, after easy eating, only vegetables and fruit from the dietary guide also involve new green juices. Your leafy vegetables primarily contain green fluids. During cleaning and detox, the less stable the diet, the smoother and more successful the healing process.

5. Once you have eliminated herpes from the body, even then, keep consuming only items from the dietary guide.

6. Nuts, grains, and seeds must be avoided while recovering from herpes. Whereas mangoes, citruses, leafy greens, and berries are recommended.

When questioned, Dr. Sebi replied very correctly that the healing time depends on the degree of body toxicity, fluid, weight, and health condition. In addition, everyone has a different fitness stage, and therefore the duration of recovery differs. Hence, the healing time varies between people.

You can detoxify herpes from a body, but the results also depend on your dedication to the procedure. Herpes is not the most straightforward virus to get clear because it sets up residency in the central nervous system's spinal cord and often remains inactive for an extended period. Basically, your body needs to 'wake it up' and usher it back. The herpes virus must be inaccessible to the body. An alkaline body is essential to keep the body alkaline by washing and treating the body through alkaline plants and alkaline food, and fasting to become rid of herpes. This is Dr. Sebi's method.

What Does the Dr. Sebi Diet Consist of?

Alkaline diets are those which do not contain foods that contain acids.

Acidic foods contain high acid content, and they are most times detrimental to human health. When there is an increased amount of acid in the body, infectious diseases find it easy to thrive, grow, and develop. Therefore, Dr. Sebi does not encourage these kinds of foods in his diet, as they might hinder the effectiveness of his recommended herbal products and foods.

The Dr. Sebi diet is a vegetarian, plant-based regimen and a basic eating routine (National Institute of Health). While following the eating regimen, numerous additional take herbs to sustain the cell, help rinse them and recuperate them from many years of frightful eating.

Dr. Sebi believes soluble nourishments to be "electric nourishments" for your cell, which are live and crude nourishments that are for the "recuperating of the country." when all is said and done, Dr. Sebi separates nourishment into six classes:

1. Live

2. Crude

3. Dead

4. Half breed

5. Hereditarily changed

6. Drugs

He used to say that you should concentrate on numbers 1 and 2 (live and crude) while avoiding 3 – 6. This incorporates maintaining a strategic distance from seedless organic products, climate-safe harvests, for example, corn, and anything with included nutrients or minerals, which can be hard for individuals thinking about that there are such a large number of crossbreed and hereditarily altered (G.M.O.) leafy foods offered in supermarkets.

As per Dr. Sebi, foods prescribed for individuals who need to live sound incorporate ready organic products, non-bland vegetables, crude nuts and margarine, and grains. Verdant greens, quinoa, rye, and Kamut can likewise assume a huge job in the Dr. Sebi diet.

Acidic foods, including meat, poultry, fish, or items containing yeast, liquor, sugar, iodized salt, or anything seared, negatively impact the human body.

Supplanting acidic foods with electric choices will assist with mending you from the negative impacts that corrosive produces.

To a great extent, crude weight control plans can appear distasteful to acidic people. Yet, you gradually become accustomed to a simple eating routine as you purge your poisons cells, prompting the disorder to fix.

Limiting corrosive in nourishments assists with diminishing bodily fluid in the body, which makes a soluble situation that makes it extremely hard for sickness to frame. Remembering herbs for your purging methodology is stunningly better.

Advantages of an Alkaline Diet

Weight Loss

This part is clear as crystal. Weight reduction will undoubtedly happen when following the eating routine because the Dr. Sebi diet comprises regular vegetables, natural products, grains, nuts, and vegetables.

Immune System Boosting

A feeble-resistant framework is the aftereffect of ailments and disorders. In some cases, they have fortified their insusceptible framework. They have been recuperated from specific infirmities by reliably following the Dr. Sebi diet. We, as a whole, realize that medication doesn't fix infections.

Decreased Risk of Disease

Acidic nourishments disintegrate the mucous layer of the cells and inward dividers of the body, which prompts an undermined framework that makes infection conceivable and a fix unimaginable. Subsequently, eating basic nourishments can lessen the danger of sickness and help your body get what it needs to take care of the great cells.

Vitality

Diets overwhelming in meat, dairy, and white sugar can delay your body and vitality levels. Concentrating on plant-based living is a superior approach and can improve the vitality that you show all the time.

Expanded Focus

Following Dr. Sebi's lessons will assist with clearing cerebrum mist to keep you engaged and less disturbed by unpleasant circumstances that emerge.

Whether you are not wiped out, utilizing a plant-based philosophy will help you carry on with a long and solid life.

Chapter 5: Dr. Sebi's 3-Step Method

Detoxification and Cleansing

As I said before, Dr. Sebi thought that every disease's source is the excess of mucus that slowly builds up in different parts of our bodies because of the acidic environment the 'standard' diets create.

As Dr. Sebi stated, human bodies can face six stages of over-acidity if the body is not nourished with alkaline foods and herbs:

1. **Sensitivity** → You know you are in this stage if you start suffering from low energy, acne, or bad odor.

2. **Irritation** → The next one is where you start facing bowel diseases such as IBS, constipation, diarrhea, or skin problems

3. **Mucous Formation** → Here's where your body can't tolerate living in an extra-acidic environment anymore and start producing mucus to try to protect itself

4. **Inflammation** → As soon as the mucus starts to build up, your body reacts by starting the inflammation process. That might cause you to start suffering from Arthritis or Fibromyalgia

5. **Indurations** → This stage's most dangerous complication is Atherosclerosis, also known as "the hardening of arteries". When mucus starts depositing into them, it takes the name of 'plaques'. Over time, these plaques can narrow or block the arteries and cause unforeseen problems, such as strokes.

6. **Degeneration** → Mucus builds up into the brain, bones, and around nerves in the last stage. If that happens, dangerous diseases may arise, such as cancer, Multiple Sclerosis, or Osteoporosis.

As strategies to remove pollutants from the body, reduce weight, or improve wellbeing, several "detoxification" or "cleansing" regimens have been introduced.

The words cleanse & detox are also used synonymously. Although both eliminate contaminants from the body, detox and a cleanse are two separate items. It is clean at the core of the term "cleanse," and you must think of washing as a way to clean the body. To specifically remove toxins, cleanse frequently utilizes vitamins or tablets, and cleanses typically concentrate mostly on the digestive system. On the other side, Detox services aim to help the normal toxin-eliminating cycles in the body. Because the liver & the kidneys are the key detoxing centers in the body, successful detox programs concentrate on helping the kidneys and liver by supplying them with the vitamins and nutrients they have to operate optimally.

What are poisons anyway, then? Of course, heavy metals are top of the mind, like arsenic. However, chronic chemical contaminants, chemicals, & pesticides are still included in the report. Toxins are simply toxic compounds that will reside in the bloodstream, disturbing cells, triggering irritation, & interacting with the body's usual functions.

Indications of toxins or a heavy toxin load (and hence the need for detoxification or cleansing) provide the following:

1. fatigue

2. headaches

3. joint pain

4. depression

5. anxiety

6. constipation

The Cleansing Journey

Making the stomach safe is linked with cleansing. The digestive system is the system the body that receives its nutrients from. It becomes inefficient in performing its tasks as it gets unstable. In the stomach, the pile-up of the dump will turn poisonous, contributing to pain and disease. Bloating is among the symptoms of a dysfunctional stomach. When the body cannot get rid of waste, that's due to gas accumulation. The food continues to decompose then. Food, as meant by default, must be natural and organic.

There are both positive and destructive microbes in the digestive system. It contributes to problems if the equilibrium of such bacteria is disrupted. Purging, in which a laxative is used to eliminate human waste, parasites, and other unnecessary material, is the essential cleansing method. The concern with this technique is that it would be non-selective & clears up the harmful benefits. It may also be harmful since, during the phase, you may lose extra water, which would make you drained. One of its reasons is that the body system gets a strip of toxic chemicals to consume lots of water.

A vice president & dietician of the Sports Education Society, Marie Spano, claims that workouts and adequate sleep play a vital role in making your function on the detox regimen.

By curing the gut by noting what goes through it. Unfortunately, it's considered fast food, and it doesn't have the nutrition your body requires. Instead, clogging things up appears to screw with the digestive tract. Soy, gluten, dairy, sugar, & caffeine-containing foods can be removed and substituted with unprocessed agricultural substitutes & additives.

The cleansing method is complete with the clearance of waste from the digestive system. Instead, it should be cured by supplying nutritious food that makes the gut function at its peak. That requires balanced food with adequate nutrition, which tends to maintain the stomach's safe levels in the stomach, such as good bacteria—organic beverages, such as unflavored probiotic yogurt, often aid.

Minneapolis Running's Sara Welle speaks about her advantages as a competitor from the cleansing plan. You must go through a well before-cleanse process to start the detox method, where you'll have to strip out alcohol & different highly processed foods. Her program's early days were unpleasant. However, she noticed that her stress levels increased as the system matured and operated properly.

The Detox Route

Another approach to clear the body of destructive chemicals is to detox. Normally, through the liver, skin, and kidneys, the body requires the removal of pollutants. Detox can strengthen the contributions of these organs. So, what toxins are attacked by the process? For example, contaminants in the atmosphere you breathe in to make their way through your bloodstream, where they settle and create pain. Chemicals such as toxins, preservatives, & additives are still used in many products. During this time, meat must be avoided.

One of the actors whose detox was performed is Gwyneth Paltrow. Over a 21-day duration, it is circulated. It's named The Safe Method by the psychiatrist who developed it. To clear the contaminants' body, he recommends a diet of shakes, nutritious foods, and vitamins—any of his patient's record post-program weight loss.

Your skin is often loaded with a mixture of chemicals hidden on the lotions of creams and other products you use. Often, the organs associated with detoxifying get overloaded.

What Are The Dr. Sebi Approved Detoxification/Cleansing Approaches?

Many detoxification programs are offered in an integrative health care model. The following are the approved methods to eliminate toxins in your body:

1. Water Fast

2. Liquid Fast

3. Smoothie Fast

4. Fruit Fast

5. Raw Food Fast

Why You Should Detox

Detoxing or detoxification is a process of ridding the body of toxins and other harmful substances that have accumulated through time. Most toxins come from the food we eat, but they can also enter the body through the air we breathe and the medicines we take. Regardless of how these toxins came about, they can be harmful to the body and pose serious threats that need to be addressed if you want to stay healthy and at your peak.

Weight Loss

Weight loss is one of the biggest reasons why people go through detoxification or why they even think about the idea. Detox for weight loss is fairly straightforward to understand, as this involves eating natural and unprocessed foods. That means less, or even no, junk foods and unhealthy food options make you put on those extra pounds. In addition, going on a detox diet means taking in fewer calories and, therefore, potentially losing weight if coupled with a good exercise program. While weight loss is perhaps the most publicized benefit of detox, most detox programs involve short-term solutions that lead to short-term results. Nevertheless, detox can help you lose weight, especially if you make it a regular part of your lifestyle.

Boosts Energy

Many detox programs result in increased energy levels for participating individuals. While it is hard to quantify energy or just how much of it a person has, the results pretty much speak for themselves, as people who undergo detox programs generally feel more energetic. They report feeling less sluggish and having an overall feeling of just wanting to be out and about and doing things rather than just lying around all the time. That can be attributed to the fact that detoxification releases the toxins that lower the body's energy levels.

The body is free from such substances ' sluggish effects by steering clear of the things that provide toxins such as sugars and trans fats. Moreover, replacing such negative foods with natural energy boosters such as fruits and vegetables can increase a person's energy levels in the best way possible. Added to this is that detoxification means keeping the body hydrated at all times, resulting in more energy and better efficiency when performing daily tasks.

Stronger Immune System

The health benefits of detox or detoxification also include a stronger immune system. Toxins are naturally harmful to the body, or at the very least, they prevent the body's systems from functioning the way they should be. Therefore, the different systems can function more efficiently and effectively by going through cleansing programs that rid the body of these toxins. In addition, the immune system specifically is given a boost, allowing a person to be less prone to sicknesses and diseases once detoxification has been completed.

The removal of toxins allows the body to absorb nutrients better, including Vitamin C, vital for the immune system. A stronger immune system and the removal of harmful toxins and contaminants help the body fight off diseases more easily. Furthermore, detox programs use herbs that help the lymphatic system function better.

What Are the Benefits of Dr. Sebi's Detoxifying Process?

1. Provides energy for the body.

2. Revitalize the body.

3. Remove toxic waste from the body.

4. Multiply cells in the body.

5. Provide the body with irons, which is very important for curing the herpes virus.

6. Cleanses and promotes blood.

How Many Days Does It Take to Cure Herpes Virus?

In one of his lectures, Dr. Sebi stated that the sufferer's weight and health condition would determine the number of days it will take to be cured. The curing time for an individual varies as everyone has a different health condition.

He also stated that the liver, gut, body fluids, and pancreas' health condition would determine how long a sufferer will take to completely cure this disease.

Furthermore, practice fasting; plan it and go for it. The more you fast, the quicker you receive your cure. You can consume dates if you are very weak during fast.

Dr. Sebi's Official method for getting rid of herpes, such as any other disease, is composed of 3 main steps. Please note that any of these parts CAN'T be passed over to succeed in your healing journey.

The three steps I'm talking about are:

1. **Cleansing** → The body must be cleaned on an intra-cellular level through detoxification to purify each cell and remove mucus excess.

2. **Revitalizing** → After cleansing, you need to nourish your body to regenerate your cells and strengthen the immune system.

3. **Avoiding Outbreaks** → Follow Dr. Sebi's nutrition guide and adopt healthy lifestyle habits every day to keep your mind and body in good shape.

CLEANSING

How to Prepare Cleansing Herbs?

Preparing your cleansing herbs would depend greatly on the form you purchased them. It's easier to prepare cleansing herbs in powder forms. You can easily make herbal teas with them in the specified or recommended dosage. However, for other forms form herbs, especially roots or leaves, it is better to use a ratio of 1 teaspoon to 1 cup (8 oz) of spring water for each herb.

However, I recommend preparing herbs in batches of mixtures for easier batch preparation and storage. That would mean mixing them up according to function and benefit. Again, this will depend on the state of your health and what minerals are most important for you. You can combine similar herbs with similar functions into a batch. Like our healer, Dr. Sebi would say: "If you want calcium, you know where to go for (sea moss), if you want Iron, you go for Burdock, and if you want a mix of both Iron and Fluorine, you go for Lily of the Valley".

In all, try not to mix more than 2 or 3 herbs. Remember, these herbs are electric, and it's best to preserve their organic carbon, hydrogen, and oxygen nature as much as we can. But, again, if you mix more than that, you may not get their accurate concentrations per ml of water, so try to limit it to 3, possibly 2.

For a clearer understanding, you can use the following mix:

- Mix **Colon and gallbladder** cleansing herbs together

- Mix **liver and kidney** cleansing herbs

- Mix **respiratory and mucus cleansing** herbs

- Mix **lymphatic and heavy-metal** cleansing herbs.

Since these herbs perform a whole-body cleanse (not just colon), including the skin, eyes, colon, liver, lymphatic system, and gallbladder, you can decide to choose how to combine them. Also, note that when you make larger batches of these herbs for storage, try not to make batches that last more than 7 to 14 days.

For pre-purchase cleansing packages
Please follow the recommended dosage or instructions that are provided for that cleansing package

For fresh Green leafy herbs
- Place in spring water and boil on low heat for 5 to 7 min

- For dried leafy herbs, boil longer – 10 to 15 min

For Dried ground (or powder) herbs
For dried ground or powder leaves or roots, mix in recommended ratios for the herb. Powder herbs are the easiest to mix in dosage proportions, so you can simply follow the package instructions

For Chunks of Dried Root herbs
If you've purchased chunks of roots or stems, you can prepare them in the following way:

- Cut or break up chunks

- Place in spring water and boil for 15 minutes

- Let cool and serve

- Alternatively, prepare in larger batches and place in jars to store in the refrigerator.

For bulk purchase herbs
If you have purchased herbs in bulk and are making your teas, find out the recommended dosage for each herb. You should prepare each herbal tea ratio of 1 teaspoon to 8 ounces of spring water as a general rule.

For capsules
I recommend that you do research and find out what the recommended dosage is for each herbal capsule

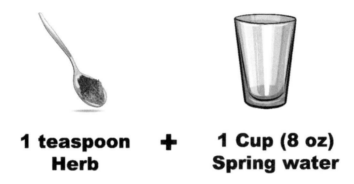

1 teaspoon + 1 Cup (8 oz)
Herb   Spring water

How To Take The Prepared Cleansing Herbs

If you are on medication, I recommend taking the herbs one hour before taking your meds; Dr. Sebi recommended this. Your colon cleansing herbs should not be consumed for longer than 30 days because your body may become dependent on them, and you want to start to reduce the dose during your last 3 to 5 days, depending on how long you've been taking them.

Routine:

- **Twice a day** - morning and night

- **Daily Consistency** - Try to stay consistent both in timing and duration. That is, try not to skew the duration. Make it consistent, and take the cleansing herb throughout the cleanse. For example, for a 14-day cleanse, the cleansing herbs can be taken twice daily, and you should take them around the same time you do take them on both mornings and evenings.

- **Gradual Wean Off** – Just like medications, it is not the best to go cold-turkey when it comes to herbal detox. Towards the end of the cleanse duration, wean off your herbs by gradually reducing the dosage and duration. The duration of the wean will depend on the length of the fast you choose. For example, I usually start weaning a week towards closure one-month fast. For a 14 day fast, I begin weaning on day 11 or 12. You can begin the wean by reducing it from twice a day to once a day. Or simply take half the dosages each for mornings and night.

You must do this because you need to signal your body to start functioning independently without dependence on herbs' cleansing. And no other way to do this than to take it slow and gradual, without bringing too much "shock" to your body.

CLEANSING HERBS

MULLEIN

Mullein is a flavorful beverage flowering plant that has been used for centuries to treat various ailments. Research shows that this herb is an effective anti-microbial, anti-inflammatory, anti-cancer, anti-hepatotoxic, antioxidant, and anti-viral herb with potency to prevent many health disorders. In addition, it helps to cleanse and detoxify the lungs and lymph system and destroy cancer.

The benefits of consuming Mullein include:

- It helps treat and prevent various types of cancer by destroying cancerous cells and preventing them from mutating.

- It helps to eliminate mucus from the small intestine

- It helps to activate healthy lymph circulation in the chest and neck

- It helps neutralize the negative effects of free radicals by protecting the cells from damages caused by free radicals.

- It helps treat and prevent various bacterial and virus infections like herpes viruses, HIV etc.

- It helps to treat and prevent respiratory tract infections.

- It helps to treat and prevent tuberculosis.

- It helps to treat earaches.

- It helps treat various health disorders like bronchitis, stroke, heart diseases etc.

- It helps prevent some chronic brain diseases like Alzheimer's, Parkinson's etc.

- It helps to treat atherosclerosis and others in the biological systems.

- It helps treat and relieve pain caused by inflammation and tumor.

- It also helps treat various ailments like asthma, bronchitis, migraine, congestion etc.

There are no negative side effects attributed to mullein consumption by mouth when writing this book. however, since there is no information

When writing this book, there are no medications that interact with mullein. Therefore, it can be combined with other herbs and drugs without issues.

Quantity Needed and Procedure

For the dosage and how to prepare Mullein tea/infusion, kindly take the following steps:

- Get some handful of fresh Mullein from a nursery farm or garden and dry it, or you can order for prepackaging Mullein tea bags online.

- Once the new leaf is dried, pour some cups of water into a saucepan and boil it.

- Once the water is boiling, measure 8.12ounce or 240ml of the boiling water, add a handful of Mullein dried leaves to the boiling water, and steep it for 20–25 minutes.

- Please keep it cold and strain it using a strainer or filter to remove the tea leaves.

- For the dosage, if you are using the flower, take 3–4g of mullein flowers daily, and if it is the fresh leaves, take 15 to 30 mL of fresh leaves 2–3 times daily.

EUCALYPTUS

The eucalyptus tree is a fast-growing evergreen tree native of Australia. This plant's leaves and bark are used for medicinal purposes like joint and muscle pain, cold, cough, congestion, etc. However, the Chinese, Greek, and Indian Ayurvedic people have incorporated this amazing herb to treat various conditions for thousands of years before now.

This plant/tree has more than 400 different species. The most used is the Eucalyptus globulus or the Australian fever tree, also known as Blue Gum.

Eucalyptus leaves cineole that is also known as eucalyptol, in which the leaf's gland contains essential oil (eucalyptus oil) and also; flavonoids and tannins, which are plant-based antioxidants that aid in reducing inflammation, controlling blood sugar, fighting against the activities of bacteria and fungi and the oil can help in relieving pain and inflammation as well as blocking chemicals that usually cause asthma.

The benefits of using or consuming eucalyptus tea/infusion include:

- It helps in cleansing the skin through steaming/sauna.

- Eucalyptus helps in relieving common cold symptoms like cough lozenges and inhalants and also sore throat and sinusitis

- It helps in relieving symptoms of bronchitis. In addition, inhaling the vapor of eucalyptus tea helps serve as a decongestant by loosening phlegm and easing congestion.

- It aids in relieving asthma: research showed that eucalyptus has the potency to break up mucous in people who have asthma.

- It aids in dental plaque and improves gingivitis: research carried out on eucalyptus shows that eucalyptus leaf has the potency to reduce dental plaque and improve gingivitis.

- It helps improve bad breath: research showed that eucalyptus has the potency to improve bad breath.

- It also helps to relives some health like; skin disease, bladder diseases, gallbladder and liver problems, bleeding gums, diabetes, burns, ulcer, stuffy nose, wounds, etc.

<u>The precaution to be note-full of before using eucalyptus tea or infusion include:</u>

- It is 100% safe for pregnant and breastfeeding mothers to consume eucalyptus tea/infusion, but the oil is unsafe.

- The tea is safe for children, but the oil might lead to seizures

- Because of eucalyptus leaves' potency leaves to lower blood sugar levels, it is advisable to consult with your doctor before using the tea with any diabetes medication

<u>**Quantity Needed and Procedure**</u>

For the dosage and how to prepare eucalyptus tea/infusion, kindly take the following steps:

- Boil water to (90-95)0 or 194-205 Fahrenheit. Alternatively, you can boil the water and drop it down for a minute or two to reduce the temperature.

- Pour a teaspoon of dried eucalyptus leaf into a teacup/mug.

- Pour 6 ounces of water (from the first step) inside the teacup/mug and allow the leaves to be steep for 10-15minutes. (you can enjoy breathing the vapors of the steeping tea)

- Get a filter to strain the loose leaves of the eucalyptus.

- You are a god. You can now enjoy the cup of eucalyptus tea/infusion at a go.

- For the dosage, take 3-4 cups per day.

.

KALE

Kale is a cruciferous vegetable family member.

Some of the benefits of consuming kale are listed below. For example:

- It is loaded with powerful antioxidants, such as quercetin and kaempferol, that have powerful heart-protective, blood pressure-lowering, anti-inflammatory, anti-viral, anti-depressant, and anti-cancer effects

- It is one of the world's best sources of vitamin C. A cup of raw kale contains even more vitamin C than a whole orange.

- Kale contains bile acid sequestrants, which can lower cholesterol levels. It might lead to a reduced risk of heart disease over time

- It is one of the world's best sources of vitamin K, which is critical for blood clotting, and does this by "activating" certain proteins and giving them the ability to bind calcium

- It is also a good source of important minerals that most people don't get enough of, such as calcium, potassium, and magnesium

- Being a high nutrient-dense food with a low-calorie and high-water content, kale provides significant bulk that helps make you feel full and avoid overeating

Precautions and Side Effects

- Consuming too much kale, high in potassium, can be harmful to people whose kidneys are not fully functional.

RED CLOVER

Red clover, scientifically known as '*Trifolium pretense,* is a wild plant belonging to the legume family. It has been used medicinally to treat several conditions, including cancer, whooping cough, respiratory problems, and skin inflammations, such as psoriasis and eczema.

Below are some of the main benefits of this herb:

- It lowers the loss of bone mineral density in postmenopausal women

- It may help reduce the risk of prostate cancer

- It may help relieve the discomforts of menopause, especially hot flashes

- Red clover ointments have been applied to the skin to treat diseases such as psoriasis, eczema, and other rashes.

- It has also been used as a cough remedy for children.

How to prepare Red Clover tea/infusion:

- Add 4 grams of dried flower tops to 1 cup (250 mL) of boiling water

- Steep for 10 minutes

- Enjoy!

Note: it's best to limit your daily intake to 1–3 cups.

Be happy if you relate to these symptoms during the cleansing stage. That's because your body is pushing out all the toxins and mucus you have been keeping inside for so long. These symptoms are only temporary and usually resolve after the first one to two weeks.

BURDOCK ROOT

Burdock root is the root of a delicious plant called Burdock, which all its body or parts are useful as either food or medicine. This plant can be found all over the world. I called this plant the wonder plant because everything about it is important as we consume its root as food and use it for medicinal purposes. Both its leaf and seed are used for medicinal purposes.

People worldwide have been using burdock root orally to treat and prevent various health disorders for over five centuries.

Because of Burdock root's chemical composition, such as; quercetin and luteolin, research has shown that it can serve as a great effective antioxidant that can treat and prevent cancer by preventing cancerous cells from growing and mutating combat aging. A compound like 'Phytosterols' helps scalp and hair follicles grow healthy hair even from baldheads. The vitamins-C helps in boosting the immune system and combat bacterial. It also helps cleanse or detoxify the liver and lymphatic system, etc.

The potassium helps reduce blood sugar levels and filter the blood by removing impurities through the bloodstream and eradicating toxins through the skin and urine.

The benefits of using or consuming burdock root tea/infusion include:

- cleanse/detox the liver and lymphatic system.

- Treat and prevent diabetes by reducing blood sugar levels in the body.

- Eliminate toxins from the body by inducing sweetness and urine.

- Purify the blood by removing heavy metals from the bloodstream.

- Treat various skin disorders and combat aging.

- Treat and prevent cancer by inhibiting the growth and mutation of cancerous cells.

- Boost the immune system and enhance circulation.

Until writing this book, there have been no side effects recorded by researchers or people who have used these herbs.

However, research has it that applying this root to your skin might cause rashes.

Quantity Needed and Procedure

For the dosage and how to prepare Burdock root tea/infusion, kindly take the following steps:

- Scrub the uprooted root of burdock heartily under running water to remove all the dirt that accompanied it from the soil.

- You should chop the Burdock root into smaller pieces (less than 1 inch). Please note that it will come dried and already chopped if you order it online.

- Pour 2-3 cup of water into your saucepan and add ¼ cup of the chopped burdock root and boil it.

- Lower your gas once the water is boiling, re-boil it for 30-40 minutes, and put off your gas.

- Once it is cold, strain it and consume it.

- For the dosage, drink one glass cup daily

CHAPARRAL

Chaparral, also called 'Larrea Tridentate', is an herb from the creosote bush, a desert shrub native to southern areas of the United States and northern regions of Mexico. This flowering plant has bright yellow flowers and thick green leaves with a resinous coating. However, despite its pretty appearance, chaparral is a controversial herb that's even been banned in many countries. However, this herb is claimed to help treat many ailments, including cancer, arthritis, and skin conditions.

The consumption of Chaparral has several benefits, such as:

- It contains a powerful antioxidant that helps the shrinkage of tumors

- It may prevent the spreading of HPV and HIV

- It prevents heart diseases by reducing levels of free radicals

- It helps to boost the immune system

- It relieves joint and muscle pain thanks to its anti-inflammatory quality

The Side Effects and note-full precautions before Consuming Chaparral are:

- Nursing mothers should avoid this herb because it has been reported to have abortifacient effects

- Although chaparral is a potent antioxidant, it has been found to have serious negative health effects, including hepatotoxicity, which is a chemically-induced liver injury

Quantity Needed and Procedure

For the dosage and how to prepare Chaparral tea/infusion, kindly take the following steps:

- Boil water to (90–95)0 or 194–205 Fahrenheit. Alternatively, you can boil the water and drop it down for a minute or two to reduce the temperature.
- Pour a teaspoon of dried chaparral leaf into a teacup/mug.
- Pour 6 ounces of water (from the first step) inside the teacup/mug and allow the leaves to be steep for 10–15minutes. (You can enjoy breathing the vapors of the steeping tea).
- Get a filter to strain the loose leaves.

You can now enjoy the cup of chaparral tea/infusion at a go.

DANDELION

Dandelion is a flowering plant known as 'yellow gowan' or 'lion's tooth. This plant is native to Eurasia and today. It is common in over 60 countries worldwide in the mild climates of the northern hemisphere. For centuries, these flowering plants have been used for the treatment of swelling (inflammation) of the pancreas, relieve pains that are caused by inflammation, treat and prevent cancer, tonsils (tonsillitis), skin disorder, bladder or urethra disorder, digestive and liver problems and enhance the general health of the liver and digestive system.

Researchers proved that it is a very effective cleansing/detoxification herb because of the chemical compositions and nutrients.

The benefits of using or consuming Dandelion include:

- It helps to detoxify or cleanse the liver and the kidney.

- It helps to treat and prevent diabetes by regulating blood sugar levels.

- It helps to fight against and relieve pains that are caused by inflammation.

- It helps to deactivate and inhibit the negative effects of free radicals in the body because of its antioxidant properties.

- It reduces the level of cholesterol.

- It lowers blood pressure by getting rid of excess fluid in the body.

- It helps to naturally shed excess weight gain by improving the metabolism of carbohydrates.

- It helps in boosting the digestive system.

- It helps to boost the immune system.

- It helps to keep the skin healthy and treat and prevent skin diseases.

Till at the time of writing this book, Dandelion is 100% safe, but consuming an overdose of it can result in some side effects like:

- Experiencing stomach upset or irritation

- Allergic reactions

The special precautions before using/consuming dandelions are:

- Pregnant and breastfeeding mothers should stay off dandelion as there is no research to know if it is harmful to them or not.

- If you are suffering from Eczema, stay off dandelion as more than 85% of people with eczema suffer an allergic reaction to dandelion.

Quantity Needed and Procedure

For the dosage and how to prepare Dandelion tea/infusion, kindly take the following steps:

- Get some fresh leaves of dandelion and wash them under running water to remove all the dirt.

- After washing it, pour ½ - 1 cup of the washed dandelion into your saucepan.

- You should boil 4-5 cups of water and pour the boiled water inside the saucepan. Next, you pour the dandelion and cover it for 12-15 hours or throughout the night (overnight).

- The next day, strain out the dandelion leaves, and you will be left with the dandelion tea/infusion.

- For the dosage, take ½ tablespoon of Dandelion per ¾ cup of water three times daily. And if you ordered your dandelion online, you can take 4-10 grams of dry leaf of dandelion three times daily.

ELDERBERRY

Elderberry is a dark purple berry from the elder tree, also known as European Black Elderberry or Sambucus Bacchae. This plant is a flowering plant from the family of Adoxaceae and native to Europe. Both the leaves and fruit (berries) of elderberry have been used for centuries to treat pain and swelling arising from inflammation. It also helps to stimulate urine production and induce sweat to detoxify the body system.

Because of how rich elderberry is with various compounds and nutrients like vitamin-C, dietary fiber, phenolic acids, which is a great and powerful antioxidant that helps to prevent and decrease the damage that is caused by oxidative stress in the body, it also contains some compounds like flavonols such as kaempferol, quercetin, isorhamnetin and anthocyanins which gives the fruit the black-purple color and makes it a strong antioxidant and anti-inflammation agent.

Elderberry also contains some nutrients, like:

- Calories

- Carbs

- Minute amounts of protein and fat

- And anthocyanins, making the plant a strong and effective antioxidant with anti-inflammatory properties.

The benefits of using/consuming elderberry include:

- It helps cleanse and detoxify the lungs and respiratory system by eliminating mucus from the upper respiratory system and the lungs.

- It helps to treat constipation.

- It helps to treat flu and cold in less than 24hours.

- It combats harmful bacteria in the body by preventing bacterial growth through its antibacterial properties.

130

- It boosts and supports the immune defense system by increasing white blood cell production.

- It protects and keeps the skin healthy.

- It helps to relieve chronic fatigue syndrome and depression.

Till at the time of writing this book, there is no record of any side effects from researchers and people who have used elderberry, but because of the compound that is present in elderberry, it will be wise to use it for not more than 12 weeks and take a break for at least a week before using it again.

The special precautions before using elderberry include:

- Ensure children below 12 years do not use/consume elderberries, and children above 12 and under 18 should not use them for more than 10days.

- Since there is no reliable information to know if elderberries are safe or not for pregnant and breastfeeding mothers, I strongly advise that they stay off elderberries.

- People who have a history of suffering from an autoimmune disease like; multiple sclerosis, lupus, rheumatoid arthritis, etc., should stay off elderberry as it has the potency to boost the immune system to become more active which could worsen their situation.

- Since elderberries have the potency to increase or boost the immune defense system, any medications designed to decrease the immune system's function will certainly interact with Elderberry.

Quantity Needed and Procedure

For the dosage and how to prepare Elderberry tea/infusion, kindly take the steps below:

- Boil 8-12oz of water in your saucepan.

- Once the water is boiling, measure one tablespoon of dried elderberries and add it to the boiling water.

- Reduce your gas and allow it to boil for at least 15 minutes.

- After the 15 minutes timing, allow it to get cold and strain it using a filter.

- For the dosage, consume 3-4 cups daily.

ELDER FLOWER

The berries and the elder plant's flowers have been used for medicine for thousands of years. while but, while having similar affinities for

Some of the benefits of consuming elderflower are listed below. For example:

- It is widely used for colds and flu, sinus infections, and other respiratory disturbances due to its antiseptic and anti-inflammatory properties.

- It also has diuretic and laxative properties and helps relieve occasional constipation

- Elderflowers have relaxing properties.

- It is rich in bioflavonoids, mostly flavones and flavonols, that are most commonly known for their antioxidant

- It has antibacterial and antiviral properties

- It can be used for its antiseptic properties as a mouthwash and gargle

Some special precautions before using elderflower include:

- **Pregnancy and breast-feeding**: There isn't enough reliable information to know if elderflower is safe to use when pregnant or breast-feeding

- **Diabetes**: If you have diabetes and use an elderflower, carefully monitor your blood sugar levels.

- **Surgery:** Stop using elderflower at least two weeks before a scheduled surgery.

One thing that seems certain is that you should not brew up any other part of the elder tree. This is because the leaves, sticks, and roots can cause a build-up of cyanide levels in the body.

Quantity Needed and Procedure

For the dosage and how to prepare Elderberry tea/infusion, kindly take the steps below:

- Put Loose Elderflower Tea into a tea infuser
- Brew freshwater using either filtered or bottled water.
- Place the Tea-filled accessory into a cup or mug.
- Fill the cup with hot water
- Let it infuse for 5-10 minutes

CILANTRO

Cilantro is a popular herb around the globe that comes from the 'Coriandrum sativum' plant. It resembles flat-leaf parsley at first glance, but it transports you to the Mediterranean, Mexico, Asia, and India at first sniff. In some parts of the world, people call it 'coriander'.

Some of the benefits of consuming cilantro are listed below. For example:

- It has been shown to bind arsenic, aluminum, and mercury together (which are toxic metals), loosening them from tissue and facilitating their elimination from the body.

- A recent study has shown that due to its natural sedative properties, this herb can help calm the nerves and improve sleep quality, almost at the same level as the popular medication Valium

- A study published in the *International Journal of Food Microbiology* found that cilantro is particularly protective against 'Salmonella', a bacteria that often causes what we know as food poisoning

- Its leaves and steams help lower blood sugar levels and improve the overall health

- Its antibacterial compounds could help keep the urinary tract healthy and free from unhealthy bacteria in an alkaline environment.

- Thanks to its antioxidant properties, cilantro may help protect your brain from serious diseases such as Alzheimer's and Parkinson's

Quantity Needed and Procedure

For the dosage and how to prepare Cilantro tea/infusion, kindly take the steps below:

Ingredients

- 1 cup water
- 3 sprigs of cilantro

Instructions

- Boil the water in a kettle or on the stovetop. Pour it into a teapot.
- Steep the cilantro leaves in hot water for 5-7 minutes.
- Remove the leaves, and drink!

How to break a detox fast?

- Slowly reintroduce solids

If you are doing water or a liquid fast, you will need to reintroduce solid foods slowly. You can begin by introducing solids like high water-content fruits. These include watermelon, apples, and berries. After that, you can introduce softer fruit solids like bananas and avocados. Later, you can incorporate harder solids like veggies. All foods must be listed on the nutrition guide. However, if doing a fruit or raw veggie fast, you can break the fast right away on solid foods.

- Drink 1-gallon spring water daily

Drink spring water daily together with the revitalizing herbs and sea moss.

How long should you detox/cleanse?

How long you should detox depends on your state of health, that is, your body's toxification level (the less healthy you are, the more toxic your body is) and tolerance level. Typically, it is recommended to fast for 7-14 days, but Dr. Sebi recommends a minimum of at least a 12 day fast. Dr. Sebi himself fasted for 90 days to cure diabetes, asthma, and impotence. It is great to cleanse at least once a year for seven days if you consume an alkaline diet. If you are not consuming an alkaline diet, then you should cleanse/detox every three months

I fasted for 14 days, and I recommend fasting for between 14 days and one month if you have high blood pressure. Again, your body's tolerance level will ultimately determine the length, so watch your body and study its reaction as you begin the fast. We are all different, and you may find that you cannot handle a basic liquid fast (water or juice). In that case, you can get started with fruit or raw vegetables fast. But make sure all foods and fruits are listed in the Dr. Sebi Nutrition Guide. Whether liquid, juice or raw food fast, the results are virtual all the same – the only major difference is when it takes to begin to see results. While raw food fasts take longer, liquid fasts are much faster. So do not worry; the most important thing is to stay committed and focused on whatever fasting method you choose.

Common Symptoms Expected During Detox Cleanse

1. Cold and Flu symptoms

2. Changes in Bowel movements

3. Fatigue and Low Energy

4. Difficulty sleeping

5. Itching

6. Headaches

7. Muscle aches and pains

8. Acne. Rashes and breakouts

9. Mucus expels (catarrh, etc.)

10. Lower blood pressure

Be happy if you relate to these symptoms during the cleansing stage. That's because your body is pushing out all the toxins and mucus you have been keeping inside for so long. These symptoms are only temporary and usually resolve after the first one to two weeks.

REVITALIZING HERBS

These are herbs, oils, foods, and things of that nature that will target the herpes virus specifically. I also recommend that you take the revitalizing herbs after your detox.

So, when you are detoxing, you'd want to take your cleansing herbs and things like that to clean your body out. Then you'd want to reintroduce the revitalizing herbs - this is when you're eating your alkaline foods and things like that. So, you would want to go ahead and take the revitalizing herbs. However, suppose your body can handle a prolonged fast. In that case, you can take the revitalizing herbs after you have done your cleanse and then take that while you are still fasting, and it should give you faster results. But you want to make sure that you are taking your sea moss during that time to rebuild up some of the things you have flushed out during your cleanse that are beneficial to your body. Revitalizing herbs are herbs and oils that target the herpes virus specifically. So, it is important you take these revitalizing herbs after cleansing and detoxifying your body so that the herbs can completely clean your body.

PAO PEREIRA

Pao Pereira is a tree that belongs to the Apocynaceae family and is native to South America. This tree's bark is rich in compounds that effectively destroy, eliminate, and inhibit cancerous cells. Because of how effective this tree's bark is, Dr. Sebi recommends this herb to revitalize the body system after cleansing.

The benefits of consuming Pao Pereira include:

- treating malaria and other infections caused by parasites.

- It effectively suppresses the Herpes Simplex Virus

- It helps treat and prevent cancer by destroying cancer and preventing cancerous cells from mutation.

- Soothing and relieving liver pain.

- It helps to treat and prevent stomach disorders like constipation and irritation.

- It helps to boost sexual arousal

Till at the time of writing this book, no side effect is attributed to the consumption of Pao Pereira; but since there is no vital information to show that this herb is 100% safe for pregnant and breastfeeding mothers, I advise that they avoid this herb's consumption.

For the dosage and how to prepare Pao Pereira tea, kindly take the steps below:

- Harvest some Pao Pereira by cutting some of its bark down the tree, chopping it, and drying it.

- Once it is dried, boil 1liter of water and pour two tablespoons of the dried Pao Pereira into the boiling water.

- Lower the heat of the fire to a medium-low and place the lid on the pot.

- Boil the mixture at medium temperature for 20 minutes.

- Allow it to get cold and train it using a strainer or filter.

You are done!

For the dosage, consume 1 cup of tea times daily.

PAU D'ARCO

Some of the benefits of consuming Pau d'Arco tea are listed below. For example:

- It has the power to naturally reduce pain in patients suffering from serious conditions, such as cancer
- It helps in fighting Candida
- It inhibits pancreatic lipase, an enzyme that helps the body better digest and absorbs fat
- It has a strong antioxidant property that protects against oxidative damage triggered by inflammation
- It works as a detoxifier since it has a laxative effect
- It has been used for thousands of years as an antiviral herb, effectively fighting Herpes, Leukemia, and AIDS.

Side Effects

If eaten in high quantity, it may cause some issues like nausea, vomiting, and anemia

Quantity Needed and Procedure

For the dosage and how to prepare Pau d'Arco tea/infusion, kindly take the steps below:

- Put 2 tsp of barks into 3 cups of boiling water
- Let it sit for 15 minutes
- Let it cool for at least 1 hour
- Strain the water
- Enjoy your tea!

HOLY BASIL

This green leafy plant, also known as 'queen of the herbs' or 'tulsi', is native to Southeast Asia. Still, it has a history within Indian medicine as a treatment for many conditions, from eye diseases to ringworms.

Some of the benefits of consuming holy basil tea are listed below. For example:

- It helps prevent certain respiratory illnesses ranging from cold and cough to bronchitis and asthma
- It helps in maintaining normal levels of cortisol hormone, which correlates to stress and anxiety
- It is widely used to treat gastrointestinal disorders and menstrual cramps
- It helps with adrenal fatigue, which can trigger herpes outbreaks
- It helps combat harmful bacteria and germs in the mouth
- It has anti-inflammatory properties that may help in relieving chronic pain
- It facilitates the metabolism of carbs and fats, ensuring that the blood's sugar is utilized for energy.

Side Effects

- If consumed in high quantities, it may temporarily decrease fertility in both men and women
- It is recommended for women to avoid consuming tulsi tea while breastfeeding
- When consumed in high quantities, some people may experience nausea or diarrhea

Quantity Needed and Procedure

For the dosage and how to prepare Holy basil tea/infusion, kindly take the steps below:

- Boil 1 cup of filtered water
- Pour it over 1 tsp of fresh leaves, ½ tsp of dried leaves, or 1/3 tsp of powder
- Cover and let it steep for at least 20 minutes

Strain the leaves, and enjoy!

BLUE VERVAIN

Blue Vervain is a perennial flowering plant that belongs to the family of Verbenaceae. It is rich in iron fluorine, which purifies the blood, phosphorus, phosphate, zinc, potassium, magnesium, etc. Because of this potency, Dr. Sebi recommends this herb for revitalizing your body after cleansing.

The benefits of using or consuming Blue Vervain include:

- It helps to treat and prevent anxiety and sleeplessness and enhance mood.

- It helps to treat and calm the central nervous system.

- It helps soothe the nerves and relaxes the mind, treating migraine headaches.

- It helps boost and protect the heart's health treat and prevent myocardial ischemia, chest pain, and heart failure.

- It helps to fight against both internal and external inflammation.

- It helps to treat menstrual cramps or pain and stomach pain.

- It improves digestive health and protects the livers and kidneys by cleansing/detoxifying the kidney and liver.

The note-full precautions before consuming blue vervain tea include:

- Because there is no information to show if these herbs are good for breastfeeding mothers or pregnant women, I advise avoiding these herbs' consumption.

- Till at the time of writing this book, there were no medications that interacted with blue Vervain.

Quantity Needed and Procedure

For the dosage and how to prepare Blue Vervain tea, kindly take the following steps:

- Get some fresh leaves and flowers of blue Vervain and dry them.

- Once it is dried, pound or chops it, or you can order it online, and it will come dried and chopped.

- Boil a cup of water (8ounce) in a saucepan.

- Once the water is boiled, pour it into a cup, measure 1 teaspoon of the Blue Vervain, and add it to the water.

- Allow it to steep for 10-15 minutes and strain it.

- You are done! For the dosage, take 2-4 cups daily.

SARSAPARILLA

Sarsaparilla root is the root of a tropical wood climbing vine that belongs to the genus Smilax family. Dr. Sebi recommends it as a revitalizing herb for many diseases, including cancer, rich in iron, calcium, and phosphate.

The benefits of consuming Sarsaparilla roots are:

- It helps to destroy and prevent cancerous cells from mutating.
- It binds the endotoxins responsible for the lesions in psoriasis patients and eliminates them from the body system.
- It helps to fast-track healing and recovery.
- It treats and prevents health issues caused by inflammations like joint pain, swelling of body parts, arthritis, rheumatoid, etc.
- It soothes and heals sexually transmitted diseases such as syphilis, herpes, gonorrhea etc.
- It helps to treat and prevent leprosy
- It helps protect and reverse damages done to the liver to function perfectly.
- It makes the body absorb nutrients and other herbs easily

There are no side effects attributed to this herb's consumption when writing this book. However, because of the 'saponins' that it contains, I advise you to consult your doctor before using this herb, as saponins can cause stomach irritation.

Quantity Needed and Procedure

For the dosage and how to prepare sarsaparilla root tea, kindly take the following steps:

- Get the root of fresh sarsaparilla.
- After getting it, pill it and remove the outer skin.
- You should now dry the outer skin in a well-ventilated place (indoors), but it will dry if you get it online. So you won't have to disturb yourself with these steps.
- Ensure you turn the root daily for 6–7 days to dry it until it is completely dried.
- Ensure that you store your dry sarsaparilla in a paper bag or cardboard box once it is dry.
- For the dosage of Sarsaparilla root, boil water and add 1–4 grams of sarsaparilla root in 8–12oz of the boiling water and allow it to simmer for 15–20 minutes.

You are good. You can now enjoy your sarsaparilla root tea/infusion three times daily.

GUACO

Guaco is a climbing plant with different names like Huaco, Guace, or Vejuco. This climbing plant belongs to the Asteraceae and cordifolia species' family and is rich in numerous minerals and compounds. Its leaves are very medicinal and nutritional. The people of Aztecs used them to clean the blood system and clear heavy metals from the bloodstream.

There are a lot of benefits that one can benefit from using or consuming Guaco. Some of them are:

- It lessens the effect or symptoms of snake poison.

- It is used to thin the blood through the coumarin activities it contains (anticoagulant and blood-thinning.)

- It helps to combat inflammation through its anti-inflammatory properties.

- It treats stomach irritation through the effect of its cleansing activities.

- It helps treat respiratory disorders like coughs, rheumatism, bronchitis, etc.

- It enhances quick recovery from the wound.

- It helps to cleanse or detoxify the blood and skin by clearing heavy metals from the blood.

- It boosts and builds the immune defense system.

- It can treat some infections diseases such as; candida yeast infection, herpes, etc.

Researchers or uses have recorded no severe side effects until writing this book.

Like I said earlier, Guaco is 100% safe for consumption by mouth, but if you are taking or using any Coumadin drugs, please consult with your doctor before using it.

And if you have any history of bleeding, do not use Guaco unless your doctor approves of it. Like I said earlier, Guaco helps to thin the blood, so any medications that can thin the blood or slow blood clotting do interact with Guaco.

Quantity Needed and Procedure

For the dosage and how to prepare Guaco tea/infusion, kindly take the following steps:

- Get some handful of fresh Guaco and wash it under running water or 2 ounces of its dried leaves if you have the dried ones.

- Pour about 6cups of water in your saucepan with the Guaco leaves and boil it until it is reduced to 2 cups.

- You can add some brown sugar (optional) if you count the brown sugar; allow it to boil for another 20 minutes.

- Strain the syrup with a strainer.

- It would help if you bottled it and stored it in a refrigerator.

For Guaco dosage, take one soupspoon 3–4 times daily.

When Should I Start Consuming the Revitalizing Herbs?

The best time to consume the revitalizing herbs is the next day after finishing your cleanse. For instance, if you fast for 14days, on the 15day, you should start consuming your revitalizing herbs.

What Are the Things That I Shouldn't Forget?

Drink at least a gallon of spring water daily.

Eat foods only on Dr. Sebi's nutritional guide once you are done with your detox /cleanse.

Never forget to use sea moss during the revitalization process

Ensure you do an intra-cellular cleanse once per year for at least seven days if you follow only the alkaline diet from Dr. Sebi's nutritional guide. Still, if you are not, you should always do an intra-cellular cleansing after every three months to cleanse your body from mucus and toxins.

Please note that consuming acidic food can only put your body at risk of outbreaks.

Herbal treatments with dr. Sebi essential oils

Some Dr. Sebi herbs are highly effective when used to treat herpes. They work well by speeding up the healing process, numbing discomfort, and relieving itching.

These herbal products are essential oils and should be handled with utmost care. If essential oils are not diluted, they can burn through the skin. So, it's advisable to dilute them with carrier oils such as coconut oil. Also, the mixture should be tested before use.

Steps to test essential oil solution

1. First, apply the mixture to the firearm.

2. Wait for about 24 hours.

If there is no adverse effect on the skin, you can use it. But if you notice any negative effects, please discard them and never use them.

Essential Oils made from Dr. Sebi Approved Herbs

Olive leaf extract

Herpes is an illness brought about by an intelligent infection (Herpes Simplex Virus). In general, it will play so savvy in the body that it never gets captured by any medication or the safe framework. It turns out to be extremely hard to fix this ailment and isn't a simple errand to do. Be that as it may, there has been exploring distinctive approaches to fix Herpes, one of which incorporates Olive Leaf extricates.

Olive leaf separate originates from the leaves of the olive plants. The concentrate contains phenolics, for example, oleuropein, which keeps up glucose digestion and skin wellbeing. It is said to be perhaps the best fixing to fix herpes. Moreover, it has mending powers and has been utilized to treat different ailments.

Olive leaf removes are assembled from the Olive plant, which contains hostile to viral, mitigating against the tumor, hostile to microbial, cell reinforcement, and progressively different properties. Olive leaf separation is a cure that battles a wide range of infections. It has been demonstrated to be a superior strategy to other drugs that don't influence well-being. In addition, it has been demonstrated

The compound called Oleuropein tends to execute the available infections. Herpes begins developing in our framework when our insusceptible framework gets feeble by stress or when our body neglects to deliver protein. Oleuropein present in the Olive leaf is the primary segment that battles the infection and secures the invulnerable framework.

Even though herpes doesn't dispense appropriately, it helps forestall the infection to episode further. When we devour the olive leaf, it assaults and harms the infection in our body and forestalls further reason. Along these lines, the odds are less of the infection getting repeated; however, it will likely experience the host's demise.

Instructions to Use Olive Leaf Extract for Herpes:

1. Three to four tablets before 6 hours of your supper. The dose must be just a single tablet at regular intervals.

2. Take the prescription until you see a change

On the off chance that a change happens, that implies the medication is working. On the other hand, if you take a greater amount of the tablets, you will confront certain side effects like weakness, influenza, migraine, and so forth.

Take less measure of tablet on the off chance that you see manifestations and on the off chance that these side effects don't leave; at that point, quit taking the tablets.

See a specialist who will set up a legitimate calendar for taking the medication and tell the best way to take it and fix the progressions.

You can join olive leaf removes with Aloe Vera, upgrading the activity for quicker outcomes.

You can likewise utilize Oregano Oil with olive leaf extricate together for better-restored results.

How Much Of Olive Leaf Extract Should I Take?

The olive leaf contains oleuropein, which contains 20 mg that aids in better assimilation and expels the infection that causes herpes in our body. That is the best home-grown drug one can settle on. Some olive leaves are not transformed into cases.

Instead, they are dried, and afterward, they are placed in a glass of warm water and devoured legitimately. That is useful in restoring herpes. 500 mg must be expended every day, and that too four times each day. You are to take dried leaves per drink alongside the tablets on the off chance you need to expend three times each day.

Are There Any Side Effects of Using Olive Leaf Extract?

There is no such damage, yet more utilization may prompt minimal symptoms. On the other hand, the overdose may make the infection increasingly confounded and prompt genuine disease. The prescription must be taken appropriately since it might mess the heart up when a greater amount is taken. The heart may diminish its pulsates, and circulatory strain may go down. It may likewise bring detoxification issues simply like: Diarrhea, Nausea, and so on. In this way, legitimate consideration must be taken.

If one experiences brevity of breath, a quick move should be made as many individuals can be touchy towards a specific type of oil like olive oil.

So, we can reason that olive leaves are the best medication for restoring herpes. The dried leave or the cases both give an advantage to the body and assault the infection of herpes. An appropriate amount must be taken to guarantee great wellbeing.

<u>**Lavender oil**</u>

Lavender oil contains aggravates disinfectant, is antibacterial and is hostile to contagious. That essentially implies Lavender executes and represses germs and infections.

If you have a virus bug experiencing your home or office, at that point, utilize Lavender

Essential oil to help stop it. Diffuse it to clean and filter the air and stop those airborne germs.

That is such a great amount more advantageous than to splash however frightful unpronounceable synthetic disinfectant showers. Those by themselves could make you wiped out!

Lavender likewise inspires one's temperament, and this will enable the insusceptible framework to help its safeguards.

Approaches to Help Stop the Germs Using Lavender

You can add drops to a splash container of water and spritz down territories of transmission, for example, the telephone, door handles, and counter. Dry with a spotless material.

Diffuse it in an Aromatherapy Diffuser to chop down the airborne germs and inspire feelings.

<u>**Oregano Essential Oil**</u>

Oregano essential oil is antiviral, best at 90% concentrate. Anything less than 90% will not benefit you to heal from the herpes virus. You'd want to apply it to your lower spine, which is where the HSV2 herpes virus is dormant. It can also be applied under the tongue and the genital area. You would want to use it two to three times per day. I recommend you put ten drops into two ounces of extra-virgin olive oil, or you can also use coconut oil because you want to dilute this, or it will burn your skin. Oregano essential oil is a great antiviral that can suppress the herpes virus. It works best at ninety percent concentration. Apply essential oregano oil to your lower spine because your lower spine is the point where HSV-2 is dormant. You can also apply it to your genital area and under your tongue. Oregano essential oil is a great antiviral that can suppress the herpes virus. It works best at ninety percent concentration. Apply essential oregano oil to your lower spine because your lower spine is the point where HSV-2 is dormant. You can also apply it to your genital area and under your tongue.

Ginger Essential Oil

You can also use ginger essential oil. It is very similar to the effects of oregano oil; it can kill the herpes virus on contact. It must be diluted as well with a carrier oil.

How to Extract Essential Oils for Herpes?

There are numerous oils for herpes. The one thing that we have to consider is the extraction process.

The proper extraction of these oils from their natural sources is a delicate process that requires a lot of experience and the right materials.

There are numerous methods of extracting essential oils. Still, we are going to cover the two most important techniques, which are:

Steam distillation

The process of steam distillation makes use of steam and pressure for the extraction process. This process is simple, but it can go wrong without expertise.

The raw materials are placed inside a cooking chamber made of stainless steel. When the material is steamed, it is broken down, removing the volatile materials behind it.

When the steam is freed from the plant, it moves up the chamber in gaseous form through the connecting pipe, which goes into the condenser.

Once the condenser is cool, the gas goes back into liquid form, the essential oil collected from the water's surface.

Cold Pressing

The cold press process extracts oils from the citrus rind, and the seeds oil the carrier oil. This process requires heat but not as much heat as the steam distillation process with a maximum temperature of 120F for the process to go as planned.

The heated material is placed in a container punctured by a device that rotates with thorns. Once puncturing is complete, the essential oils are released into a container below the puncturing region. These machines then use centrifugal force to separate the essential oil from the juice.

Both processes are essential. It has to be done properly with the right level of information from experts who know a lot about the process; if not a lot of harm, good can and will be done.

Avoiding Flare-ups

Once you can no longer see any of the symptoms you suffered from, you can consider the 'Revitalizing' process ended. At this point, you need to focus on living your life the healthy way, following the Dr. Sebi nutritional guide to avoid outbreaks and maintaining your body in its natural alkaline state, where disease can't manifest itself.

I'll give you some lifestyle tips to living a herpes-free life, but before that, let's see 4 of the most common factors that may trigger a flare-up:

Sexual intercourse ➔ As for genital herpes, some people find that the friction of sexual intercourse irritates the skin and brings on symptoms. Using a water-based lubricant can help reduce irritation.

Sunlight and Colds ➔ Exposure to sunlight or cold may trigger flare-ups of cold sores (HSV-1)

Weak Immune System ➔ People whose immune system is weakened by HIV or chemotherapy, for example, tend to experience outbreaks more often

Hormone Imbalance ➔ Quick hormonal changes in women during menstrual may cause genital herpes outbreaks.

Most importantly, the number one factor that correlates to herpes outbreaks is stress.

Managing stress is the number one thing you need to focus on to avoid flare-ups, implying that you will follow Dr. Sebi's nutritional guide and eliminate over-acidity from your body.

Here are five lifestyle tips you can follow to manage stress better and keep herpes away:

Sleep enough

When you don't get good sleep, you drain your entire body and brain of vital functioning energy. In response, your body and brain are reduced to anxiety; it may be hard for you to focus and make logical thoughts. On the other hand, anyone experiencing an anxiety episode is advised to get a maximum of 8 hours of uninterrupted sleep. I know I say 8 hours, and it may be hard even to make them fall asleep. You can try and prepare the environment in which they will sleep, make it cozy, warm, and secure; you can even sleep by their side so that they know you are there. When you do all these, the person's brain starts adjusting from anxiety mode to relief mode, and thoughts like, 'I think I am safe in this room, I think she will make me safe' is what will be crossing their minds.

Exercise

While exercise has been clinically proven to reduce anxiety and improve mood, it can also treat many other health problems. Health issues can be a major anxiety trigger, and easing the symptoms of those ailments can further reduce anxiety symptoms.

Also, exercising can help people relax. When a person exercises, their body releases hormones that produce a calming effect. Exercise also increases body temperature, which can be very relaxing. Working up a sweat is tiring, but it's a great way to calm down.

When some people hear the word "exercise," they picture a gym full of lifting weights. However, many fitness activities can provide the exercise someone with anxiety needs. Even everyday activities like gardening or washing a car can elevate the mood.

Many people think they don't have time for exercise, but exercise doesn't take hours. Instead, people can find little ways to increase physical activity throughout the day. For example, they might stretch at their desk at work or take a quick walk during their lunch break.

Studies suggest that 30 minutes of exercise a day, three days a week, can dramatically reduce anxiety symptoms. However, those same studies show that even small amounts of activity can positively affect. So if someone doesn't have time for lengthy workouts, they should still find ways to exercise their body needs.

While increased physical activity provides several health benefits, they aren't lasting. For exercise to improve anxiety, it must be done consistently. That makes it all the more important for people to find exercise routines they can stick with and physical activities that they enjoy.

Beginning an exercise routine is the hardest part for many people who suffer from anxiety. However, once they get started, they find these physical activity periods one of the most enjoyable parts of the day. Sticking with an exercise routine can be very easy if planned out well.

Anyone beginning an exercise routine should think about the physical activities they enjoy most. Do they enjoy playing with their children? Riding a bicycle? Gardening in their backyard? When it comes to reducing anxiety symptoms, any activity that gets the body moving counts as exercise.

No one should feel like they have to decide on a workout plan and stick to it forever. Sampling a variety of different activities can help keep motivation levels high. Different kinds of exercises have different benefits, and switching between them gives people the chance to experience them all.

If the thought of joining a gym is enough to bring on a panic attack – you're probably not alone. You don't need to have a social phobia (or any other kind of anxiety disorder) to have an aversion to the gym! However, healthy exercise has surprising implications for anxiety disorders and other psychological conditions, including depression. The mechanisms by which exercise and mental health are related are not fully understood. Many medical experts worldwide now acknowledge that exercise has a major impact on many psychological conditions. For example, it is believed that exercise can effectively combat depression as many commonly prescribed drugs.

There is no need to join a gym for the good news. If you want to, then there is certainly no harm in signing up. However, "exercise", in this context, means simple, easy exercises that anybody should be able to manage. A few times a day, short bursts of activity are the type of exercise that experts recommend. For example, a brisk walk lasting only ten minutes is believed to be enough to raise your emotional state for a couple of hours. It can be hard for those with anxiety disorders to get out and about occasionally. For some, with severe conditions, it can seem impossible. However, exercise will help improve your emotional state and take your mind off the anxiety. Use the following tips to increase your chances of successfully incorporating exercise into your life.

Don't start with the intention of completing a 10K run. Instead, use small bursts of activity – the type that gets you a little out of breath and sweating – into the day. Ten minutes every so often is better than half an hour in one go.

Moderate level intensity exercise is recommended as perfect for improving physical and mental health. That includes walking briskly, cycling, jogging, or swimming. Walking and jogging should not need any investment, and if you're uncomfortable alone, partner up with a friend or relative. Ideally, buddy up with someone who addresses the same issues or has a good understanding of them for extra support.

Psychologists recommend that the exercises you choose should be rhythmic and repetitive. That helps to clear the mind and focus it on the task at hand. Walking, again, is the simplest of these and should be easy to achieve for many people.

If you begin to experience anxiety during a period of exercise, focus your mind on your breathing. Use a meditation technique like "mindfulness meditation" (described briefly in the next chapter) to become aware of your body, breathe simply, and limit the impact of negative or nervous thoughts. Experience the moment you are in, not the fears in your mind. Alternatively, count each step (out-loud if necessary) to distract your mind from the feelings of anxiety.

Talk About Your Problems with Other People

It helps if you have a trusted friend or relative willing to listen to your worries. Trying to contain your feelings can be very challenging. It will just allow your panic to snowball. When a person is willing to listen to your problems and vulnerabilities, you will be more at ease and realize that you are not alone. Secondly, things aren't as bad as they seem.

Do not always expect that the other person will comfort you completely. It is highly unlikely that the other person will be able to erase all your worries. However, talking about worries will prevent them from becoming bigger and bigger. It will prevent you from snapping in an unexpected situation. Talking about your problems will prevent you from exploding and may assist you in maintaining perspective.

Work with a Therapist

Don't be afraid of working with a therapist if your stress or anxiety severely interferes with your quality of life. Holistic help is only taking the edge off the problem. Therapists are experienced individuals trained to understand what you are going through and provide unconditional support to prevent you from descending into more serious anxiety disorders, depression, or stress-related disorders.

Having a Little Fun Killed Nobody

Laughing is a great relaxation technique and stress reliever. It increases lots of good feelings and serves to discharge tension. One major problem with people prone to anxiety is that they tend to take life so seriously that they appear to be melancholy all the time, and they eventually stop creating fun moments in their life. Fun and play are essential for the brain's proper functioning; it is a technique that stimulates the brain to come up with creative ideas rather than concentrating on little worries and fears. Within the fun and play, you may develop various ways to apply in situations when you are rendered anxious and helpless. Remember that rigidity limits you to a certain scope of ideas that will directly influence your take on the world.

Conclusion

So, all of these put together will give you just a massive number of herbs and foods that should help kill the herpes simplex virus while healing your body. Herpes ailment is a drawn-out corruption acknowledged by the herpes simplex virus (HSV). The body's areas influenced by this sullying are the genital locale, the oral area, the skin, and the butt-driven district. This ailment is known for its incredibly drawn-out stretch. It commonly assaults people causing several tribulations; some are smooth, and some are perilous.

Genital herpes is one of the most by and large saw kinds of herpes simplex sickness. Genital herpes pollution is an explicitly transmitted affliction that results in genital and butt-driven disturbs. In addition, there might be wounds that likewise sway the mouth and face. Dr. Sebi was a notable cultivator that restored many individuals experiencing herpes, and different disorders, for example, disease, aids, hypertension, fibroid, diabetes, body torment, illicit drug use, and so forth.

You know now what Dr. Sebi herpes fix is. Dr. Sebi's answer for herpes constantly appears on each side of the world. The purpose behind the so fiery widespread is genuinely not a colossal number of dollars spent on pills or worldwide eminence, considering how some huge name is getting a handle on it. Instead, it is to reach the hearts of herpes patients in such a case that its adequacy.

Overall, Dr. Sebi's herpes fix is compelling with zero symptoms. When you eat well nourishments, your insusceptible framework will have the quality it needs to fend off intruders. Dr. Sebi's herpes cure is a perpetual solution for herpes, which keeps you away from herpes episodes and encourages the different reactions that antivirals may give you. Dr. Sebi's herpes cure can work appropriately with the right spices and the best quality items, so ensure you read the book and investigate different assets to ensure you are prepared to begin the procedure. In any case, there's as yet an opportunity that this treatment won't work for you and could conceivably work for your companion, relative, neighbor, or who else because your body is not quite the same as their body. Your body may respond an alternate way, so it's smarter to make an arrangement and counsel your doctor if things don't beat that.

I hope you will be able to implement in your life what you have learned in this book!

BOOK 4: <u>DR. SEBI AUTOIMMUNE SOLUTION</u>

THE EFFECTIVE METHOD TO FREE YOURSELF FROM CHRONIC PAIN AND FATIGUE WITHOUT MEDICATION. HOW TO NATURALLY REVERSE LUPUS, RHEUMATOID ARTHRITIS, PSORIASIS AND MORE

Chapter 1: Immune System Made Simple

What Is the Immune System?

Sickness is caused by bacteria, toxins, or viruses that enter the body and cells in the body that mutate. Without any type of defense against these at all, we'd die very quickly from even the simplest of elements. Our defense comprises a complex system of organs, cells, and tissues that function together to form our Immune System, which first *defends* against intruding bacteria or viruses and then *attacks* if anything should get through.

Your immune system is made up of three different types of immunity. These are innate immunity, acquired immunity, and passive immunity.

These immunities make up two immunity systems, which each gives its response. These are the adaptive and innate immune responses. Two separate systems interact in complex and critical ways, yet one immune system. If their balance is off, there can be dire consequences.

Innate System (Innate Immunity)

The innate system creates your innate immunity. That is the immunity with which you were born. It's your body's second line of defense, as it immediately tackles anything that it sees as a threat. This system responds similarly to every threat and is known as nonspecific. It also responds to every infection in the same way. That makes the innate system also known as non-adaptive. The components of the non-adaptive system include:

Stomach acid

Phagocytic white blood cells

Fever

Enzymes in your skin oils

Enzymes in your tears

Inflammation

Cough reflex

Antimicrobial chemicals.

Mucus (traps tiny particles and bacteria)

Adaptive System

The adaptive system creates an acquired immunity. It is your body's third line of defense. Not only is it adaptive, but it's also specific. That means that it knows the difference between one pathogen and the next and responds in a specific way to each one. So although it may take your adaptive immune system a little while fighting off a pathogen the first time it encounters it, after defending against it once, it learns that pathogen's weaknesses. As a result, it can quickly eradicate it the next time if your immune system lets it take hold again at all.

The adaptive system's core components are lymphocytes, which, as we have seen above, are a class of white blood cells. First, your B cells target an antigen (a pathogen fragment). Then TH cells release cytokines to activate the B cell (immune cell). That starts a chain reaction leading to antibodies to eradicate the pathogen. Finally, after the crisis has passed, your body transforms a small bit of the activated B and TH cells into memory cells, which immunize you against that pathogen.

Passive Immunity

Passive immunity is produced when you build immunity by using antibodies produced outside of your body. Examples of passive immunity would be a baby's immunity from the antibodies through the breastmilk. Another example of passive immunity is that which can be gained through an immunization (antiserum injection), such as the tetanus antitoxin. Unfortunately, passive immunity, though it provides immediate protection, must be repeated. The effects wear off.

How Does the Immune System Function?

As you go throughout the day, your immune system is always on high alert for something called antigens. Antigens are anything foreign invaders the body recognizes as harmful. These can be viruses, bacteria, or fungi. Chemicals, toxins, drugs, and even eyelashes can be recognized as antigens. They can be proteins (occasionally, they can be something else) on the cells' surface. But that's not all your immune system has to be on the lookout for. There are also damaged cells called free radicals in your bloodstream that steal the electrons from your healthy cells, damaging them and possibly leading to cancer.

Your body, however, has antigens called HLA antigens that are supposed to be there. These are proteins that are a natural part of your cells. Your immune system recognizes those antigens as normal and leaves them alone. So, here's the question:

How does it tell what to attack and what to leave alone?

Our body is amazing. First, unhealthy cells use "danger" cues to signify their presence. These are called danger-associated molecular patterns (DAMPs). When your immune system recognizes a DAMP, which comes in several different varieties, it knows to attack that cell and how to attack it. And being that unhealthy cells can be caused by many things, from sunburn to infection to cancer, your body has its work cut out for it.

Besides this, contact with infectious microbes, or pathogens, sets off a completely different set of signals. Infectious microbes are things like bacteria and viruses. These signals are called pathogen-associated molecular patterns (PAMPs). Each PAMP is also responded to differently.

The immune system also deals with allergens, such as fungi, pollen, and foods. How your body responds to each of these depends on how much of an invader it decides that particular allergen is to your body. That is why some people get away with hardly any allergies at all.

After your body knows what's a friend and foreign, then what?

What Is an Immune Response?

The immune response is how your body responds to the antigens in your system. A healthy immune system kicks into gear right away, battling the virus, bacteria, or fungi when it's first assaulted. However, suppose it can't be triggered when needed or doesn't have the resources to sufficiently eradicate the foreign intruder. In that case, you end up with problems like infection and sickness. However, when the immune system is triggered without cause or refuses to "shut off" after the danger has passed, you end up with different complications, such as autoimmune disease and allergic reactions.

Part of the reason a healthy immune system works so well is that it's so extensive. It utilizes nearly every part of the body.

Let's look at each part of the immune system and how it responds to invaders:

Skin

As always, your skin is your first line of defense. It's like the wall and mote around the castle. Your skin cells defend against bacteria, viruses, and other microbes by secreting antimicrobial proteins, which attack the microbes upon contact. Immune cells themselves also develop within the different layers of skin.

Bone Marrow

Though they differ greatly, every immune cell begins life from stem cells in the bone marrow. From there, they travel to their destination. Then, they mature into the necessary immune cells. Though they originate from the same source, these mature cells can perform the immune function for that part of the body.

The myeloid progenitor stem cell matures into innate immune cells responsible for fighting infection. The adaptive immune cells (B cells and T cells), which fight specific viruses and bacteria, mature from the lymphoid progenitor stem cell. The natural killer cells (NK cells) also mature from the lymphoid progenitor cell. NK cells perform the function of both adaptive and innate immune cells.

Bloodstream

Immune cells endlessly patrol the bloodstream, ready to attack at the first hint of trouble. The immune cells in your bloodstream are white blood cells or leukocytes. Doctors can tell if a bacterial infection has activated your immune system by checking neutrophils, a certain type of leukocyte.

There are two families of leukocytes—phagocytes and lymphocytes. Phagocytes beat up on the pathogens and destroy what they can. At the same time, Lymphocytes write invading pathogen information into the cell to be remembered and then eradicated.

These two families are made up of five leukocyte classes, all of which perform their immunity task.

The one mentioned earlier (neutrophils) is the first immune defense on the scene in response to microbial infection.

Monocytes are also one of the first responders to microbial infection. They're slower to react but last longer than neutrophils. They're also the first response to a pathogenic infection.

Eosinophils are the immune cells that battle multicellular parasites.

Basophils are the first response to inflammation. They release the chemicals heparin and histamine upon activation.

Lymphocytes include the B lymphocytes (B cells) and T lymphocytes (T cells). B cells and T cells join forces to start a chain reaction leading to the production of antibodies in the presence of viruses and bacteria. Cytotoxic T cells NK cells join forces to eradicate virus-infected cells.

Relative Proportions of White Blood Cells in a Healthy Human Body

Neutrophils	60-70%
Monocytes	1-6%
Eosinophils	1-3%
Basophils	Less than 1%
Lymphocytes	20-30%

Antibodies

The Lymphocytes that create the antibodies can then recognize the infected or damaged cells and tag them for eradication. However, it can't do the destroying. That's the job of the NK cells.

Antibodies also counteract toxins (pathological or biological) and activate the complement system, a group of proteins that help eradicate viruses, bacteria, or infected cells.

Complement

The complement system comprises over thirty proteins that unite to eradicate antigens, specifically infectious microorganisms. The liver is responsible for producing the majority of the complement system. These proteins circulate through the body via the extracellular fluid and blood until they're needed.

Then, and only then, the immune system gives two signals. One signal is triggered by molecules embedded in the microorganism. The other signal is triggered by antibodies bound to the microorganism's surface. The next two complements are triggered when one complement is triggered in the sequence. In this way, they create two pathways, both leading toward the same pivotal protein. Finally, the pivotal protein is activated when the pathways converge, triggering a gruesome attack on the microorganism.

Lymphatic system

It plays a major role in the immune system. The lymphatic system is a network of lymph, lymphoid organs, extracellular fluid, and lymphatic vessels. It is one of the main highways for travel between bloodstream and tissue.

The lymphatic vessels span the body and carry waste products from the body. They also contain tissue fluid and immune cells, which use the lymph organs as their home base.

The immune cells travel this highway to play reconnaissance. As the lymphatic system carries the other cells' waste products, the immune cells scan it for PAMPs and DAMPs. If something is found, the immune response in the cell will be triggered. It will reproduce, and cells will leave in masses to crush, kill, and destroy.

Lymph Nodes

Several small " pathogen traps are located along this highway of lymphatic vessels, lymph, and immune cells are several small "pathogen traps." Built specifically for trapping and eradicating pathogens and other invaders or damaged cells as they flow through, these "traps" are called lymph nodes. The lymph nodes are merely bean-shaped clusters of immune cells that are chockful of white blood cells—every "invader's" worst nightmare.

Thymus

The immune cells in your thymus are T cells. Your thymus is one of the smaller organs located in your upper chest near your thyroid.

Spleen

Though the spleen isn't directly tied into the lymphatic system, it still does the same basic job, entitling it to be part of it just the same. It's a vital part of the body's defenses as it filters the blood and sends the information it collects. The spleen is also rich with immune system cells ready to activate and attack the minute a blood-borne pathogen is recognized.

Mucosal Tissue

One of the easiest access points for any virus or bacteria is by way of mucosal surfaces, which include the lips, ears, nostrils, genital area, eyelids, and anus. Our immune system has that covered. In addition, our respiratory, digestive, and reproductive tracts are lined with mucosal tissue. This tissue is what keeps the insides in and the outside out. But what's to keep the viruses and bacteria from crossing that threshold? That would be your handy mucosal tissue, which not only provides a barrier but also have even cells at standby. Different areas gut also have access areas, where the immune cells check the gastrointestinal tract contents for a reason for alarm.

Inflammation

When your tissues are damaged by trauma, bacteria, heat, toxins, or any kind of antigen, the inflammatory response will be triggered. That causes your body to release several different kinds of chemicals. A few of these are prostaglandins, histamine, and bradykinin. When these chemicals are released into your system, your blood vessels will begin to leak into the damaged tissues. That causes swelling around the antigen, which helps to quarantine it from your other tissues.

The chemicals released during the inflammatory response also attract phagocytes, eradicating germs and " eating" damaged or dead cells. This process is called phagocytosis.

What Is an Altered Immune Response?

Your immune system can have one of three responses—an efficient immune response, an inadequate immune response, and an overactive immune response. If your immune system is healthy, protecting you adequately, you have an efficient immune response.

If your immune system allows you to develop diseases, it's inefficient. Unless it's caused by an outside source, such as medication, an inefficient immune system is typically caused by an immune deficiency disease. An immune deficiency disease can be primary, meaning you were born with it or acquired, which means another illness causes it.

There is also an overactive immune system. For example, an allergic reaction or hypersensitivity can cause your immune system to be overactive. That can cause an autoimmune disease to develop when your immune system begins attacking your body. Both an inefficient and overactive immune system is altered immune responses.

Why Does Your Immune System Begin Attacking Your Body?

Until the beginning of the 20th century, Paul Ehrlich proposed that autoimmune tissue attacks might be possible. However, he didn't believe that the autoimmune response could become pathological. The 1950s finally allowed us to understand autoimmune diseases and autoantibodies as we understand them today.

We've come a long way, but doctors have no real answer to that question. However, they have noticed that certain autoimmune diseases are more prevalent in certain groups of people.

A 2014 study found on sciencedirect.com stated that two women tend to get an autoimmune disease to every one man.

Autoimmune diseases typically kick in between 15 and 44 years old.

They typically favor one ethnic group over the next. For example, Lupus tends to be more prevalent among Hispanic and African Americans than Caucasians.

Some autoimmune diseases tend to be genetic. For instance, if one family member has Lupus or multiple sclerosis, the other family members are susceptible to developing an autoimmune disease. However, it may not be the same.

Researchers believe you might be more likely to develop an autoimmune disease if exposed to certain solvents, chemicals, or environmental factors.

A study performed in 2015 by Lisa A. Reynolds, Leah T. Stiemsma, B. Brett Finlay, and Stuart E. Turvey theorizes that a lack of exposure to germs might cause an overreactive response to harmless antigens.

A diet high in sugar and fat and many processed foods are thought to trigger inflammation, which sets off an autoimmune response and heightens the risks of developing an autoimmune disease. Thus, the scope of this book.

A healthy immune system is vital to a healthy body. When the immune system is out of balance, it not only fails to defend against antigens, but it can begin to attack itself, causing an autoimmune disease, which can be devastating. At this point, the immune system becomes sensitive to life itself. Simple things, such as strenuous exercise, the stress of personal problems, travel, and even a simple diet change, can affect your overall health. Besides this, years of exposure to even low-level inflammation can raise the risks of developing other diseases, such as cardiovascular disease and cancer.

Chapter 2: Autoimmune Diseases

In the world of medicine, the field of autoimmunity is still in the embryonic stages.

The first historical mention of autoimmunity goes back in our recent history to the German biologist and pathologist Paul Ehrlich. They won the Nobel Prize for Medicine in 1908. Around the turn of the last century, Ehrlich coined the term *horror autotoxicus* (fear of self-poisoning) as the phenomenon that could occur when a person's defenses turned against them. At the time, horror autotoxicus was largely a clinical observation about findings made in certain patients. Ehrlich was much involved in describing antigens and their chemical structure and looking at something new called *antitoxins*.

He realized that an antigen and foreign matter could also be a part of our tissues but perceived as foreign by the immune system. In short, he put forth the now-well-accepted theory that our immune systems can react to something that is native to our bodies in addition to seeking out strangers. However, he did not know how or with what.

Around the same time, the great internist William Osler, a contemporary of Ehrlich, studied skin diseases that he thought were related to tuberculosis (TB) but were autoimmune diseases. Although he eventually concluded that these diseases were unique and not TB, he did not have the tools to prove their biological origins. It would be another fifty years until the immune system was defined and Ehrlich and Osler's observations were substantiated. Antibodies were not identified until the 1950s, so all these investigators dreamed creatively about what "might be," which is much the same process that all medical researchers use today.

A decade later, in the sixties, the concept of autoimmunity as a cause of human illness became part of the medical lore when doctors Gerald Edelman of Rockefeller University and Rodney Peters at Oxford University defined the structure of an antibody. That resulted in the development of laboratory tests to help recognize autoimmune diseases. Soon after, T cells and B cells were identified. The discovery of the origins of antibodies and autoreactive cells made autoimmunity an active science and medicine research field.

Considering that all of this happened in the last forty years, we have made astonishing progress.

The human immune system collects certain chemicals and cells that fight and protect our bodies against the infections that cause bacteria and viruses. As such, the immune system plays a vital role in protecting us against microbial infections. However, in autoimmune disorders, the immune system fails to function properly. It mistakenly takes the body's cells and tissues as foreign invaders and starts killing them. What happens when the immune system fails to differentiate between its cells and foreign invaders? When this happens, the affected body forms autoantibodies that mistakenly attack the body's cells. On the other side, the regulatory T cells fail to do their job in keeping the immune system in line. That results in a mistaken attack on your body's cells.

The damage that results from this process is known as an autoimmune disease. Autoimmune disorders are mainly divided into two categories: Organ-specific autoimmune disorders. One organ is mainly affected by the disorder; the other is a non-organ-specific autoimmune disorder that can affect multiple organs and systems. There are about 80 autoimmune disorders, ranging from minor to disabling in severity, based on the type of affected organ and the degree of disability. Due to some unknown reasons, women are more likely to get autoimmune disorders than men, especially during childbearing periods; it is assumed that sex hormones might be one reason amongst the others. To date, there is no cure for autoimmune disorders. Still, with some treatment options, the symptoms of autoimmune disorders can be managed.

Autoimmune diseases are very common, affecting more than 23.5 million people in the USA alone. Autoimmune disorders are one of the leading causes of disability and death. As we all know, there are many (about 80) autoimmune disorders, and some are very common, yet some autoimmune disorders are rare.

What Is an Autoimmune Disease?

Have you ever been to the grocery store and seen an acquaintance that you haven't seen in a while? You go up to the person to say "hi", tap them on the shoulder, and when they turn around, you notice you've never met this person in your life. They are a stranger. You have that moment of panic where you try to think of what to say, and then the awkward explanations begin.

Autoimmune diseases are a lot like this illustration. Our body has developed an intricate and amazing security system to protect itself from germs and viruses: our immune system. The hardworking security guards. Of this system are the white blood cells. They patrol the highways of the body called the vascular system. The vascular system is a series of veins and arteries that circulate blood from the heart, through the body, and back to the heart. They patrol the vascular system searching for invading bodies like viruses and germs. When they find these "bad" cells floating around, the white blood cells attack them. However, when a person has an autoimmune disease, the white blood cells mistake their cells for a harmful, invading cell. So, the white cells swarm those cells and attack them. The white cells can mistake any number of our types of cells, organs, or systems. Once your white cells have identified these as dangerous, they will continue to attack those cells.

Close-up of a Neutrophil Antibody (white blood cell)

 When this happens, you have an autoimmune disease. More than eighty diagnosed autoimmune diseases affect more than 23 million Americans suffering from them. 80% of those diagnosed are women. Each autoimmune disease is a different system, organ, or cell that the white cells have mistaken for a dangerous foreign body. For example, in the case of my disease, Psoriatic Arthritis, my body attacks both my skin and joint cells.

But why are autoimmune diseases so much more prevalent in women? Are women just weaker and more prone to disease?

The opposite is true. Women have a double X chromosome. The X chromosome has more than 1000 kinds of genes housed on it. Whereas the Y chromosome has only just over 100 genes. That means there is a defective gene on one of their X chromosomes. Anytime a female's redundant gene on the other X chromosome can step in and replace the defective gene. It makes females less prone to X gene-linked hereditary diseases and infectious diseases. It causes them to live longer statistically and healthier lives than men. However, in the case of autoimmune diseases, the XX chromosomes are the issue.

The X chromosome is where you find the genes for the immune system. So why do women have autoimmune disease issues? Isn't more of an immune system a good thing? No, it isn't. The X chromosome is the only chromosome not doubled in both men and women. To prevent a woman from having a double expression of the X chromosome's genes, her body naturally shuts down (inactivates) the chromosome's redundant genes. The body is smart does this inactivation in a pattern (usually 50/50 per X chromosome). But sometimes, it fails to shut down a redundant gene. Or it will it the redundant genes in a wonky way (60/40 or 80/20). The body inactivates the genes in a wonky way. It is called "skewed gene inactivation". The biology of women works against them when it comes to autoimmune diseases. However, researchers and doctors aren't sure why female hormones often seem to trigger autoimmune diseases somehow. It is normal for the onset of autoimmune disease symptoms to occur during puberty.

In my case, the first time my hands froze, and I couldn't use my fingers was when I was 17 years old, during my first year of college. I had had small flares of "rashes" on my skin, attributed to dry skin throughout my childhood. It wasn't until later that I learned those occasional "rashes" were psoriasis, not just dry skin. When my fingers froze, I knew exactly what it was. I had watched my grandmother suffer and eventually die of complications from the same disease. Instead of getting help, I ignored my symptoms and pretended fine. Had I gone to the doctor then, I may have been able to avoid the breakdown of my body that would come thirteen years later. The earlier you treat autoimmune diseases, the better. Quite often, doctors can significantly slow down or even halt the progress of these diseases. That is important because autoimmune diseases are degenerative.

You should look for signs if you are concerned that you have an autoimmune disease. Some of these signs are:

- Swelling of the Joints
- Pain in the Joints
- Abdominal Pain
- Chronic Diarrhea or Constipation
- Swollen Glands
- Other Chronic Digestive Issues

- Chronic Fevers
- Trouble swallowing Food or Drinks
- Unexplained Weight Loss or Weight Gain
- Skin Rashes or Other Skin Issues
- Chronic Exhaustion or Fatigue

If you have these symptoms, please discuss them with your doctor.

Cause and Treatment

Many people complain that it is difficult to get an autoimmune disease diagnosis. Unfortunately, this can be true for several reasons. Diagnosing an autoimmune disease is not a cut and dry process. There isn't a specific blood test that you can run that says you have or don't have most of these diseases. Rather it is a process of looking for markers in the blood, noting symptoms, and taking tissue samples in some cases. It also can be complex because many of the symptoms can be caused by other illnesses and viruses. It sometimes takes time and patience to receive the correct diagnosis. I have found having the right doctor to be imperative. My rheumatologist was able to diagnose me, whereas my other doctors failed.

Doctors and researchers do not know the causes of autoimmune diseases. However, they do have a list of things they know are contributing factors or commonalities between patients.

These things are:

- Genetics
- Lifestyle
- Environmental Factors
- Stress

- Weight
- Diet
- Smoking

Autoimmune diseases can vary drastically in how severely they affect the person suffering from them. One person's life may be relatively unaffected, whereas the next person is severely affected. In many of these cases, the severity of the disease has to do with lifestyle and environmental issues. Smoking and being overweight statistically make diseases worse. Also, someone with a strong genetic link seems to have drawn the unlucky straw when it comes to the severity of the disease.

How Autoimmune Diseases Cause Inflammation

An autoimmune disease causes the overproduction of chemokines and cytokines, leading to inflammation of the body tissues. For instance, an excess of cytokines in the joints can cause rheumatoid arthritis. This condition worsens when chemokines bring more destructive components of the immune system, like T cells, macrophages, and neutrophils, to the affected joints, intensifying the inflammatory response.

Who is at Risk of Getting Autoimmune Diseases?

Anyone can get autoimmune disorders, but certain people are at more risk, for example:

Childbearing Women

Due to some unknown reasons, more women (of childbearing age) than men suffer from autoimmune diseases.

People Having a Positive Family History for Autoimmune Diseases

Some autoimmune diseases run in families, like multiple sclerosis and Lupus. It is a common trend that some autoimmune diseases affect different family members. If a person inherits some family genes, that person has more chances of developing an autoimmune disease. However, a combination of genes and other factors can increase the development of an autoimmune disease.

People Who Are Constantly Exposed to Certain Substances

Exposure to certain environmental triggers and exposures can lead to or worsen autoimmune disorders. For example, sunlight, certain solvents, bacterial and viral infections are associated with autoimmune diseases.

People of Certain Races

Some autoimmune diseases affect certain races more severely than others. For instance, Lupus is more common and severe in Hispanic people and American Africans. Similarly, type 1 diabetes is more prevalent in white people than others.

How are Autoimmune Diseases Treated?

Traditionally, autoimmune diseases are treated in one or a combination of several ways. First, doctors prescribe corticosteroids (steroids), immunosuppressants, and nonsteroidal anti-inflammatory drugs. There are many drugs in each classification of drugs. The doctor will prescribe will depend on your disease, its severity, and what your body will tolerate.

Corticosteroids

Corticosteroids (aka steroids) are synthetic medications that emulate the hormone cortisol that your body produces. These medications are used to decrease inflammation (the body's process to attack foreign or dangerous cells in the body) and decrease the immune system's activity by knocking back someone's immune system with an autoimmune disease. But unfortunately, it also leaves the person with a compromised immune system. Common corticosteroids prescribed are prednisone and cortisone.

Immunosuppressants

Immunosuppressants are prescribed to suppress the immune system exactly as the name suggests. They are prescribed for various reasons, including autoimmune diseases and anti-rejection medications for organ transplants. There are many types of immunosuppressants (including corticosteroids). What is prescribed depends on your disease and your body's tolerance.

A few types of immunosuppressants are:

- Corticosteroids
- prednisone

- prednisolone
- Janus kinase inhibitors
- tofacitinib
- Calcineurin inhibitors
- cyclosporine
- mTOR inhibitors
- sirolimus
- methotrexate
- IMDH inhibitors

- leflunomide
- Biologics
- adalimumab
- certolizumab
- etanercept
- infliximab
- rituximab
- Monoclonal antibodies
- basiliximab

That is by no means a complete list of the medications available. Rather it is a brief overview. Often, doctors will prescribe dietary changes and lifestyle modifications as well.

Types of Autoimmune Diseases

This section will include a small list of the most common autoimmune diseases and information about each one. This is by no means a way to diagnose a disease, as a qualified doctor must do that. However, that is simple information that could help identify possible disease symptoms and encourage you to talk to your qualified doctor.

Celiac disease

 Celiac Disease is an autoimmune disease that causes the sufferer to not eat gluten. If you eat any gluten, your body responds with an autoimmune reaction that causes damage to your small intestine. Gluten is a protein found in grains. It can also be found in medicines and household products like Chapstick and even on stamps in the glue.

Crohn's disease

Crohn's disease is an autoimmune disease that affects the bowels. It causes inflammation of the lining and walls of the gastrointestinal tract. It is a very painful disease but is not usually life-threatening.

Endometriosis

Endometriosis is an autoimmune disease of the uterus. Endometriosis causes the uterine lining tissue to grow in other parts of the uterus, reproductive system, or other organs. It can cause severe pain, infertility, heavy menstrual flow, and miscarriages.

Eosinophilic esophagitis (EoE)

 Eosinophilic esophagitis is an autoimmune disease associated with food allergies. It causes inflammation of the esophagus and eosinophilic cells' growth, a type of white blood cell-specific to the esophagus. When these cells build up too much, they create swelling and other autoimmune reactions.

Fibromyalgia

Fibromyalgia causes widespread pain, tenderness, insomnia, and fatigue. It is not classified as an autoimmune disease but is co-morbid with several autoimmune diseases. Fibromyalgia is also known to cause or exasperate depression.

Graves' disease

Graves' disease is an autoimmune disease that affects the thyroid gland. It causes the gland to produce too much of its hormone. . It causes an inability to tolerate heat, nervousness, and weight loss. It affects women at a much higher rate than men.

Lupus

Lupus is an autoimmune disease that causes inflammation of many different systems in the body. There are three common types of Lupus: Systemic Lupus Erythematosus (SLE), Discoid Lupus, and Drug-induced lupus *Lyme disease*

Lyme disease is an autoimmune disease caused by the bite of a deer tick.

Multiple sclerosis (MS)

Multiple sclerosis (MS) is an autoimmune disease that affects the brain and spinal cord. The autoimmune reaction is that the body attacks the myelin sheathing of the nerves, slowing down the brain's messages to other parts of the body.

PANDAS (Pediatric Autoimmune Neuropsychiatric Disorders Associated with Streptococcus).

PANDAS is an autoimmune disorder that affects children and teens after strep throat or scarlet fever. The autoimmune response is psychiatric, causing OCD, Tourette's style tics, and even aggression.

Psoriasis

Psoriasis is an autoimmune disease of the skin. The autoimmune response causes red scaly patches caused by the overproduction of skin cells.

Psoriatic Arthritis.

Psoriatic arthritis is an autoimmune disease where the body's autoimmune response to psoriasis causes joint inflammation, pain, and mobility issues.

Rheumatoid arthritis (RA)

Rheumatoid arthritis (RA) is an autoimmune disease that causes pain, swelling, and mobility issues in the joints.

Type 1 diabetes

Type 1 diabetes is an autoimmune disease that causes the pancreas not to produce enough insulin. Insulin is a hormone that helps to move blood sugar into cells. Without insulin, glucose will build in the body and lead to coma and even death.

Diagnosis of Autoimmune Disorders

It is generally very hard to diagnose an autoimmune disease, especially in its initial stages. This is because autoimmune diseases involving many organs and systems are very difficult to diagnose.

Based on the type of autoimmune disorders, diagnostic methods can involve:

☐ X-rays

☐ Biopsy

☐ Certain blood tests, including those that can detect autoantibodies

☐ Physical examination

☐ Patient history

☐ Antinuclear Antibody Test

☐ Protein Electrophoresis

☐ Complement Test

☐ C Reactive Protein Test

Chapter 3: Complications That Can Arise Because of an AD

Cancer

Cancer may begin anywhere within the body. It starts when the cells multiply rapidly and occupy the space of normal cells. That makes it impossible for the body to act the way it ought to.

That several people will handle cancer well. More people lead long lives after cancer care than ever before.

We'll clarify here what cancer is and what its causes are. Cancer isn't just one disorder; there are several tumors. It is not about a single disorder. Cancer may begin in the breast, in the lungs, in the colon, or in the blood. In specific ways, cancers are similar but vary in how they develop and propagate.

How does cancer look alike?

Our cells do have some things to perform in our bodies. Regular cells break in an ordered manner. They die when stretched out or injured, and new cells arise. Cancer occurs when the cells start developing out of balance. The cancer cells begin to expand and shape new cells. They clutch off normal ones. That creates complications in the section of the body where cancer starts.

Cancer cells are often spread to other areas of the body. For example, lung cancer cells may migrate to the bones and expand. It is called metastasis (meh-TAS-uh-sis), as cancer cells disperse. If lung cancer progresses to the bones, it is also considered a tumor of the lungs. The cancer cells, mostly in bones, seem to doctor, much like the lungs. If it began with the bones, it is considered bone cancer.

Some tumors are easy to develop and propagate. The other will expand gradually. Often, they react to care in numerous ways. For example, some cancer forms are best handled with surgery; others respond favorably to Chemotherapy. Usually, 2 or 3 procedures are used to produce optimal outcomes.

The specialist may like to figure out what type of cancer it is. People living with cancer require care that fits their cancer form.

Many tumors develop a lump called a growing tumor. However, the lumps aren't always cancer. So health care professionals are pulling a piece of the swelling out and searching to observe cancer. Non-cancer bumps or lumps are named benign. Cancer-causing lumps are called malignant.

Such tumors, such as leukemia (blood cancer), do not develop tumors. Instead, they mature in the body's blood cells or other cells.

"There is anxiety running inside you when you're told you're getting cancer. In the beginning, it is so impossible to care for something more than the illness. Every morning, this is the first thing you think or talk about. I want people with cancer to feel it's getting easier. Thinking about cancer lets you cope with all the different feelings you experience. Remember, getting upset is natural. -Delores, "cancer survivor

What induces cancer?

Cancer can be caused by gene damage, which has accumulated. Such changes could be because of chance or exposure to the substance that causes cancer.

The cancer-causing compounds are known as carcinogens. Carcinogens, like some compounds of cigarette smoke, can be chemical elements. Cancer may also be triggered by bacterial, environmental, or genetic causes.

However, we should remember that we cannot assign the illness to a source in most cancer situations.

We may segment risk factors for cancer in approximately the below groups:

Factors related to lifestyle

Environmental

Bacteria and viruses

Factors related to lifestyle include:

• Alcohol

• Tobacco

• Several factors related to food, such as barbecue-generated polyaromatic hydrocarbons and nitrites.

Some cancer-causing factors related to the living environment and work include:

• Pitch and tar

• U.V. radiations

• polynuclear Hydrocarbons (e.g., benzopyrene), and asbestos fibers

• Certain compounds made of metal

• Certain toxic plastic chemicals (e.g., vinyl chloride)

Bacteria and viruses can induce cancer:

• Helicobacter pylori (blamed for gastritis)

• HCV, HBV (hepatitis virus causing hepatitis)

• HPV (human papillomavirus, papillomavirus inducing modifications, for example, in the cervical cells)

• Epstein-Barr virus (herpes virus triggering lymphoid gland inflammation).

Ischemic heart disease, or cardiovascular failure

Ischemic heart disease is chronic chest pain or distress when a heart does not have enough oxygen. This disease most often happens through exertion or agitation when the heart needs a more massive blood flow. Ischemic heart disease is expected in the U.S... However, it is a leading cause of mortality globally, also called coronary heart disorder.

Ischemic heart disease develops when blood cholesterol particles pile up on the arteries' walls and supply the heart with blood. Deposits, which are called plaques, can eventually form. These deposits shorten the arteries and end up restricting blood flow. This reduction in blood flow reduces the oxygen supplied to the heart muscle.

The symptoms and signs of ischemic heart disease can develop slowly as arteries are blocked. However, if an artery unexpectedly becomes blocked, it may occur quickly. Many patients with cardiovascular disease show almost no signs. In contrast, others may experience shortness of breath and extreme chest pain (angina) that may cause a risk of a heart attack.

Luckily ischemic heart disease can be successfully treated through lifestyle changes. And further, through practicing heart-healthy practices, such as consuming a low-sodium diet, a low-fat diet, getting physically active, not smoking, and maintaining a healthy diet.

If left untreated, ischemic heart disease can cause severe heart failure. Cardiac damage can cause heart attack and pain, as well as life-threatening

Causes

Ischemic heart disease is caused by decreased blood flow into either blood vessels that pump oxygen (coronary arteries). As a result, the heart muscle does not get the oxygen it needs to work correctly, while blood flow is reduced.

Cardiac Ischemic can develop slowly; when plaque builds up with time, or when an artery is completely blocked, it can occur quickly. For this cause, ischemic heart disease occurs most commonly in individuals with atherosclerosis (plaque build-up on the coronary artery walls), coronary artery spasm, blood clots, or severe illnesses that intensify the need for oxygen in the core.

What are the risk factors for cardiac ischemia?

The risk of developing ischemic heart disease rises with several factors. Not every person with risk factors gets ischemic heart disease. Risk factors for cardiac ischemia include:

• History of familial cardiac problems

• High cholesterol level in the blood

• Hypertension

• High level of Triglycerides in blood

• Diabetes Mellitus

• Body high in fats

• No exercise or physical movement

• Tobacco and many other applications

Diabetes mellitus

Diabetes mellitus, generally referred to as Diabetes, is a metabolic condition producing elevated blood sugar levels. The hormone insulin transfers the glucose from the blood into the cells for energy absorption or usage. Diabetes means the body either doesn't produce sufficient insulin or can't utilize the insulin it produces efficiently.

Untreated high diabetes blood sugar will affect your skin, your nerves, your kidneys as well as other organs.

There are several types of Diabetes:

• **Type 1 diabetes**, which is an autoimmune disorder. The body's immune system harms the pancreatic cells, where insulin is produced. What triggers the assault is unknown. Around 10 percent of people living with Diabetes have this kind.

• **Type 2 diabetes** occurs when your body becomes insulin resistant and blood sugar builds up.

• **Prediabetes** usually occurs when the body's blood sugar level is higher than average but not high enough for a type 2 diabetes diagnosis.

• **Gestational Diabetes**. This form is induced by insulin suppressing hormones released by the placenta during pregnancy.

A rare condition named diabetes insipidus, although it has a similar name, is not linked to diabetes mellitus. That is common when the kidneys absorb most of the body fluid.

Every diabetes condition has its signs, causes, and therapies.

Causes of Diabetes

Each form of Diabetes has various causes.

Type 1 diabetes

Healthcare professionals do not realize what is responsible for Diabetes type 1. The immune system wrongly targets and kills the insulin-producing beta-cells in the pancreas for whatever reason.

In certain people, genes may play a part. A virus may also set off an assault on the immune system.

Type 2 diabetes

Diabetes type 2 arises from various conditions related to physiology and lifestyle. Being obese or overweight often heightens the risk. Carrying extra fats, particularly in the belly, makes the cells highly immune to insulin's impact on your blood glucose.

Gestational Diabetes

Gestational Diabetes is the outcome of changes in hormone levels during pregnancy. The placenta releases hormones, which render the cells of a pregnant woman less vulnerable to the insulin effects. That may induce elevated sugar levels in the blood during gestation.

Women who become overweight during pregnancy or carry far too much weight during pregnancy are more prone to have gestational diabetes.

Dr. Sebi and Diseases

What Is The Source Of Disease And How To Get Rid Of The Root Cause?

According to Oxford learners dictionaries, "disease is an illness affecting humans, animals or plants, often caused by infection." In contrast, Dr. Sebi defines disease as "compromising the mucous membrane".

When I said the mucous membrane is compromised, the mucous membrane has been broken. So, wherever the mucous membrane gets broken or compromised determines the sickness that will manifest.

He further states that there is only one disease, which is the mucus (inflammation)." So take it or leave it, there is only one disease, and mucus is the source of all the types of diseases.

Below is a table showing you where the mucous membrane gets compromised and the sicknesses that will manifest:

S/No.	Point f Membrane Compromised	Sickness
i.	Lungs	pneumonia, cystic fibrosis (COPD), chronic obstructive pulmonary disease
ii.	bronchial tubes	Bronchitis
iii.	Trachea	Hemoptysis, wheezing and Stridor
iv.	Reproductive organ	Fibroid or low sperm count, infertility, endometriosis, etc.
v.	Pancreatic duct	Diabetes
vi.	The retina of the eye	Blindness or blur sight
Vii	kidney	Kidney stone, acute kidney injury, etc.
Viii.	Brain	Parkinson, paranoia, insomnia, etc.
Ix	Joint	Arthritis
x	heart	Heart failure, high/low blood pressure etc.
And	A lot	More

This is why Dr. Sebi disagrees with the idea of cleansing only one part of the body, which is the colon but believes in cleansing the entire body system. According to late Dr. Sebi, the only way to eliminate the root cause of hypertension is through an intracellular cleansing (cleansing/detoxification) of the whole cells because the whole body is interconnected. Therefore, cleansing one cell without the others is as good as not cleansing as the un-cleanse cells will infect the cleanse cells.

So, undergoing an intracellular cleansing means that you are resetting your entire cells from the Colon to the Lymph glands, Liver, Gallbladder, Kidney, and the skin back to their original state (alkaline environment) where no disease will be able to withstand and revitalize the body system to recover from the energy that it has loosed due to the presence of the disease.

What Are The Basis To Heal Yourself From ADs?

In other to treat autoimmune diseases naturally, the following rules must be respected:

1) Follow Dr. Sebi's nutritional guide religiously

2) Consume at least 1 gallon of spring water daily.

3) Consume only moderate sea salt and avoid table salt completely.

4) Make sure you don't consume more grain, including alkaline grain.

5) Ensure you are not suffering from any kidney or thyroid disorder

Approved Alkaline Foods

You can't heal from diseases if you don't fight mucus, but you can't get rid of it if you constantly feed your body with bad acidic foods.

Following Dr. Sebi's diet will allow your body to return to its original alkaline state and repair the damaged mucus membrane, slowly but surely.

Below are listed the 'what to eat' and ' what not to eat' in Dr. Sebi's nutritional guide:

The list of alkaline vegetables recommended by Dr. Sebi includes:

Kale	Okra
Bell Peppers	Mushrooms
Garbanzo Beans (chickpeas)	Onions
Lettuce (no Iceberg)	Squash
Mexican Squash (Chayote)	Amaranth Greens
Mexican Cactus (Nopales)	Wild Arugula
Zucchini	Tomato (plum and cherry)

The list of Fruits recommended by Dr. Sebi includes:

Grapes seeded	Bananas (smallest and burros)
Apple	Chirimoya sugar apple

Cherries	Prunes
Plums	Raisins (seeded)
Figs	Berries
Tamarind	Curants
Limes and key limes w/seed	Pears
Mangoes	Soursops
Prickly Pear	Peaches
Orange Seville or sour	dates
Cantaloupe	Soft jelly coconuts
Papaya	Melons (seeded)

Nuts and seeds recommended by Dr. Sebi are, for example:

Walnuts	Brazil Nuts
Hazelnut	Hemp Seed
Raw Sesame Seeds	

Alkaline oils you can use include:

Olive oil	Grapeseed Oil
Coconut oil	Hemp seed Oil
Avocado Oil	

The list of spices and seasonings that Dr. Sebi recommended are:

Pure Sea Salt	Onion Powder
Cayenne	Cloves Dill
Thyme	Oregano
Basil	Habanero
Sage	

The lists of approved grains are:

Kamut

Wild rice

Amaranth

Quinoa

Flours approved by Dr. Sebi are:

Quinoa flour

Tef flour

Rye flour

Ultimately, the lists of things that Dr. Sebi recommends that we should avoid are:

All types of meat, including white and red meat.

Dairy products like milk, cheese, yogurt, butter, etc.

All types of sugar (including cube and powdery)

Do not use microwave

Garlic

All human-made food (can and package food)

Chapter 4: Healing Your Immune System with Dr. Sebi's Teachings

As I said before, Dr. Sebi thought that the source of every disease is the excess of mucus that slowly builds up in different parts of our bodies because of the acidic environment the 'standard' diets create.

As Dr. Sebi stated, human bodies can face 6 stages of over-acidity if the body is not nourished with alkaline foods and herbs:

Sensitivity → You know you are in this stage if you start suffering from low energy, acne or bad odor.

Irritation → The next one is where you start facing bowel diseases such as IBS, constipation and diarrhea

Mucus Formation → Here's where your body can't tolerate living in an extra-acidic environment anymore and start producing mucus to try to protect itself

Inflammation → As soon as the mucus starts to build up, your body reacts by starting the inflammation process. That might cause you to start suffering from Arthritis or Fibromyalgia

Indurations → This stage's most dangerous complication is Atherosclerosis, also known as "the hardening of arteries". When mucus starts depositing into them, it takes the name of 'plaques'. Over time, these plaques can narrow or block the arteries and cause unforeseen problems, such as strokes.

Degeneration → In the last stage, mucus starts to build up into the brain, bones and around nerves. If that happens, dangerous diseases may arise, such as cancer, Multiple Sclerosis or Osteoporosis.

Dr. Sebi's Official method for treating autoimmune diseases is composed of 3 main steps. Please note that any of these parts can't be passed over to succeed in your healing journey.

The three steps I'm talking about are:

Cleansing → In this first stage, your body must be cleansed on an intra-cellular level through detoxification to purify each cell and remove the excess mucus.

Revitalizing → After cleansing, you need to take time to nourish your body, regenerate your cells and strengthen the immune system.

Keeping the Immune System Healthy → By Following Dr. Sebi's nutrition guide and adopting healthy lifestyle habits every day, you will be able to keep your mind sharp and strengthen the immune system.

STAGE 1: CLEANSING

How to Prepare Cleansing Herbs?

Preparing your cleansing herbs would depend greatly on the form you purchased them. It's easier to prepare cleansing herbs in powder forms. You can easily make herbal teas with them in the specified or recommended dosage. However, for other forms form herbs, especially roots or leaves, it is better to use a ratio of 1 teaspoon to 1 cup (8 oz) of spring water for each herb.

However, I recommend preparing herbs in batches of mixtures for easier batch preparation and storage. That would mean mixing them up according to function and benefit. Again, this will depend on the state of your health and what minerals are most important for you. You can combine similar herbs with similar functions into a batch. In all, try not to mix more than 2 or 3 herbs. Remember, these herbs are electric, and it's best to preserve their organic carbon, hydrogen, and oxygen nature as much as we can. Again, if you mix more than that, you may not get their accurate concentrations per ml of water, so try to limit it to 3, possibly 2.

For a clearer understanding, you can use the following mix:

- Mix **Colon and gallbladder** cleansing herbs together

- Mix **liver and kidney** cleansing herbs

- Mix **respiratory and mucus cleansing** herbs

- Mix **lymphatic and heavy-metal** cleansing herbs.

Since these herbs perform a whole-body cleanse (not just colon), including the skin, eyes, colon, liver, lymphatic system, and gallbladder, you can decide to choose how to combine them. Also, note that when you make larger batches of these herbs for storage, try not to make batches that last more than 7 to 14 days.

For pre-purchase cleansing packages

Please follow the recommended dosage or instructions that are provided for that cleansing package

For fresh Green leafy herbs

- Place in spring water and boil on low heat for 5 to 7 min

- For dried leafy herbs, boil longer – 10 to 15 min

For Dried ground (or powder) herbs

For dried ground or powder leaves or roots, mix in recommended ratios for the herb. Powder herbs are the easiest to mix in dosage proportions, so you can simply follow the package instructions

For Chunks of Dried Root herbs

If you've purchased chunks of roots or stems, you can prepare them in the following way:

- Cut or break up chunks

- Place in spring water and boil for 15 minutes

- Let cool and serve

- Alternatively, prepare in larger batches and place in jars to store in the refrigerator.

<u>**For bulk purchase herbs**</u>

If you have purchased herbs in bulk and are making your teas, find out the recommended dosage for each herb. You should prepare each herbal tea ratio of 1 teaspoon to 8 ounces of spring water as a general rule.

<u>**For capsules**</u>

I recommend that you do research and find out what the recommended dosage is for each herbal capsule

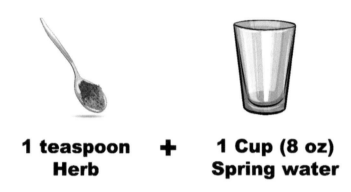

1 teaspoon Herb **+** **1 Cup (8 oz) Spring water**

<u>How To Take The Prepared Cleansing Herbs</u>

If you are on medication, I recommend taking the herbs one hour before taking your meds; Dr. Sebi recommended this. Your colon cleansing herbs should not be consumed for longer than 30 days because your body may become dependent on them, and you want to start to reduce the dose during your last 3 to 5 days, depending on how long you've been taking them.

<u>ROUTINE:</u>

- **Twice a day** - morning and night

- **Daily Consistency** - Try to stay consistent both in timing and duration. That is, try not to skew the duration. Make it consistent, and take the cleansing herb throughout the cleanse. For example, for a 14-day cleanse, the cleansing herbs can be taken twice daily, and you should take them around the same time you do take them on both mornings and evenings.

- **Gradual Wean Off** – Just like medications, it is not the best to go cold-turkey when it comes to herbal detox. Towards the end of the cleanse duration, wean off your herbs by gradually reducing the dosage and duration. The duration of the wean will depend on the length of the fast you choose. For example, I usually start weaning a week towards closure for a one-month fast. For a 14 day fast, I begin weaning on day 11 or 12. You can begin the wean by reducing it from twice a day to once a day. Or simply take half the dosages each for mornings and night.

You must do this because you need to signal your body to prepare to start functioning independently without dependence on herbs' cleansing. And no other way to do this than to take it slow and gradual, without bringing too much "shock" to your body.

Cleansing Herbs to Boost Lupus Healing Process

CASCARA SAGRADA

It is a natural laxative, purgative shrub plant from Rhamnaceae's family that Dr. Sebi recommended because of its potency to cause muscle contractions in the intestine, detox/cleanse the colon, and stimulate the colon the colon liver and pancreas secretion, and moves stool through the bowel. In addition, this herb is rich in glycosides, Vitamin-A, B, C, and D, emodin, and anthracoid, making it effective in cleansing and revitalizing herbs.

The benefits of Consuming Cascara Sagrada include:

- It helps to get rid of toxins from the colon.

- It serves as a laxative for constipation.

- It helps to soothe and dissolve gallstones.

- It helps to treat and prevent liver problems.

- It helps to destroy and inhibit cancerous cells from mutation.

- It helps to soothe and treat digestive problems.

- It relieves joint and muscle pain and other pains caused by inflammation.

- It treats transmitted diseases caused by viruses and bacterial

When writing this book, there are no side effects attributed to healthy adults who consume Cascara sagrada for a short period.

The note-full precautions before Consuming Cascara Sagrada are:

- Nursing mothers should avoid these herbs because they can inflict their babies with diarrhea.

- If you suffer from disease or health disorders like; stomach irritation or upset without knowing the cause, colitis, kidney disorders, intestinal blockage, or Crohn's disease, please do not use this herb without medical supervision.

For the dosage and how to prepare cascara sagrada tea, kindly take the steps below:

- Get Cascara Sagrada plants, remove some of the bark, and chop it.
- Once you have chopped it, dry it until it is dried, or you can order it online, and it will come chopped and dried.
- Pour 8-10 ounces of water into your saucepan and add 1-1½ teaspoon of cascara sagrada bark in the saucepan.
- Steams the mixture for 15-20 minutes on your cooker.

- After 15-20 minutes, steam, allow it to reduce its hotness and strain it to remove the chopped bark of cascara sagrada.

You are done. For the dosage, consume1cup (8-10ounce) of Cascara Sagrada tea 2-3 times daily.

SARSAPARILLA

Sarsaparilla root is the root of a tropical wood climbing vine that belongs to the genus Smilax family. Dr. Sebi recommends it as a revitalizing herb for many diseases, including cancer, because it is rich in iron, calcium, and phosphate.

The benefits of consuming Sarsaparilla roots are:

- It helps to destroy and prevent cancerous cells from mutating.
- It binds the endotoxins responsible for the lesions in psoriasis patients and eliminates them from the body system.
- It helps to fast-track healing and recovery.
- It treats and prevents health issues caused by inflammations like joint pain, swelling of any parts of the body, arthritis, rheumatoid, etc.
- It soothes and heals sexually transmitted diseases such as syphilis, herpes, gonorrhea etc.
- It helps to treat and prevent leprosy
- It helps protect and reverse damages done to the liver to function perfectly.
- It makes the body absorb nutrients and other herbs easily

There are no side effects attributed to this herb's consumption when writing this book. However, because of the 'saponins' that it contains, I advise you to consult your doctor before using this herb, as saponins can cause stomach irritation.

For the dosage and how to prepare sarsaparilla root tea, kindly take the following steps:

- Harvest some sarsaparilla plant roots and wash them under running water to remove all the dirt that accompanied them from the soil.
- After washing it, pill off the outer skin, chop it into smaller pieces and dry it in a well-ventilated place (indoors) for at least seven days (ensure you turn the drying root daily for the seven days until it is completely dried.) iii. Once it is dried, store it in a paper bag or cardboard box. (Ensure you don't store it in a plastic container as it will get mold).
- Measure 1teaspoon of the dried chopped Sarsaparilla root and add it to your saucepan and add 8 ounces of water. Boil it for 15-20minutes v. Strain it using a filter. You are done!
- For the dosage, consume 1cup (8ounce) 3 times daily.

CHAPARRAL

Chaparral, also called 'Larrea Tridentate', is an herb from the creosote bush, a desert shrub native to southern areas of the United States and northern regions of Mexico. This flowering plant has bright yellow flowers and thick green leaves with a resinous coating. However, despite its pretty appearance, chaparral is a controversial herb that's even been banned in many countries. However, this herb is claimed to help treat many ailments, including cancer, arthritis, and skin conditions.

The consumption of Chaparral has several benefits, such as:

- It contains a powerful antioxidant that helps the shrinkage of tumors

- It may prevent the spreading of HPV and HIV

- It prevents heart diseases by reducing levels of free radicals

- It helps to boost the immune system

- It relieves joint and muscle pain thanks to its anti-inflammatory quality

The Side Effects and note-full precautions before Consuming Chaparral are:

- Nursing mothers should avoid this herb because it has been reported to have abortifacient effects

- Although chaparral is a potent antioxidant, it has been found to have serious negative health effects, including hepatotoxicity, which is a chemically-induced liver injury

Dosage and Administration:

Chaparral tea has traditionally been prepared with 1 teaspoonful of chaparral leaves/flowers steeped in 1 pint of boiling water for 15 minutes. You can drink up chaparral teas to 3 times a day.

MULLEIN

Mullein is a flavorful beverage flowering plant that has been used for centuries to treat various ailments. Research shows that this herb is an effective anti-microbial, anti-inflammatory, anti-cancer, anti-hepatotoxic, antioxidant, and anti-viral herb with potency to prevent many health disorders. In addition, it helps to cleanse and detoxify the lungs and lymph system and destroy cancer.

The benefits of consuming Mullein include:

- It helps treat and prevent various types of cancer by destroying cancerous cells and preventing them from mutating.
- It helps to eliminate mucus from the small intestine
- It helps to activate healthy lymph circulation in the chest and neck
- It helps neutralize the negative effects of free radicals by protecting the cells from damages caused by free radicals.
- It helps treat and prevent various bacterial and virus infections like herpes viruses, HIV etc.
- It helps to treat and prevent respiratory tract infections.
- It helps to treat and prevent tuberculosis.
- It helps to treat earaches.
- It helps treat various health disorders like bronchitis, stroke, heart diseases etc.
- It helps prevent some chronic brain diseases like Alzheimer's, Parkinson's etc.
- It helps to treat atherosclerosis and others in the biological systems.
- It helps treat and relieve pain caused by inflammation and tumor.
- It also helps treat various ailments like asthma, bronchitis, migraine, congestion etc.

There are no negative side effects attributed to mullein consumption by mouth when writing this book. However, since there is no information to show whether this herb is harmful to pregnant and breastfeeding mothers, I advise them to avoid its consumption.

When writing this book, there are no medications that interact with mullein. Therefore, it can be combined with other herbs and drugs without issues.

For the dosage and how to prepare Mullein tea, kindly take the steps below:

- Harvest some fresh mullein leaves, dry them until they are dried, and chop them into smaller pieces. Alternatively, you can place an order online, and it will come dried and chopped.
- Once the fresh leaves are dried, measure 1-2 teaspoons and pour them into your teacup or mug.
- Measure 8-10 ounces of water and boil it.
- Once the water is boiling, pour it inside your teacup or mug where the mullein leaves are and allow it to steep for 15-20 minutes.
- Strain it, and you are done!
- Take 1 cup (8-10ounce) 2-3 times daily for the dosage.

BURDOCK ROOT

Burdock root is the root of a delicious plant called Burdock, which all its body or parts are useful as either food or medicine. This plant can be found all over the world. I called this plant the wonder plant because everything about it is important as we consume its root as food and use it for medicinal purposes. Both its leaf and seed are used for medicinal purposes.

People worldwide have been using burdock root orally to treat and prevent various health disorders for over five centuries.

Because of Burdock root's chemical composition, such as; quercetin and luteolin, research has shown that it can serve as a great effective antioxidant that can treat and prevent cancer by preventing cancerous cells from growing and mutating combating aging. A compound like 'Phytosterols' helps scalp and hair follicles grow healthy hair even from baldheads. The vitamins-C helps in boosting the immune system and combat bacterial. It also helps cleanse or detoxify the liver and lymphatic system, etc.

The potassium helps reduce blood sugar levels and filter the blood by removing impurities through the bloodstream and eradicating toxins through the skin and urine.

The benefits of using or consuming burdock root tea/infusion include:

- It cleanse/detox the liver and lymphatic system.
- Treat and prevent diabetes by reducing blood sugar levels in the body.
- Eliminate toxins from the body by inducing sweetness and urine.
- Purify the blood by removing heavy metals from the bloodstream.
- Treat various skin disorders and combat aging.
- Treat and prevent cancer by inhibiting the growth and mutation of cancerous cells.
- Boost the immune system and enhance circulation.
- Until at the time of writing this book, there have been no side effects recorded by researchers or people who have used these herbs.
- However, research has it that applying this root to your skin might cause rashes.

For the dosage and how to prepare Burdock root tea/infusion, kindly take the following steps:

- Scrub the uprooted root of burdock heartily under running water to remove all the dirt that accompanied it from the soil.
- You should chop the Burdock root into smaller pieces (less than 1 inch). Please note that it will come dried and already chopped if you order it online.
- Pour 2-3 cup of water into your saucepan and add ¼ cup of the chopped burdock root and boil it.
- Lower your gas once the water is boiling, re-boil it for 30-40 minutes, and put off your gas.
- Once it is cold, strain it and consume it.
- For the dosage, drink one glass cup daily

DANDELION

Dandelion is a flowering plant known as 'yellow gowan' or 'lion's tooth. This plant is native to Eurasia and today. It is common in over 60 countries worldwide in the mild climates of the northern hemisphere. For centuries, these flowering plants have been used for the treatment of swelling (inflammation) of the pancreas, relieve pains that are caused by inflammation, treat and prevent cancer, tonsils (tonsillitis), skin disorder, bladder or urethra disorder, digestive and liver problems and enhance the general health of the liver and digestive system.

Researchers proved that it is a very effective cleansing/detoxification herb because of the chemical compositions and nutrients.

The benefits of using or consuming Dandelion include:

- It helps to detoxify or cleanse the liver and the kidney.
- It helps to treat and prevent diabetes by regulating blood sugar levels.
- It helps to fight against and relieve pains that are caused by inflammation.
- It helps to deactivate and inhibit the negative effects of free radicals in the body because of its antioxidant properties.
- It reduces the level of cholesterol.
- It lowers blood pressure by getting rid of excess fluid in the body.
- It helps to naturally shed excess weight gain by improving the metabolism of carbohydrates.
- It helps in boosting the digestive system.
- It helps to boost the immune system.
- It helps to keep the skin healthy and treat and prevent skin diseases.

Till at the time of writing this book, Dandelion is 100% safe, but consuming an overdose of it can result in some side effects like:

Experiencing stomach upset or irritation

Allergic reactions

The special precautions before using/consuming dandelions are:

Pregnant and breastfeeding mothers should stay off dandelion as there is no research to know if it is harmful to them or not.

If you are suffering from Eczema, stay off dandelion as more than 85% of people with eczema suffer an allergic reaction to dandelion.

For the dosage and how to prepare Dandelion tea/infusion, kindly take the following steps:

- Get some fresh leaves of dandelion and wash them under running water to remove all the dirt.
- After washing it, pour ½ - 1 cup of the washed dandelion into your saucepan.
- You should boil 4-5 cups of water and pour the boiled water inside the saucepan. Next, you pour the dandelion and cover it for 12-15 hours or throughout the night (overnight).

- The next day, strain out the dandelion leaves, and you will be left with the dandelion tea/infusion.
- For the dosage, take ½ tablespoon of Dandelion per ¾ cup of water three times daily. And if you ordered your dandelion online, you can take 4-10 grams of dry leaf of dandelion three times daily.

GUACO

Guaco is a climbing plant with different names like Huaco, Guace, or Vejuco. This climbing plant belongs to the Asteraceae and cordifolia species' family and is rich in numerous minerals and compounds. Its leaves are very medicinal and nutritional. The people of Aztecs used them to clean the blood system and clear heavy metals from the bloodstream.

There are a lot of benefits that one can benefit from using or consuming Guaco. Some of them are:

- It lessens the effect or symptoms of snake poison.

- It is used to thin the blood through the coumarin activities it contains (anticoagulant and blood-thinning.)

- It helps to combat inflammation through its anti-inflammatory properties.

- It treats stomach irritation through the effect of its cleansing activities.

- It helps treat respiratory disorders like coughs, rheumatism, bronchitis, etc.

- It enhances quick recovery from the wound.

- It helps to cleanse or detoxify the blood and skin by clearing heavy metals from the blood.

- It boosts and builds the immune defense system.

- It can treat some infections diseases such as; candida yeast infection, herpes, etc.

There are no severe side effects that researchers or uses have recorded until writing this book.

Like I said earlier, Guaco is 100% safe for consumption by mouth, but if you are taking or using any Coumadin drugs, please consult with your doctor before using it.

And if you have any history of bleeding, do not use Guaco unless your doctor approves of it. Like I said earlier, Guaco helps to thin the blood, so any medications that can thin the blood or slow blood clotting do interact with Guaco.

For the dosage and how to prepare Guaco tea/infusion, kindly take the following steps:

- Get some handful of fresh Guaco and wash it under running water or 2 ounces of its dried leaves if you have the dried ones.
- Pour about 6cups of water in your saucepan with the Guaco leaves and boil it until it is reduced to 2 cups.
- You can add some brown sugar (optional) if you add the brown sugar; allow it to boil for another 20 minutes.
- Strain the syrup with a strainer.
- You should bottle it and store it in a refrigerator.

183

- For dosage, take 1 soupspoon 3-4 times daily.

Cleansing Herbs that Help Relieve Multiple Sclerosis Symptoms

EUCALYPTUS

The eucalyptus tree is a fast-growing evergreen tree native of Australia. This plant's leaves and bark are used for medicinal purposes like joint and muscle pain, cold, cough, congestion, etc. However, the Chinese, Greek, and Indian Ayurvedic people have incorporated this amazing herb to treat various conditions for thousands of years before now.

This plant/tree has more than 400 different species. The most used is the Eucalyptus globulus or the Australian fever tree, also known as Blue Gum.

Eucalyptus leaves cineole that is also known as eucalyptol, in which the leaf's gland contains essential oil (eucalyptus oil) and also; flavonoids and tannins, which are plant-based antioxidants that aid in reducing inflammation, controlling blood sugar, fighting against the activities of bacteria and fungi and the oil can help in relieving pain and inflammation as well as blocking chemicals that usually cause asthma.

The benefits of using or consuming eucalyptus tea/infusion include:

- It helps in cleansing the skin through steaming/sauna.

- Eucalyptus helps in relieving common cold symptoms like cough lozenges and inhalants and also sore throat and sinusitis

- It helps in relieving symptoms of bronchitis. In addition, inhaling the vapor of eucalyptus tea helps serve as a decongestant by loosening phlegm and easing congestion.

- It aids in relieving asthma: research showed that eucalyptus has the potency to break up mucous in people who have asthma.

- It aids in dental plaque and improves gingivitis: research carried out on eucalyptus shows that eucalyptus leaf has the potency to reduce dental plaque and improve gingivitis.

- It helps improve bad breath: research showed that eucalyptus has the potency to improve bad breath.

- It also helps to relives some health like; skin disease, bladder diseases, gallbladder and liver problems, bleeding gums, diabetes, burns, ulcer, stuffy nose, wounds, etc.

The precaution to be note-full of before using eucalyptus tea or infusion include:

- It is 100% safe for pregnant and breastfeeding mothers to consume eucalyptus tea/infusion, but the oil is unsafe.

- The tea is safe for children, but the oil might lead to seizures

- Because of eucalyptus leaves' potency leaves to lower blood sugar levels, it is advisable to consult with your doctor before using the tea with any diabetes medication

For the dosage and how to prepare eucalyptus tea/infusion, kindly take the following steps:

- Boil water to (90-95)0 or 194-205 Fahrenheit. Alternatively, you can boil the water and drop it down for a minute or two to reduce the temperature.

- Pour a teaspoon of dried eucalyptus leaf into a teacup/mug.

- Pour 6 ounces of water (from the first step) inside the teacup/mug and allow the leaves to be steep for 10-15minutes. (you can enjoy breathing the vapors of the steeping tea)

- Get a filter to strain the loose leaves of the eucalyptus.

- You are a god. You can now enjoy the cup of eucalyptus tea/infusion at a go.

- For the dosage, take 3-4 cups per day.

PRODIGIOSA

Prodigiosa, also known as 'Prodijiosa or Hamula, is a perennial plant with large bushy leaves and flowers, and it's from the daisy family and native to Mexico and California. These plants have a grey-purple hue on the underside and dark green leaves on the upper side and grow up to 5 feet in height, with their flowers growing in clusters. This plant has a long history with the Mexicans. It has been used for centuries to treat diabetes, arthritis, diarrhea, and stomach disorder and relieve aching joints.

Because of the chemical and compound composition of Prodigiosa, research has shown that it is very effective for the treatment of diabetes II because it aids in stimulating the pancreatic gland to secret and reduces or lowers blood sugar level and burn down fat in the gallbladder. The irony is that Prodigiosa can cause more damage to people suffering from Type I diabetes. Furthermore, consuming Prodigiosa's tea/infusion helps boost the digestion of fat, improve bile synthesis in the liver, dissolve tiny gallstones, and treat chronic gastritis and other digestive systems disorders. Although there is no research to prove its effectiveness in treating cataracts, it is believed that it can cure cataracts.

Prodigiosa is used for several reasons, including:

- Treatment of diabetes (type II).
- Treatment of diarrhea.
- Treatment of stomach pain.
- Treatment of gallbladder disease.
- Enhancing the digestion of fat and boosting the digestive system's healthiness.

The note-full precautions to beware of before using or consuming Prodigiosa includes:

- Pregnant and breastfeeding mothers should not use or consume Prodigiosa as there is no research to back it to whether it is safe or not.
- It is a no-go area for people suffering from diabetes I. People with diabetes II should control their sugar levels while consuming this herb.

How to prepare Prodigiosa tea/infusion:

- Dry the fresh leaves until it is dried.
- Once the fresh leaves are dried, or the one you ordered for is available, boil 8 or 16ounce of water and brew 1 or 2 tablespoons of Prodigiosa leaves in the warm water for 15minutes.
- After brewing it, strain the Prodigiosa leaves.
- Take a cup (8ounce) of Prodigiosa tea/infusion two times per day for the dosage.

ELDERBERRY

Elderberry is a dark purple berry from the elder tree, also known as European Black Elderberry or Sambucus Bacchae. This plant is a flowering plant from the family of Adoxaceae and native to Europe. Both the leaves and fruit (berries) of elderberry have been used for centuries to treat pain and swelling arising from inflammation. It also helps to stimulate urine production and induce sweat to detoxify the body system.

Because of how rich elderberry is with various compounds and nutrients like vitamin-C, dietary fiber, phenolic acids, which is a great and powerful antioxidant that helps to prevent and decrease the damage that is caused by oxidative stress in the body, it also contains some compounds like flavonols such as kaempferol, quercetin, isorhamnetin and anthocyanins which gives the fruit the black-purple color and makes it a strong antioxidant and anti-inflammation agent.

Elderberry also contains some nutrients, like:

- Calories

- Carbs

- Minute amounts of protein and fat

- And anthocyanins, making the plant a strong and effective antioxidant with anti-inflammatory properties.

The benefits of using/consuming elderberry include:

- It helps cleanse and detoxify the lungs and respiratory system by eliminating mucus from the upper respiratory system and the lungs.

- It helps to treat constipation.

- It helps to treat flu and cold in less than 24hours.

- It combats harmful bacteria in the body by preventing bacterial growth through its antibacterial properties.

- It boosts and supports the immune defense system by increasing white blood cell production.

- It protects and keeps the skin healthy.

- It helps to relieve chronic fatigue syndrome and depression.

Till at the time of writing this book, there is no record of any side effects from researchers and people who have used elderberry, but because of the compound that is present in elderberry, it will be wise to use it for not more than 12 weeks and take a break for at least a week before using it again.

The special precautions before using elderberry include:

- Ensure children below 12 years do not use/consume elderberries, and children above 12 and under 18 should not use them for more than 10days.

- Since there is no reliable information to know if elderberries are safe or not for pregnant and breastfeeding mothers, I strongly advise that they stay off elderberries.

- People who have a history of suffering from an autoimmune disease like; multiple sclerosis, lupus, rheumatoid arthritis, etc., should stay off elderberry as it has the potency to boost the immune system to become more active which could worsen their situation.

- Since elderberries have the potency to increase or boost the immune defense system, any medications designed to decrease the immune system's function will certainly interact with Elderberry.

For the dosage and how to prepare Elderberry tea/infusion, kindly take the steps below:

- Boil 8-12oz of water in your saucepan.
- Once the water is boiling, measure one tablespoon of dried elderberries and add it to the boiling water.
- Reduce your gas and allow it to boil for at least 15 minutes.
- After the 15 minutes timing, allow it to get cold and strain it using a filter.
- For the dosage, consume 3-4 cups daily.

RHUBARB ROOT

Rhubarb Root is a very effective laxative that Dr. Sebi recommended because it boosts the digestive tract's health. However, Rhubarb roots are rich in various nutrients, making them a perfect herb for cleansing the body.

The benefits of Consuming Rhubarb Root are:

- It helps treat various types of sores like; canker sores, cold sores, etc.
- It helps to destroy various viruses like; herpes simplex virus, HIV, etc.
- It helps to enhance and relieve the symptoms of menopause.
- It helps to serve as a remedy for treating pancreatitis (swelling of the pancreas).
- It helps boost and enhance people's respiratory system suffering from ARDS to breathe healthier.
- It helps to soothe and cure menstrual pain (dysmenorrhea).
- It helps to treat and stop blood bleeding in the stomach.
- It helps to treat and prevent gastrointestinal (GI) bleeding.
- It helps to shed excess body weight (cholesterol) naturally.

When writing this book, there are no side effects attributed to consuming Rhubarb root and its rhizome for over two years, except it leaves that contain oxalic acid, which is unsafe.

For the dosage and how to prepare Rhubarb root tea, kindly take the steps below:

- Uproot some roots of the Rhubarb plant (make sure that the plants uprooted are above four years, in autumn).
- Wash the uprooted roots under running water to remove all dirt from the soil, remove the external fibers, and dry it on a plane surface.
- Once it is dried, chop it into smaller pieces. (Not more than 0.5 inches) or pound it and store it in a tightly closed container. Alternatively, you can order it online, and it will come dried and chopped.
- Pour 8 ounces of water in a saucepan, add 1tablespoon of the pounded or chopped rhubarb root, and boil the mixture for 15-20minutes v. After the timing, reduce the heat of the gas for about 10 minutes and put off the fire.
- Allow it to get cold for at least 10-15minute and strain out the root.
- You are done. Take 1 cup (8ounce) of the infusion three times per day for the dosage.

Cleansing Herbs that Help Relieve Rheumatoid Arthritis Symptoms

BLADDERWRACK

Bladderwrack is a type of brown algae or seaweed typically found in the chilly waters of the Northern Atlantic and Pacific coasts of the United States and on the Atlantic and Baltic coasts of Europe.

Although bladderwrack has been growing in cold ocean waters for thousands of years, its use as a health-supportive supplement is relatively recent.

Some of the known benefits of this algae are the following:

- Promotes healthy mineral levels
- Supports a healthy hormone balance
- Supports healthy metabolism and a healthy weight
- Seeks to support the immune system
- Boost the energy levels

Dosage and administration:

Bladderwrack may be eaten whole or made into a tea using 1 teaspoon per cup of hot water, allowing each cup to sit at least 10 minutes before drinking. You can drink up to three cups of tea per day.

BLUE VERVAIN

Blue Vervain is a perennial flowering plant that belongs to the family of Verbenaceae. It is rich in nutrients like iron fluorine, which purifies the blood, phosphorus, phosphate, zinc, potassium, magnesium, etc. Because of this potency, Dr. Sebi recommends this herb for revitalizing your body after cleansing.

The benefits of using or consuming Blue Vervain include:

- It helps to treat and prevent anxiety and sleeplessness and enhance mood.
- It helps to treat and calm the central nervous system.
- It helps soothe the nerves and relaxes the mind, thereby treating migraine headaches.
- It helps boost and protect the heart's health treats and prevents myocardial ischemia, chest pain, and heart failure.
- It helps to fight against both internal and external inflammation.
- It helps to treat menstrual cramps or pain and stomach pain.
- It improves digestive health and protects the livers and kidneys by cleansing/detoxifying the kidney and liver.

The note-full precautions before consuming Blue Vervain tea include:

Because there is no information to show if these herbs are good for breastfeeding mothers or pregnant women, I advise avoiding these herbs' consumption.

Till at the time of writing this book, there were no medications that interacted with blue Vervain.

For the dosage and how to prepare Blue Vervain tea, kindly take the following steps:

- Get some fresh leaves and flowers of blue Vervain and dry them.
- Once it is dried, pound or chops it, or you can order it online, and it will come dried and chopped.
- Boil a cup of water (8ounce) in a saucepan.
- Once the water is boiled, pour it into a cup, measure 1 teaspoon of the Blue Vervain, and add it to the water.
- Allow it to steep for 10-15 minutes and strain it.
- You are done! For the dosage, take 2-4 cups daily.

NETTEL

Also known as 'Stinging nettle', it is a perennial plant originally native to Europe, North Africa, and Asia. Its name comes from its hairs all over the surface that actually "sting" you. These hairs act like miniature hypodermic needles, injecting you with histamine, folic acid, and other substances that cause localized redness and pain.

These properties are believed by some to have a beneficial effect. For example, in ancient medicine, stinging nettle was used to treat rheumatism, flu, gastrointestinal and urinary tract disorders. In some cases, the plant would be used to make a medicinal tonic; in others, the leaves and stems were applied to the skin to treat muscle or joint pain.

The benefits of using or consuming Nettel include:

- It helps relieve muscle and joint pain
- It treats urinary tract infections
- It relieves symptoms of an enlarged prostate gland
- It helps boost and protect the heart's health treats and prevents myocardial ischemia, chest pain, and heart failure.
- Since it lowers blood sugar levels, it is also used to treat diabetes
- Polyphenols from nettle extract have shown exciting potential for treating breast cancer

Side Effects

Stinging nettles are generally considered safe and side effects are relatively mild. However, you may experience stomach upset and sweating if taken by mouth. In addition, if used topically, it is not uncommon to develop skin irritation and rash.

For the dosage and how to prepare Nettel tea, kindly take the following steps:

- Add water to the leaves.
- Boil the water
- Turn off the stove and let it sit for 6 minutes.
- Pour the mixture through a small strainer.

NOPAL CACTUS

Also known as 'the prickly pear cactus, it is a plant native to Mexico. It is famous for offering health benefits due to its high antioxidant, vitamin, and mineral content.

It is usually eaten whole, but if you cut the pads (Nopales) into small dice, you can easily turn them into juice, jams or tea.

The consumption of Nopal Cactus has several benefits, such as:

- It is a plant rich in antioxidants, flavonoids and vitamin C
- It protects your body from heart disease
- It lowers cholesterol levels
- It is a natural diuretic that helps you treat water retention problems
- The antioxidant compounds of the nettle cactus restrict the growth and development of cancer cells

Side Effects

Potential side effects of nopal cactus supplements include:

headache

nausea

bloating

diarrhea

Pregnant women should not take nopal cactus supplements because there isn't reliable information about whether or not it is safe.

Dosage and Administration:

300 grams of steamed nopal fruits or 500 grams of broiled stems.

Supplements usually come in tablets or capsules containing 650mg of pure nopales extract. The dosage for these is one per day with your meal.

How to break a detox fast?

- Slowly reintroduce solids

If you are doing water or a liquid fast, you will need to reintroduce solid foods slowly. You can begin by introducing solids like high water-content fruits. These include watermelon, apples, and berries. After that, you can introduce softer fruit solids like bananas and avocados. Later, you can incorporate harder solids like veggies. All foods must be listed on the nutrition guide. However, if doing a fruit or raw veggie fast, you can break the fast right away on solid foods.

- Drink 1-gallon spring water daily

Drink spring water daily together with the revitalizing herbs and sea moss.

How long should you detox/cleanse?

How long you should detox depends on your state of health, that is, your body's toxification level (the less healthy you are, the more toxic your body is) and tolerance level. Typically, it is recommended to fast for 7-14 days, but Dr. Sebi recommends a minimum of at least a 12 day fast. Dr. Sebi himself fasted for 90 days to cure diabetes, asthma, and impotence. It is great to cleanse at least once a year for seven days if you consume an alkaline diet. If you are not consuming an alkaline diet, then you should cleanse/detox every three months

I fasted for 14 days, and I recommend fasting for between 14 days and one month if you have high blood pressure. Again, your body's tolerance level will ultimately determine the length, so watch your body and study its reaction as you begin the fast. We are all different, and you may find that you cannot handle a basic liquid fast (water or juice). In that case, you can get started with fruit or raw vegetables fast. But make sure all foods and fruits are listed in the Dr. Sebi Nutrition Guide. Whether liquid, juice or raw food fast, the results are virtual all the same – the only major difference is when it takes to begin to see results. While raw food fasts take longer, liquid fasts are much faster. So do not worry; the most important thing is to stay committed and focused on whatever fasting method you choose.

Common Symptoms Expected During Detox Cleanse

- Cold and Flu symptoms
- Changes in Bowel movements
- Fatigue and Low Energy
- Difficulty sleeping
- Itching
- Headaches

- Muscle aches and pains
- Acne. Rashes and breakouts
- Mucus expels (catarrh, etc.)
- Lower blood pressure

Cleansing Herbs To Treat Hypertension and Arteriosclerosis

Arteries become clogged when plaque forms inside them. It makes arteries harden. If untreated, this condition will sooner or later lead to a heart attack or a stroke because blood will, over time, flow more and more slowly. As a result, blood may not reach the vital organs in quantities those organs need to function well. The additional danger lies in that sometimes, parts of the soft plaque break free of the artery walls and create blood clots. Suppose a clot blocks blood flow. Death is imminent.

This condition is known as arteriosclerosis, and it occurs when too much plaque accumulates in the arteries. Plaque buildup is caused by a diet high in saturated fats, obesity, smoking, and a sedentary lifestyle. These are major risk factors for this condition. Additionally, those with type 1 and type 2 diabetes and arthritis seem to be more prone to arteriosclerosis.

Conventional medicine recommends anticoagulants for blood thinning to protect the body from heart attacks and stroke. However, like most medications, they come with certain side effects, e.g., they can cause you to bleed more when you cut yourself than you would if you didn't take this medication.

There are two types of medication:

One is called **anticoagulants**, and they prevent the blood from clotting.

The other one is called **antiplatelets**.

However, blood thinners don't make your blood thinner. Nor can they break up clots. Instead, what they do is keep blood from forming new clots.

Blood transports nutrients throughout the body. If it flows smoothly, your organs and tissues will be healthy; if it doesn't, they'll starve. Therefore, to maintain healthy blood pressure, keep your cells healthy, and maintain healthy pH levels, you need good circulation. You will know your circulation is not great if your hands and feet are often cold, or if you often feel dizzy, breathless, have chest pains, develop varicose veins, *etc.*

Blood circulation can be affected by aging and high blood pressure because, as you age, your arteries become less elastic and gradually become narrower. That results in higher blood pressure or that your heart has to work much harder to circulate blood through the body.

Fortunately, certain lifestyle changes can help you improve your blood flow without medication.

The first step to take if you want to heal from this condition naturally is to eat a healthy alkaline diet. Regular exercise is also crucial.

I will describe to you some herbs that I found useful on myself when I used to suffer from bad circulation:

FLOR DE MANITA

Also called 'Hand Flower Tree' or 'Devil's Hand Tree', it is a flower that grows on evergreen trees in Central and South America.

Some of the main benefits of this herb are:

- It helps with lower abdominal pain
- It has great effects on heart problems
- It helps reduce edema
- It lowers high blood pressure
- It helps lower cholesterol levels

Dosage and administration

- Use 2 tsp of herbs with 8 oz of water twice a day

LILY OF THE VALLEY

Listed below are some of the health benefits of using Lily of the Valley:

- It may help to improve heart health
- It is used for treating congestive heart failure, valvular heart disease, dropsy and cardiac debility
- It has been shown that it can improve the functioning of the nervous system
- By easing blood flow, it helps lower blood pressure levels
- It has diuretic properties that help in flushing out the toxins and infection-causing bacteria from the urinary tract
- It has therapeutic properties that help with anxiety symptoms

Precaution and Side Effects

- Overdose may lead to nausea, vomiting, gastrointestinal irritation and dehydration

Dosage and administration:

- **Tincture:** 3g twice a day.
- **Liquid Extract:** 200 mg three times a day.
- **Dried Extract:** 75 mg twice a day.

RED CLOVER

Below are some of the main benefits of this herb:

- It lowers the loss of bone mineral density in postmenopausal women

- It may help relieve the discomforts of menopause, especially hot flashes

- It may help treat diseases such as psoriasis, eczema, and other rashes.

- It has also been used as a cough remedy for children.

How to prepare Prodigiosa tea/infusion:

- Add 4 grams of dried flower tops to 1 cup (250 mL) of boiling water

- Steep for 10 minutes

- Enjoy!

It's best to limit your daily intake to 1–3 cups.

Be happy if you relate to any of these symptoms during the cleansing stage. That's because your body is pushing out all the toxins and mucus you have been keeping inside for so long. In addition, these symptoms are only temporary and usually resolve after the first one to two weeks.

STAGE 2: REVITALIZATION

The revitalizing herbs that help boost your immune system are:

SOURSOP

Soursop is the fruit of the "Annona Muricata" tree, a native of tropical regions in the Americas that belong to the Annonaceae family. Its leaves are widely used because they are rich in various nutrients like iron, calcium, phosphorus, magnesium, sodium, potassium, zinc, etc. That makes the tea very effective in fighting against the mutation of cancerous cells.

Other benefits of consuming soursops tea are:

- It helps to destroy and eliminate cancerous cells and inhibit the growth of cancer cells.
- It is a very strong and effective antioxidant that helps neutralize free radicals that damage the cells.
- It helps to soothe heart disorders.
- It helps lower blood sugar levels for people who have type 2 diabetes.
- It helps to fight against infectious diseases caused by bacterial. Such diseases like yeast infections, cholera, gingivitis, Staphylococcus, tooth decay etc.
- It helps to soothe and alleviate swelling (inflammation) etc.

The note-full precautions before consuming soursops tea include:

- Since there is no information about this herb's harmful effects on pregnant and breastfeeding mothers, I advise that they stay off this herb.
- Although this herb is tempting, please make sure you consume this herb under a medical practitioner's supervision.

For the dosage and how to prepare soursops tea, kindly take the following steps:

- Harvest some fresh Soursops leaves, dry them until it is dried, chop them, or pound them into smaller pieces. On the other hand, you can place an order online, and it will come dried and chopped.
- Measure 1 teaspoon of the chopped leaves of the Soursops and pour it into your teacup or mug.
- Boil 8 ounces of water and add it to the Soursop leaves in the teacup or mug and cover it.
- Allow the leaves to steep for 10-15 minutes and strain them.
- You are done!
- For the dosage, consume 2-3 cups of the Soursops tea daily

IRISH SEA MOSS

Irish Sea Moss is red algae that belong to the family of Florideophytes that grows on the rocky parts of the Atlantic coast of various countries, including the British Isles, Jamaica, Scotland, etc. Dr. Sebi recommends this herb for revitalizing the body after cleansing because it has over 92 out of 102 minerals that the body needs to be healthy. Some minerals are, for example:

- Phosphorus
- Iodine
- Selenium
- Calcium
- Bromine
- Iron
- Potassium

Some of the benefits of consuming Irish Sea Moss are:

- It heals and boosts the immune defense system.
- It treats and prevents hyperthyroidism and boosts the functionalities and health of the thyroid.
- It helps to soothe joint pain and swelling and treat arthritis.
- It helps to enrich the overall mood and reduce fussiness.
- It helps to combat infections caused by viruses and bacterial.
- It helps treat and prevent various skin disorders like acne, skin wrinkling, and alleviating inflammation.
- It helps to treat and prevent digestive and respiratory tract disorders.

The note-full precautions to beware of before consuming Irish Sea moss include:

- Because of how rich Irish Sea moss is with iron can trigger hypothyroidism for people suffering from Hashimoto's disease.
- Stop using the herb if you notice any allergies or reactions.

For the dosage and how to prepare Irish Sea Moss tea, kindly take the steps below:

- Measure and boil 1cups (8ounce) of water in a ceramic pot.
- Once the water is boiled, measure 2-3 tablespoons of Irish Sea moss gel (or 1teaspoon for the fine form) and add it to the boiling water.
- Allow the Irish Sea moss for 10-15 minutes to dissolve completely.
- You are done!
- For the dosage, take 1 cup of Irish Sea moss tea daily in the morning.

SHEPARD'S PURSE

Growing all over the world, it's one of the most common wildflowers on Earth. Its name comes from small triangular fruits resembling a purse, but it's also known as "lady's purse" or "mother's heart".

Among the conditions shepherd's purse is said to heal are:

- High blood pressure
- Bladder's infections
- Premenstrual syndrome
- Heavy periods
- Kidney diseases

Dosage and administration:

The British Herbal Pharmacopoeia (BHP) suggests a dose of 1-4 gms or by infusion or a dose of 1-4mls of the ethanolic extract (a well-rounded tsp is approx 1.5 grams)

VALERIAN ROOT

The benefits of consuming valerian roots include:

- It helps treat and calm the central nervous system relieving anxiety, stress, depression, and chronic fatigue syndrome (CFS).
- It helps to treat and prevent sleeplessness (Insomnia).
- It helps relieve and reduces the severity and frequency of hot flashes in postmenopausal women and relief premenstrual disorders (PMS).
- It helps soothe dysmenorrhea (menstrual cramps) and relieve pains during menstruation.
- It helps to lower blood pressure and the rate of heartbeat.
- It is used to remedy Attention-deficit hyperactivity disorder (ADHD).
- It is used to treat and relieve some health issues like headaches, convulsions, epilepsy, mild tremor, joint pains, stomach irritation, etc.

Valerian root has no side effects if used for less than 28 days, but if you consume too much of it, you might suffer some side effects like:

- Stomach irritation.
- Headache
- Swing mood
- Sleeplessness
- Sluggishness

The note-full precautions before consuming valerian root include:

Since much is unknown about this herb's safety for pregnant and breastfeeding mothers, I advise them to stay off this herb.

Because of this herb's drowsiness effect, I strongly advise you not to drive or operate any machinery after consuming valerian root.

For the dosage and how to prepare Valerian root tea, kindly take the following steps:

- Harvest some valerian plants' roots, wash them, chop them into smaller pieces, and dry them.
- Alternatively, you can order it online, and it will come dried and chopped.
- Boil 8-10 ounces of water and add 1teaspoon of the valerian root and allow it to boil for 15-20 minutes.
- Allow it to get cool and strain.
- You are done! For the dosage, take 1 cup (8-10ounce) of valerian tea 30-60minutes before going to bed daily.

ASHWAGANDHA

The benefits of using or consuming Ashwagandha also include:

- It helps to reduce stress fast by regulating chemicals in your brain
- It is widely used to fight anxiety in herbal medicine
- Being an energy booster, it helps not to feel fatigued
- It may help improve heart health by reducing cholesterol and triglyceride levels
- It may help to reduce sugar levels in people suffering from diabetes
- It acts as a pain reliever, preventing pain signals from traveling along with the central nervous system.
- May increase muscle mass and muscle strength

Dosage and administration:

Take 250mg to 3000mg daily with abundant water in the morning.

STAGE 3: 7 TIPS FOR A HEALTHY IMMUNE SYSTEM

Avoid table salt

Even if you don't have high blood pressure, you shouldn't take more than one teaspoon of salt per day. And if your blood pressure is high, you should limit your salt intake to half a teaspoon per day. To make sure you avoid hidden salt in your diet, avoid canned and processed foods as much as possible.

Avoid added sugar

Added sugar contributes to weight gain, which contributes to heart disease and high blood pressure. Avoiding sugar is not only about avoiding cakes and sweets. Sugar is added to almost anything, especially canned foods and processed foods – another reason you should eat homemade freshly cooked meals.

Exercise

Exercise strengthens your heart and lowers your blood pressure. If your occupation or hobbies make you move around, you don't need to worry. However, suppose you have a sedentary job. In that case, you should take at least two hours a week and do some serious cardio exercises or walk briskly for a few kilometers.

Maintain a healthy weight

When you put on weight, your blood sugar levels go up. So, if you are overweight, try losing at least a few pounds – your body will feel the difference. Besides, when you weigh less, there's less pressure on your heart and joints, and the easier you'll find it to exercise.

Limit or avoid alcohol

It's well-known that heavy drinking raises blood pressure. Men, especially those over 65, should not take more than two drinks a day, and women should take only one. The older you are, the less you should drink.

Eat more fresh fruits and vegetables

Fruits and vegetables are high in nutrients. So, besides lowering your blood pressure, they can help you prevent many chronic diseases, *e.g.,* cancer, heart disease, *etc.*

Quit smoking

Smoking not only raises your blood pressure, the chemicals in tobacco can damage your arteries, making them narrow and forcing your blood pressure to go up. Secondhand smoke has the same effect. The unhealthier your current lifestyle is, the longer it'll take you to adopt healthy living habits. Why not try changing your lifestyle gradually? First, reduce salt, sugar, unhealthy fats, alcohol, and cigarettes. Then, try introducing healthy living habits one at a time, e.g., take fruit for dessert instead of cake, fill yourself up with a soup or a salad before the main meal, try climbing the stairs instead of taking an elevator, stop adding salt, eat less meat, *etc.*

That way, you will gradually ease yourself into a healthy lifestyle. Besides, after you successfully lowered it, regaining high blood pressure can be very demoralizing, and you may find it difficult to motivate yourself to try again.

Conclusion

After reading this book, you are well aware of inflammation, why it is helpful and harmful simultaneously, how to decrease it, and what natural foods can help you fight against auto-inflammatory diseases and inflammation. Inflammation is the immune system's response to certain infections, injuries, and environmental triggers. Inflammation is not bad itself, and it can be helpful for the body. Simply, without inflammation, you cannot heal. But when left untreated and unmonitored, it can lead to chronic inflammation and cause serious health problems and diseases like cancer, rheumatoid arthritis, and heart diseases. This is why chronic inflammation is dangerous and should be treated with great care and attention.

Today, there are many medications on the market to treat inflammation and inflammatory diseases like steroids and NSAIDs. But the problem is that you cannot use these drugs for a long time because of associated side effects and their damaging effects on the immune system. So what should be done to battle inflammation? Nature is so wise as Nature has provided us with so many natural anti-inflammatory foods that can be used to fight against inflammation and regularly eat them. We can stop inflammation, inflammatory diseases, and conditions and keep ourselves healthy and strong.

It is essential to maintain an equilibrium in your life regardless of your path. Since acidic elements dominate our lifestyle, having an alkaline diet has become more crucial. The excessive use of chemical medicines has further weakened the commoners' immune systems, making them prone to today's world's complex diseases. Dr. Sebi worked against this lifestyle. As a result, he enjoyed some severe breakthroughs in his career, well explained in the preceding chapters. If we switch from our current way of life to nature's conduct, we can prevent many diseases and cure others. The latest developments and research in herbal medicine have endorsed Dr. Alfredo Bowman's work. The herbal elements that build up Dr. Sebi's diet plan have all the minerals and vitamins vital for our body. His medicines have also shown significant results fighting diseases that are considered severe and sometimes untreatable in the medical sciences today with minimum side effects, unlike the same subject's chemical treatments.

BOOK 5: <u>DR. SEBI KIDNEY FAILURE SOLUTION</u>

THE MOST COMPLETE MANUAL TO NATURALLY TREAT CHRONIC KIDNEY DISEASE (CKD) AND STAY OFF DIALYSIS

Chapter 1: Kidneys

Kidneys are two organs about your fist's size located near the bottom of your rib cage, on either side of the spine. Millions of tiny things called 'nephrons' in each kidney filter the blood.

Kidney disease will attack these nephrons. The damage it causes might leave the kidneys unable to get rid of the waste. There are about 26 million people in the United States affected by kidney disease. What happens when the kidneys get damaged and can't function properly. This damage might be caused by different long-term chronic conditions, high blood pressure, and diabetes. In addition, kidney disease could cause other problems such as malnutrition, nerve damage, and weak bones.

If it worsens with time, the kidneys might stop working altogether. That means that you might have to undergo dialysis to help the kidneys perform. Dialysis is a medical treatment where a machine purifies and filters the blood. This won't cure the disease, but it does help prolong life.

Understanding how a disease works is not as simple as telling someone that the letter B comes after A. We need first to recognize the functions of a kidney. That way, we might understand just how the disease affects the organ.

When they are functioning normally, kidneys are responsible for crucial jobs, such as:

- Clear out waste substances and materials from your blood
- Flush out excess water from your body
- Manage your blood pressure
- Encourage your bone marrow to produce red blood cells
- Restrict the amount of phosphorus and calcium absorbed and excreted

You might be surprised by some of the responsibilities above. For example, some people raise their eyebrows in surprise when they realize that our kidneys are responsible for stimulating our bone marrow to produce red blood cells or RBCs. But that is how versatile our kidneys are.

The feature that interests us is that our kidneys help filter blood. There are a million filtering units in the bean-shaped organs. In turn, these units, called nephrons, have a filter known as a glomerulus along with another component called "tubule". Those are pretty complex terms but don't worry; I shall not drop a biology explanation.

To put it simply, a glomerulus is a modified blood vessel. Typically, your normal blood vessels transport blood throughout the body. But, on the other hand, the glomerulus filters your blood to create urine. But once the urine has been produced, what happens to it? Are glomeruli going to do all the work of transporting them to your bladder?

That's where tubules come into play. These tiny structures take the waste materials from the glomerulus, look through them to see if any useful materials might have been included by accident, then passes on the useful materials back to the blood and urine to the pelvis. Think of this arrangement as a nightclub with two bouncers. The first bouncer is dealing with a large crowd outside. You might take advantage of that fact and sneak in, only to realize that a second guard is waiting for you, who has his job made easier because the first guard has whittled down the crowd to a manageable number. This time, you better be right about the age in your ID.

It's like your body created its version of the two-step verification process that you find when you try to open your bank account online or log in to certain websites; fluids get 'verified' for good materials first by the glomerulus, then by tubules. But it is necessary because your body is trying to filter your blood properly.

How the Kidneys Work

Our kidneys are bean-shaped filters that work in teams. They have a very important job since they keep our bodies stable. They use signals from the body like blood pressure and sodium content to help keep us hydrated and our blood pressure stable.

If the kidneys don't function right, numerous problems could happen. When these toxins' filtration becomes slow, these harmful chemicals can build up and cause other body reactions like vomiting, nausea, and rashes. When the kidney's functions continue to decrease, its ability to get rid of water and release hormones that control blood pressure can also be affected. Symptoms such as high blood pressure or retaining water in your feet might happen. Reduced kidney function could cause long-term health problems such as osteoporosis or anemia.

The kidneys work hard, so we have to protect them. They can filter around 120 to 150 quarts of blood each day. This will create between 1 and 2 quarts of urine made up of excess fluid and waste products.

When Your Kidney Functions Get Kidnapped

According to the National Kidney Foundation, the two main causes of chronic kidney disease are high blood pressure and diabetes (National Kidney Foundation, n.d.). Suppose you visit a doctor, health expert, or diet consultant. In that case, you will realize that one of the major ways to manage your blood pressure and prevent diabetes is a healthy diet. But more on that later.

As the blood pressure or diabetes levels worsen, so does the amount of waste build-up. The waste goes into your blood faster than the kidneys can filter. At this point, your kidneys are like an overworked employee at a firm; there is so much work remaining, but only a small amount of time to get finished during a particular period. As a result, the kidneys begin to deteriorate over time. The filters start to leak, unable to hold on to the waste build-up anymore. As a result, only a small percentage of the entire waste gets filtered properly, with the rest entering the bloodstream. For some, the time it takes for kidney failure might be months, while for others, the kidneys could worsen across a span of years. It depends on numerous factors like diet, lifestyle choices, and even genetics.

Pretty soon, you might feel like your kidney functions have been kidnapped; they don't seem to be functioning well anymore, or they barely exist. But that is not the case. Think of the example of the overworked employee that we used earlier. At some point, the employee could collapse out of dehydration or exhaustion. Similarly, kidney disease causes the organs to fail, which causes numerous problems such as low energy, high exhaustion levels, sleep difficulties, poor appetite, swollen ankles and feet, and the need to urinate more often, especially at night.

Many people mistakenly believe the kidneys act as sponges, far from the truth. The kidneys do not absorb and hold onto waste and harmful compounds. Instead, the kidneys filter out these toxins to be completely removed from the body. They do this with a complex system consisting of millions of nephrons microscopic filters. Nephrons are comprised of two components: the glomerulus and the tubule. To cleanse the blood, the glomerulus strains the larger molecules from fluid and waste. After this passes through the glomerulus, they head to the tubule. As the blood travels through the tubule component of the nephrons, smaller waste molecules are collected. Not only that, but the tubule also collects any minerals found within the blood and then transfers them back into the bloodstream. But how are these toxins removed from the kidneys and the body so that they don't stay stuck within your organs? When the kidneys filter water from your bloodstream, it combines the water with the filtered waste and toxins, allowing them to be carried to the bladder before being expelled from the body.

Some of the waste that the kidneys remove from your blood is excess acid produced to maintain healthy minerals and water levels. This acid affects the levels of many minerals, such as potassium, sodium, calcium, and phosphorus. When these minerals are out of balance, your body will be unable to function properly. As these minerals are electrolytes, they affect the maintenance and control of your muscles, nerves, tissues, and balance. Without the proper balance of these electrolytes, you can be in a rather dangerous situation.

Athletes are frequently aware of the importance of maintaining balanced electrolytes since your body will naturally become depleted of these minerals as you sweat. It is also the main reason that sports drinks are popular. These drinks contain all the electrolytes the human body requires, allowing people to refuel on water and minerals simultaneously. However, if you consume too many sports drinks or electrolytes in other forms, you will overload your blood and kidneys. Therefore, it is important to balance electrolytes with neither too few nor too many.

Your kidney provides other functions. Some of them are:

- electrolyte levels and blood pressure maintenance
- excess acid elimination
- hydration control
- hormones and vitamin D production.

When the kidneys cannot purify and filter blood, it accumulates waste in the body, which is harmful. This condition is referred to as a renal failure, and it can even cause death unless treated on time. But, before understanding what renal failure is, you need to understand what kidneys are. The two bean-shaped organs located on either side of your spine in your back are referred to as kidneys. They help clean the blood by removing waste products from it in the form of urine. Not only this, but kidneys also help maintain the balance of certain elements in blood like sodium, potassium, and calcium, and even control the secretion of hormones that help control blood pressure and red blood cells.

Kidney or renal failure refers to the kidneys aren't functioning like they are supposed to. "Kidney failure" covers a lot of different problems, and some of these problems could be an insufficient supply of blood to your kidneys for filtration. Diseases like diabetes, high blood pressure, and any damage to the kidney's filters can+ severely damage your kidneys. In addition, any scar tissue or even kidney stones can block your kidney and result in renal failure.

Some different signs and symptoms can help you spot kidney failure. It is important to be aware of these symptoms because early detection can help timely treatment and curb the problem before it becomes severe. Keep an eye out for the following signs if there is a decrease in the output of urine over some time, retention of any fluid that results in the swelling up of your legs, ankles, or feet, extreme drowsiness, and shortness of breath, feeling of constant fatigue, confusion, seizures or even coma in some severe cases, a build-up of pressure in chest or chest pain. Also, there are cases where acute kidney failure causes no signs or symptoms and can be detected through different lab tests done for some other reason. You should immediately make an appointment with your doctor when you start noticing any of the signs or symptoms of acute kidney failure.

The Kidneys and the Endocrine System

The human kidneys play an important role in the endocrine system, which produces and controls hormones within the body. For example, the kidneys are critical in producing renin, erythropoietin, and calcitriol. Not only that, but they also synthesize prostaglandins, which affect various aspects of kidney function.

Along with the production and synthesis of hormones, the kidneys also participate in the degradation of hormones, including insulin and the parathyroid hormone.

Erythropoietin:

The erythropoietin hormone regulates the production of red blood cells. When this hormone is out of balance, a person's blood can become dangerously thin or dangerously thick, potentially lethal if left without emergency medical intervention.

For adults, an average of ninety percent of their erythropoietin is formed and synthesized by the kidneys. The liver produces the remaining ten percent. While the liver plays a vital role in erythropoietin production during the fetal stages of growth, for adults, the liver is no longer able to compensate for the kidneys' lack of production. That means that if the kidneys fail to produce adequate erythropoietin levels, the liver cannot maintain this hormone's healthy levels.

Most people who develop end-stage renal failure will experience anemia and a deficiency in erythropoietin. While doctors will sometimes administer blood thickeners to increase blood cell production, it is not always effective.

Calcitriol:

Also known as 1,25-dihydroxy vitamin D3, calcitriol is a vital bioactive form of vitamin D3. This vitamin has important roles in bone mineralization and health, phosphorus regulation, and calcium regulation. However, many calcitriol effects are yet to be discovered, as they reside in various cells.

Calcitriol is important for human health. The body cannot directly benefit from vitamin D absorbed from food or the sun. This "vitamin" is not a true vitamin but a hormone. The vitamin D we absorb from outside sources is delivered to the kidneys synthesized into the bioactive form of calcitriol. Once the calcitriol has been synthesized, the body can then use it to maintain homeostasis.

As kidney disease frequently causes a deficiency in calcitriol, many doctors will treat their patients with this hormone. In addition, it can be used to treat symptoms such as:

Hyperparathyroidism is an endocrine disorder characterized by excessive hormone production.

Low blood calcium

Osteomalacia, softening of the bone.

Osteoporosis, degradation of the bones.

Calcitriol has a couple of other purposes, as well. First, it activates cell osteoblasts. This cell secretes the matrix needed for bone formation. It synthesizes collagen required for nearly all tissues, cartilage, and other body aspects. Second, calcitriol stimulates the small intestine, allowing it to synthesize protein and absorb calcium.

Renin:

A part of the angiotensin-aldosterone system (RAAS), renin is an important component in kidney hormone health. After all, this system manages fluid balance, electrolyte balance, blood pressure, and systemic vascular resistance.

When there is a decrease in blood volume in the kidneys (causing low blood pressure) due to insufficient blood flow, your cells will begin to synthesize the renin protein and enzyme. Unfortunately, the renin releases and alters several enzymes and proteins, creating angiotensin II. That then causes the arteries to constrict, resulting in a rise of both diastolic and systolic blood pressure. Therefore, renin is vital in raising low blood pressure to a safe and manageable level.

Prostaglandins:

The cellular metabolism of arachidonic acid derives the prostaglandins from creating a series of fatty acid hormone-like products. Unlike most hormones, prostaglandins are not produced and then carried through the bloodstream to affect the body's specific functions. Instead, they are created by chemical reactions throughout the body wherever they are needed at the time. These prostaglandins' purpose is to help the body heal from both illness and injury, making them a part of the inflammation response.

While chronic high inflammation levels are damaging, as we will discuss later in this book, the inflammation response is still a vital part of the body. Without the inflammation response, we would be unable to heal or protect ourselves from harmful bacteria and viruses. They also manage blood clotting when we get a wound less likely to bleed out. Not only that, but prostaglandins play an important role in the female reproductive system. This hormone controls the menstrual cycle, ovulation, and induction of labor.

But if prostaglandins are produced throughout the body as needed, what do they have to do with the kidneys? The kidneys are one of the many locations within your body that produce this hormone. It plays an important role in kidney health. It turns out that the prostaglandins produced within the kidneys play an important role in overall kidney function. The kidneys' process of filtering waste, delivering minerals to the bloodstream, adding clean fluids back to the bloodstream, and transporting urine to the bladder is known as renal hemodynamics. Pro prostaglandins help manage this entire process. Without renal prostaglandins, the kidneys would not function properly, creating dangerous side effects.

As you can see, the kidneys play several very important roles in overall health. That means that it can be quite dangerous when something goes wrong with the kidneys, causing extreme symptoms. But what exactly could go wrong with your kidneys? First, when your kidneys cannot function correctly, it can cause a build-up of fluid and waste within the body, along with excessive levels of minerals and electrolytes. This would result in kidney disease, which can, later on, lead to high blood pressure, fluid retention, fatigue, and back pain.

Many things may cause the kidneys to become damaged or diseased. Some of the causes may be infections, various diseases, diabetes, or high blood pressure. The kidneys can also become damaged if there is a malfunction of the blood vessels leading to the kidneys, causing the organs to receive inadequate blood supply. As there is no one cause of kidney disease or damage, your doctor will have to diagnose your kidney disease itself and the cause of the disease. Your doctor must learn the initial cause; otherwise, they will not treat it properly. For instance, if your kidneys are damaged due to the inadequate blood supply, your doctor will not help if they are only treating you for diabetes. Thankfully, your doctor should be well-equipped to learn the cause of your disease if you have one.

Chapter 2: Chronic Kidney Disease (CKD)

What is Chronic Kidney Disease (CKD)?

We talk about Chronic Kidney Disease (CKD), when kidney functions decline for three months or more. There are five stages of evolution of a CRM according to the severity of the renal involvement or the degree of deterioration of its function.

Sometimes failure suddenly occurs. In this case, it is called an 'acute failure' of the kidney, which is often treated with urgency by dialysis for some time. Usually, kidney function recovers itself. Generally, this disease settles slowly and silently, but it progresses over the years. People with CKD do not necessarily go from stage 1 to stage 5 of the disease. Stage 5 is known as an end-stage renal disease (ESRD) or kidney failure in the final stage.

It is important to know that the expressions terminal, final, and ultimate mean the end of any kidneys' function (kidneys working at less than 15% of their normal capacity) and not the end of your life. To stay alive at this stage of the disease, it is necessary to resort to dialysis or a kidney transplant. Dialysis and transplantation are known as renal replacement therapy (TRS).

That means that dialysis or the transplanted kidney will "supplement" or "replace" the sick kidneys and do their job.

What Are the Causes of Chronic Kidney Disease?

There are different kinds of diseases and disorders of the kidneys. At present, we do not know for sure all the causes. Some are hereditary, while others develop with age. In addition, they are often associated with other diseases, such as diabetes, heart disease, or high blood pressure.

Most kidney diseases attack kidney filters, damaging their ability to eliminate waste and excess fluids. No treatment can cure these diseases, but it is possible to prevent them or slow down their evolution. It is especially true of diseases like diabetes and hypertension, the leading causes of kidney failure.

The CKD is defined by the presence of an anatomical and urinary indicator of renal impairment and a decrease in the rate of glomerular filtration (GFR) persisting beyond three months. This disease is classified into five stages of increasing severity, according to the GFR. A DFG within normal limits characterizes the first two stages. It requires renal impairment markers, including urinary tests (proteinuria, Haematuria, or pyuria) or morphological abnormalities renal ultrasound (contours bumpy, asymmetrical in size, small kidneys or large kidneys, polycystic, etc.).

A real decrease in GFR characterizes only the other three stages. For example, the end-stage of chronic renal failure (CRT) or stage 5 of CKD is defined by a GFR <15 ml/min / 1.73 m².

Renal impairment is defined by the presence of pathological abnormalities or biological markers of the kidney, including abnormalities of urinary or kidney morphological tests detected by imaging.

Historically, the lack of consensus in the definition of CKD (especially chronic renal failure) its severity has led to late diagnosis, inadequate medical management, and data deficiency at a global level.

It was not until 2002 that this gap was filled by adopting the DFG thresholds or the aforementioned CKD stages.

Even though people with diabetes use insulin by injection or take medication, they cannot shelter some small blood vessel lesions, like those in the eye's retina. In this case, the retina may be damaged, resulting in vision loss. Also, they are not immune to the deterioration of the fragile blood vessels of the renal filters.

Progressive deterioration of the kidneys is seen when urine tests show higher and higher protein levels. As the disease progresses, the number of proteins increases. As for treatment, the sooner it starts (for example, with drugs such as ACE inhibitors or A2 blocking agents), the more likely it is to slow the disease's progression. Kidney disease caused by diabetes can slow the evolution of the disease regardless of its stage.

Over time, diabetes can reach kidney filters at no return: the kidneys no longer function, and renal replacement therapy becomes essential. In addition, people with diabetes are prone to infections, which are changing rapidly. If these infections, especially those of the urinary tract, are not treated, they can damage the kidneys. Therefore, it is recommended that people with diabetes not overlook any condition and treat it immediately.

Hypertension

The kidneys secrete a hormone that plays an important role in increasing or reducing blood pressure. When the kidneys are so affected that they do not function properly, this hormone's secretion can increase and cause hypertension, damaging the kidneys. Therefore, it is necessary to closely monitor hypertension to avoid renal function deterioration in the long term.

Glomerulonephritis

The glomerulonephritis, or nephritis, declares when glomeruli, these tiny filters used to purify the blood, deteriorates. There are several kinds of glomerulonephritis. Some are hereditary, while others occur due to certain diseases such as strep throat. The causes of most glomerulonephritis are not yet known. Some glomerulonephritis cure without medical treatment, while others require prescription drugs. Some do not respond to any treatment and have chronic kidney disease. Some clues suggest that glomerulonephritis is due to a deficiency in the body's immune system.

Autosomal Dominant Polycystic Disease

Often in their forties, people with the disease will need dialysis or a kidney transplant. But because the loss of kidney function is changing at a different pace, depending on the individual, the time between the onset of cysts and the need for dialysis varies widely. Since the disease is hereditary, people are advised to inform other family members to carry out the required tests as they may be affected.

The Obstruction of the Urinary Tract

Any obstruction (or blockage) of the urinary tract may damage the kidneys. Blocks can occur in the ureter or at the end of the bladder. Narrowing the ureter at the superior or inferior level is sometimes due to congenital malformations, leading to chronic kidney disease in children. In adults, increased prostate volume, kidney stones, or tumors often obstruct the urinary tract.

Reflux Nephropathy

Reflux nephropathy is the new name of the former "chronic pyelonephritis."

Illegal Drugs

The use of illegal drugs can cause kidney damage. Over-the-counter medications (without a prescription) High-dose and long-term use of over-the-counter medications can cause kidney damage.

Important: Beware of medications, including herbal remedies, sold without a prescription. It would be wiser to seek your doctor's advice before buying them.

Prescription Drugs

Some medications prescribed to people with kidney disease cause renal dysfunction. The lesions are sometimes reversible and sometimes irreversible. Many medicines prescribed by prescription are safe, but the doctor makes changes accurate to the dosage. So always ask your doctor or your pharmacist for information about the potential side effects of prescribed drugs.

Other Kidney Disorders

Other issues can affect the kidneys, such as, for example, kidney stones, Syndrome Alport, Fabry disease, Wilms tumor (children only), not including infections of bacterial origin.

What are the complications of chronic kidney disease?

- Fluid in your lungs or fluid retention that might cause swelling in your legs and arms
- Blood vessel and heart disease
- High blood pressure
- Hyperkalemia
- Increased risk of bone fractures and weak bones
- Anemia
- Reduced fertility
- Erectile dysfunction

- Decreased sex drive
- Decreased immune response
- Central nervous system damage, causing seizures, personality changes, and difficulty concentrating
- Pericarditis
- Irreversible damage to your kidneys
- Pregnancy complications

Stages of Chronic Kidney Disease (CKD)

Chronic kidney disease (CKD) is not a sudden condition; it occurs in stages. Patients move from one stage of chronic kidney disease to the other as the kidneys' effectiveness decreases over time until they get to the last stage. The last stage of chronic kidney disease is kidney failure. At this stage, patients need dialysis or a kidney transplant to survive.

Stages of chronic kidney disease are identified according to a patient's estimated Glomerular Filtration Rate (GFR) - the rate at which the kidney filters toxins from the blood. GFR is considered the yardstick for measuring overall kidney functions. GFR is usually determined by examining the level of blood creatinine. This waste product is produced during muscle metabolism, in conjunction with other factors such as age, sex, body size, and race. . Let us highlight the stages of chronic kidney disease (CKD).

Stage 1

The kidneys' functions are still normal at stage one, and patients may not notice any obvious symptoms. But protein can be noticed in patients' urine if tested. This is because the kidneys' estimated glomerular filtration rate (GFR) at stage one is 90 ml per minute or above. This is similar to the GFR of a healthy kidney.

Stage 2

Stage two chronic kidney disease (CKD) characterizes a mild decrease in kidney functions. At this point, a little rise in creatinine level in the blood can be noticed if the patient is tested. The kidney's estimated glomerular filtration rate (GFR) in stage two is around 60 to 89 ml per minute.

Stage 3

Stage 3 is often the middle stage of chronic kidney disease (CKD). It is the most common category of chronic kidney disease. At stage 3, there is a moderate decrease in kidney functions, and patients must have started to sense some complications of chronic kidney disease. These complications include anemia, high blood pressure, bone weakness, and fatigue. The third stage of chronic kidney disease (CKD) occurs in two phases. The estimated glomerular filtration rate (GFR) for phase one, stage 3 of CKD, is around 45 to 59 ml per minute. In comparison, phase two features an estimated GFR of 30 to 44 ml per minute.

Stage 4

At stage four, the kidney functions will have decreased immensely, and the patient will be faced with many negative health conditions associated with chronic kidney disease (CKD). This stage is associated with severity. Doctors will already be planning for dialysis or a kidney transplant at this stage. Stage four's estimated glomerular filtration rate (GFR) is around 15 to 29 ml per minute.

Stage 5

Stage five is the last stage of chronic kidney disease. It is the stage where the kidneys finally fail. The estimated glomerular filtration rate (GFR) is below 15 ml per minute. The kidneys may still function a bit, but the kidney function level at this stage will not be enough to keep the patient alive. At stage five, the patient will need dialysis or a kidney transplant to survive.

Chapter 3: Kidney Failure

What is kidney failure?

You reach the "Kidney Failure" stage when your kidneys cannot remove toxins and waste in your blood from the foods you eat and the things you drink. Sometimes called "chronic kidney disease" or "chronic kidney failure."

It isn't a disorder that happens overnight— it's a gradual issue that can be discovered early and treated, diet modified, and it's possible to solve what causes the problem.

Partial renal failure is possible, but it typically takes a long time (or a really bad diet for a short time) to achieve full renal failure. You don't want total renal failure because it will require regular dialysis to save your life.

Specifically, dialysis procedures wash excess blood and pollutants in the blood using a device because your body can no longer do the job. Despite therapies, death could be very painful. In addition, renal failure can result from long-term diabetes, high blood pressure, irresponsible diet, and other health concerns.

A renal diet is about moderating the diet's protein and phosphorus intake. Limiting sodium intake is also necessary. By regulating these two factors, you can regulate most of your body's toxins/waste, improving your kidney function.

When you notice it early enough and control your diet with extreme care, you can avoid complete renal failure. When you notice it early, you can remove it.

It's your kidney's job to remove stuff you don't need and balance the ones your body needs. If your kidneys couldn't play this role effectively, it's high time you discover what you can do. A doctor's prescribed renal diet can help filter out toxic substances you don't need in your body.

Understanding the Different Types of Kidney Failure

In general, there are five different kidney failures that you should be aware of. So I will try to go through them one by one to clear things up.

Acute Pre-Renal Kidney Failure

It is caused by insufficient blood flow to the kidney. In this scenario, the kidney fails to filter toxins as enough blood doesn't flow through it. It is possible to treat this type of failure as long your doctor can figure out the cause of your abnormal blood flow.

Acute Intrinsic Kidney Failure

It can happen if you experience any form of direct trauma to your kidneys, such as an accident or physical impact, causing toxins to overload and might lead to ischemia (Oxygen fails to get enough oxygen).

<u>Some causes include:</u>

- Shock
- Bleeding
- Glomerulonephritis
- Renal Blood Vessel Obstruction

Chronic Pre-Renal Kidney Failure

It happens when your kidney fails to receive sufficient blood for a prolonged period. As a result, the kidney tends to shrink, eventually losing its function in this situation.

Chronic Intrinsic Kidney Failure

It occurs if your kidney has experienced long-term damage due to intrinsic kidney disease.

Intrinsic diseases can come from a lack of oxygen, bleeding, or trauma.

Chronic Post-Renal Kidney Failure

If you experience blockage in your urinary tract for a long time, then the pressure build-up might damage your kidney.

Understanding if Your Kidneys Have Failed

There are various ways to understand if your kidneys have any problems.

Some of the common ones include:

- *Urinalysis* → In this type of test, the doctor will take samples of your urine and check them for any abnormalities, such as sugar or abnormal protein that might have leaked into the urine.
- *Urine Volume Measurements* → Measuring your urine volume is possibly one of the simplest tests out there. If you have very low urine output, it might indicate that you have kidney disease caused by a urinary blockage.
- *Blood Samples* → If urine isn't doing it, the doctor might ask you to take blood tests to measure various substances filtered by the kidneys.
- *Imaging* → Various imaging tests, such as CT Scans, MRIs, and Ultrasounds, tend to provide a full image of the kidney and the urinary tract, allowing the doctor to find blockages or abnormalities.
- *Kidney Tissue Samples* → Tissue from your kidney can be taken and examined to look for scarring, toxin deposits, or infectious organism. The physician will try to take a kidney biopsy to collect your sample.

In most cases, the doctor will take a biopsy sample while you are awake; however, the doctor will give you a local anesthetic to ensure that you don't feel any pain.

Acute Renal Failure - Symptoms and Treatment

Acute renal failure (ARF) is a serious but treatable condition resulting from kidney function loss. There are various symptoms and treatments for acute renal failure, otherwise known as acute kidney failure.

Acute kidney failure, as stated earlier, is sudden kidney function loss. As you may know, your kidneys are responsible for removing body waste products and helping balance other minerals in your body and bloodstream.

They're an essential part of the body, as they can't work without them. For example, suppose your kidneys stop working in acute kidney failure. In that case, the body will quickly fill up with many waste products, contaminants, and other liquids, rendering it lethal.

How is Acute Renal Failure Caused?

Acute renal failure has various causes. Many are related to other factors in the body that can affect the kidneys, while others are directly related.

Urine-flow Blockage.

It can cause kidney failure by blocking kidney waste excretion. It can be caused by a tumor, enlarged prostate, blockage or inflammation of the urinary tract, trauma, or kidney stones.

Blood loss to the kidneys.

Any type of bodily injury, specifically localized kidney injury, can cause sudden blood flow loss, resulting in severe kidney damage.

Some medicines can cause acute kidney failure.

Some medicines can have very large side effects on the kidneys. Many of these medicines can be found in some antibiotics, blood pressure medicines, certain colors used in CT scans, and more commonly, some pain killers.

All these can have a poisoning effect on the kidneys and should not be taken for extended periods. When you suffer from any of these problems, try to find other ways to cope, including finding ways to fix the problem's first cause.

Some people may risk more acute kidney failure. For example, those suffering from chronic conditions such as heart conditions, obesity, liver disease, high blood pressure, and other organ conditions will have more acute renal failure.

Also, as mentioned earlier, it is important to explore ways of reducing pressure on the kidneys when suffering from the above condition to avoid any chances of acute renal failure or kidney disease.

What are Acute Renal Failure's common symptoms?

Before any type of kidney disease is apparent, signs can be seen and considered very mild. Some may even remain unnoticed until too late. If you have any of these common symptoms, act immediately.

Common symptoms of acute renal failure may include:

- Fluid retention (swelling in the body—usually feet and hands)
- Loss of appetite
- Urinating problems

- Some vomiting and nausea
- Dizziness
- Lower back pain
- And general restlessness.

These signs may go unnoticed in people already suffering from other long-term medical conditions. They may be thought to be related to the current disease. It is important to remember that steps should be taken to help treat the condition at the slightest sign of acute renal failure symptoms.

Simple medical tests decide how to tell if you have acute kidney failure. After consulting the doctor, urine and blood samples must be taken.

These can help show your blood and urine toxicity and help you decide if you are now at risk of acute renal failure. In addition, other measures, such as measuring fluid intake and loss, are important to determine whether fluid retention is caused.

Acute renal failure has some forms of treatment, including hospital stays and continuing procedures. All this depends on the severity of the acute renal failure and the signs and causes of renal problems.

Such therapies vary from dialysis, medicines, and surgery. Appropriate medication is selected based on how far the renal failure can go.

Nevertheless, most physicians now believe that acute renal failure is largely caused by poor diet and lifestyle factors, as with virtually all medical conditions. Some of our preferred Western foods contain preservatives and chemicals that our bodies cannot process.

They usually contain large amounts of sodium and potassium, which are not good for anyone fighting kidney disease. The kidney diet was created based on eastern diets (which now have very rare genetic-related renal failure) and has been shown to help treat and even reverse acute kidney failure.

Learning to Deal with Kidney Failure

Learning that you are suffering from kidney failure might be difficult to cope with. No matter how long you have been preparing for the inevitable, this is something that will come as a shock to you.

It might be a little bit difficult at first to get yourself oriented to a new routine, but once you get into the groove, you'll start feeling much better.

Your nurses, loved ones, doctors, and co-workers will all be there to support you.

To make things easier, though, let me break down the individual types of problems you might face and how you can deal with them

Chapter 4: Causes of CKD

Causes and Risk Factors

Many of us are not aware that the cause of kidney disease doesn't necessarily have to occur in the kidneys themselves. Problems affecting our overall health and well-being can also induce damage to the kidneys. In the same way, common health problems can also impair the function of these organs. The most frequent causes of kidney disease are hypertension and diabetes.

High blood pressure, which affects 75 million people in the US or one in three adults, can damage blood vessels in the kidney and impair their function. In other words, damage to blood vessels in the kidneys due to hypertension doesn't allow them to remove wastes and extra fluid from your body. That leads to a vicious cycle as an accumulation of waste and extra fluid increases blood pressure. Besides damaging filtering units in kidneys, high blood pressure can also reduce blood flow to these organs. As you're already aware, organs cannot function properly without a blood supply.

About 30.3 million people, or 9.4% of the United States population, have diabetes, causing several complications. Just like hypertension, diabetes also damages small blood vessels in the kidneys. As a result, the body retains more salt and water than it should. Moreover, diabetes also damages the body's nerves, making it difficult for you to empty the bladder. The pressure from a full bladder can back up and damage or injure kidneys. Let's also not forget that if urine remains in the body for a long time, it can lead to an infection from the fast growth of bacteria and high blood sugar levels. Estimates show that 30% of patients with type 1 diabetes and 10% to 40% of people with type 2 diabetes will eventually experience kidney failure.

Besides diabetes and hypertension, other causes of kidney disease include:

- Infection
- Renal artery stenosis
- Heavy metal poisoning
- Lupus

- Some drugs
- Prolonged obstruction of the urinary tract from conditions such as kidney stones, enlarged prostate, some cancers

Diagnosing Kidney Disease

Your doctor will be the first to know if you are in a high-risk group for getting kidney disease. They will do some tests to see how well your kidneys are functioning. Some of the tests might be:

Urine Test

Your doctor will ask for a urine sample to test it for albumin, a protein that gets passed into the urine if the kidneys become damaged.

Kidney Biopsy

When doing a kidney biopsy, your doctor will take out a little piece of tissue from the kidney after being sedated. This sample could help determine if you have kidney disease, what type you have, and the amount of damage that has already happened.

CT Scan or Ultrasound

A CT or computed tomography scan and ultrasound can give your doctor clear pictures of your urinary tract and kidneys, letting your doctor see if your kidneys are too large or small. They can also show any structural problems or tumors that might be there.

GFR or Glomerular Filtration Rate

This test measures how well the kidneys work and show what stage of kidney disease you might be in.

Chapter 5: Symptoms of CKD

One way to help a person know if they are suffering from chronic kidney disease is to be informed about its signs and symptoms.

When these signs and symptoms show, immediately seek the assistance of medical experts to avoid complications.

The common signs of chronic kidney disease are:

- **Nausea and Vomiting**. When you experience nausea, you sense discomfort in your upper stomach. You get a sensation of uneasiness and an urge to vomit involuntarily. Most of the time, a person vomits after experiencing nausea.

- **Loss of Appetite**. Changes in your eating habits may signify that you already suffer from a chronic kidney disorder. When you begin to notice that you are eating less than usual or are not feeling any urge or motivation to eat at all for no apparent reason, it is time that you consult your doctor. Not only is it a sign of chronic kidney disease, but a loss of appetite may also result in weight loss and malnutrition.

- **Changes in urination**. Whether you are urinating more or less than usual or are experiencing changes in your urine's color, you should seek medical assistance. We know that the kidneys are the ones responsible for the production of urine. If there are changes in urination, this means that there are changes in the functioning of the kidney as well. It may be a sign of improvement for some but can be very risky for many. You know that you are experiencing changes in urination when you frequently need to wake up in the middle of the night just to urinate; your urine has a bubble or is foamy when it contains blood, dark-colored. You urinate less frequently and in smaller amounts, or whenever you feel difficulty or pressure when urinating.

- **Swelling**. Swelling may occur whenever you are injured or accidentally bump into something hard. However, experience swelling without any external cause. This may be a sign that your kidneys are beginning to fail. Swelling occurs because the kidneys can no longer remove the extra fluids in your body. Swelling may occur in the ankles, legs, feet, hands, or face.

- **Fatigue**. The kidneys produce hormones responsible for keeping us energetic every day. But unfortunately, our bodies also fail to receive and carry oxygen when they fail, making our brains and muscles tire quickly.

- **Itching or Skin Rash**. As mentioned in the first chapter, one of the kidneys' main functions is to filter the blood and remove the bloodstream wastes when the kidneys fail to function properly; these wastes build up, causing itching and skin rash.

- **Shortness of Breath**. When the kidneys fail to remove extra fluid in our body, they can stay in the lungs and build up in there. As a result, the kidney can also trigger the development of anemia. When anemia is complicated, your body will starve for oxygen. Thus, one experiences shortness of breath.

Chapter 6: Correlation With Other Diseases

According to experts, renal disease requires early diagnosis and targeted treatment to prevent or delay both a condition of acute or chronic renal failure and the appearance of cardiovascular complications to which it is often associated.

Hypertension and diabetes can promote onset, not adequately controlled by drug therapy, prostatic hypertrophy, kidney stones, or bulky tumors. As a result, they reduce the normal urine

Or the kidney damage can be determined by inflammatory processes (pyelonephritis, glomerulonephritis) or by the formation of cysts inside the kidneys (polycystic kidney disease) or by the chronic use of some drugs, alcohol, and drugs consumed in excess.

A fundamental role in alleviating the already compromised kidneys' work is the diet, the first prevention. It must be studied with an expert nutritionist or a nephrologist to maintain or reach an ideal weight on the one hand and on the other to reduce the intake of sodium (salt), and the consequent control of blood pressure, and other substances (minerals), without creating malnutrition or nutritional deficiencies. Particular attention should also be paid to cholesterol, triglycerides, and blood sugar levels.

Understanding what causes kidney failure goes a long way to deciding just what kind of treatment you should focus on. Of course, the most important factor that you should focus on is your diet. But as you focus on your diet, make sure that you are following your doctor's instructions in the event of other complications. First, let us look at a few common causes of kidney diseases.

Diabetes

Many may already know that diabetes affects our body's insulin production rate. But what many may not know is the extent of damage that diabetes can cause to the kidneys. Insulin is essential because it regulates sugar or glucose in our blood. The inability to control the glucose damages the kidneys' function to filter fluids and waste products.

We do know that diabetes is one of the leading causes of CKD. But we have yet to understand in detail why and how it can harm the kidneys.

High Blood Pressure

When blood pressure increases and becomes uncontrollable, it causes stroke, heart attack, and chronic kidney disease. In addition, too much pressure against the blood vessels' walls can contribute to the kidney's failure to function properly.

Thus, a person must watch over his diet and the activities he engages in to avoid hypertension. Although it is a common health problem, it still poses serious risks and complications.

The risk factors for hypertension include age, obesity, family history, smoking, lack of exercise, stress, excessive alcohol consumption, high fat diet, and sodium intake.

It is important to remember that high blood pressure can be a cause and CKD symptom, similar to diabetes.

So, what exactly is blood pressure? People often throw the term around, but they cannot pinpoint what happens when the blood pressure increases.

Autoimmune Diseases

IgA nephropathy and lupus are two examples of autoimmune diseases leading to kidney diseases. But just what exactly are autoimmune diseases?

They are conditions where your immune system perceives your body as a threat and begins to attack it.

We all know that the immune system is like the defense force of our body. It is responsible for guiding our body's soldiers, known as white blood cells, or WBCs. In addition, the immune system is responsible for fighting against foreign materials, such as viruses and bacteria. When the system senses these foreign bodies, various fighter cells, including the WBCs, combat the threat.

Typically, your immune system is a self-learning system. That means it can understand the threat and memorize its features, behaviors, and attack patterns. It is an important capability of the immune system since it allows the system to differentiate between our cells and foreign cells. But when you have an autoimmune disease, your immune system suddenly considers certain parts of your body, such as your skin or joints, as foreign. It then proceeds to create antibodies that begin to attack these parts.

Before one thinks about their condition treated, it is first important to know the causes and symptoms. Knowing the causes of a particular disease is necessary for treatment and prevention.

Chronic kidney disease is most commonly caused by hypertension and diabetes. Therefore, 2/3 of the cases of chronic kidney disease are found in people suffering from these two conditions. However, other factors may account for the development of chronic kidney disease.

Malformations

Even when you are still in your mother's womb, risks of developing chronic kidney disease are already present. Mothers should be extra cautious when pregnant because preventing urine outflow may affect the baby's organs.

Lupus

Systemic lupus erythematous causes the body's immune system to attack the kidney even if it is not foreign tissue. As a result, it may take a long time before a person recovers from lupus. It eventually goes back after some time, but it is possible through proper treatments.

Obstructions

Obstructions or blockages such as tumors, kidney stones, or enlarged prostate gland can trigger chronic kidney disease development.

The causes mentioned above are just the most common of the many causes of chronic kidney disease. In addition, there are cases when CKD is caused not only by a single factor. Sometimes, a combination of these factors causes the development of chronic kidney disease.

Nonetheless, a patient needs to know the cause of their condition to be prescribed the proper treatments and medications.

Chapter 7: Conventional Treatments

Dialysis

It is an artificial way of filtering the blood that gets used when your kidneys are very close to failing or have completely failed. Most people with kidney disease might have to go on dialysis totally or until you find a kidney donor. Dialysis is a treatment performed to filter and purify the blood using a specialized machine. A dialysis machine performs the same function as the human kidneys. Depending on your condition's severity, you may be required to undergo dialysis treatment once a week or 2-3 times weekly. People should understand that dialysis treatment doesn't cure the disease; it only helps extend your life.

There are two kinds of dialysis: **peritoneal** and **hemodialysis**.

Peritoneal Dialysis

In this type of dialysis, the peritoneum starts functioning for the kidneys. The peritoneum is the membrane that outlines the abdominal wall. A tube gets implanted and is used to fill the stomach with dialysate. All the waste in the blood will flow out of the peritoneum and into this dialysate. This fluid then gets drained out of the stomach.

There are two types of peritoneal dialysis:

Continuous cycler-assisted peritoneal dialysis: for this one, a machine is used to pull the fluid in and out of the stomach while you sleep.

Continuous ambulatory peritoneal dialysis: for this one, the stomach is filled and then drained numerous times throughout the day.

The common side effects are infection of the stomach cavity or around the area where the tube was inserted. The other side effects could include hernias and weight gain. A hernia happens when a part of the intestine is pushed through a tear or weak spot in the stomach wall.

Hemodialysis

Hemodialysis is a type of dialysis that is performed using a dialysis machine. Blood will be passed into the machine via a tube connected to an "access" (we shall talk about "access" later under this subtopic). The machine will then filter the blood to eliminate excess fluid and waste products. There is a part of the dialysis machine called the dialyzer. The dialyzer acts as a filter during hemodialysis. It is modeled after the glomeruli. The dialyzer ensures that toxins and waste products are filtered out of the blood.

In contrast, protein and red blood cells, which are too big to escape the filter, are retained. After filtration, clean blood containing protein and red blood cells will be released into the blood via another tube. As a result, patients usually undergo hemodialysis thrice a week. Each hemodialysis session can last up to four hours or more, depending on the amount of waste in the blood and the dialysis machine's capacity. Hemodialysis is the most preferred dialysis treatment for most kidney failure patients.

Kidney Transplant

A kidney transplant is another option that can be used to treat kidney failure. A person who received a new kidney can go back to their normal routine, and dialysis is no longer needed. It is normally a long process before a person with kidney failure can get a compatible donor. After the transplant, you are required to take immunosuppressive drugs to prevent your body from rejecting the newly introduced kidney. A kidney transplant may not be for everyone, especially those with compromised immunity. It is best to talk to your doctor about this procedure.

One amazing thing is that our body can function well with just one kidney. When a person's kidneys fail, another person can donate one of their healthy kidneys to the kidney failure patient. After the kidney transplant, the patient and the donor can live a healthy life with one healthy kidney. In some cases, the donor may be deceased; healthy kidneys can be removed from someone who just died to replace a kidney failure patient. Thus, we have two categories of kidney transplantation: living-donor kidney transplantation and deceased donor kidney transplantation. Living donors are usually close relatives of the patient. To receive a healthy kidney from a deceased donor, you must be on a national waiting list. The procedures for benefiting from deceased donor transplantation may vary across countries.

Drugs and medication

Your doctor will either endorse angiotensin-converting enzyme (ACE) inhibitors, ramipril and lisinopril, or angiotensin receptor blockers (ARBs, for instance, olmesartan and irbesartan). However, medicines for blood pressure can slow the movement of kidney disease. Therefore, your doctor may recommend these medicines to save kidney work, regardless of whether you have hypertension.

Likewise, you may be cured with cholesterol drugs (for instance, simvastatin). These remedies can reduce blood cholesterol levels and assist kidney health. Relying upon your side effects, your doctor may also recommend medications to relieve expansion and treat anemia (decline in the number of red blood cells).

Medical Management

Suppose you have budget issues or j want to avoid dialysis or transplant altogether. In that case, there are some medical solutions that you might look into to reduce the symptoms of kidney failure.

They won't completely reverse the effects, but they might let you stay healthy until your kidneys can no longer function.

If you opt for medical management, then the first thing to do is consult with your physician, as they will point you in the right direction.

They will create a care plan to guide you on what you should and should not do. Make sure always to keep a copy of the plan wherever you go and discuss the terms with your loved ones as well.

It should be noted that most individuals who tend to go for medical management opt for hospice care.

The primary aim of hospice care is to decrease your pain and improve your final days' quality before you die.

In medical management, you can expect a hospice to:

- – Help you by providing you with a nursing home
- – Help your family and friends to support you
- – Try to improve the quality of your life as much as possible
- – Try to provide medications and care to help you manage your symptoms
- – But keep in mind that regardless of which path you take, always discuss everything with your doctor

Chapter 8: Dr. Sebi and Kidney's Health

How did Dr. Sebi address kidney diseases?

Dr. Sebi said, "Detoxification is at the heart of getting rid of kidney problems associated with mucus out of the body; there are no other ways that will bring the required result." Therefore, fasting is an essential factor that can help detoxify the body, especially the kidney. Fasting helps your body, including the blood, kidney, and liver, experience cleansing and detoxification. To achieve a cure for kidney problems, you have to be willing to make a sacrifice like the one you are about to undergo.

Detoxifying your body could end your kidney problems, depending on how serious you engage in the methods since they are not easy to eliminate.

Dr. Sebi's products used for cleansing and detoxification are Bio-Ferro, Viento, and Chelation. You can buy them at drsebiscellfood.com.

Any problem with your kidneys might lead to your blood not being purified well. It causes toxins to be accumulated in the blood. You might have a family history of kidney problems, high blood pressure, and diabetes. Recent studies show that overusing normal medications for various diseases can significantly deteriorate your kidneys' health. Many people are habitual users of medications, even for the slightest aches and pains. You have probably done it since you didn't know that these drugs could harm your health, including your heart, liver, and kidneys. Many people today have moved to a more holistic approach to their health. Dr. Sebi knew what some scientists are trying to prove today. He might have known that people today would need his help curing their kidney problems. Yes, he created an herbal remedy for kidney problems.

If you have been diagnosed with kidney disease, following Dr. Sebi's diet can help you. Make sure you talk with your doctor if you feel like something isn't quite right with your health. When you think about all the toxins being put into our bodies today, it isn't any wonder that so many people have kidney problems.

Foods to Limit to Safeguard Kidney Function

We have already seen a lot of the food that you should avoid. For that reason, I will include a few more to explain why they should be avoided. Then I will show you some incredible spice blends and seasonings that you can use on your food. And to make things even more interesting, I will show you some lip-smacking sauces and kitchen staples perfect for the renal diet.

Let's start with some foods that you should avoid.

Whole-Wheat Bread

Normally, whole-wheat bread is considered a healthy option. But for people with kidney diseases, that is not the case. The reason for this is that the more whole-wheat and bran in bread, the more potassium and phosphorus content you are likely to find in them.

A 30 gram (or 1 ounce) serving of whole-wheat bread could contain around 68 mg of potassium and 57 mg of phosphorus. If you eat plenty of it, that would potentially be too much for your kidneys.

Brown Rice

The case for avoiding brown rice is similar to the one made to avoid whole-wheat bread; it contains too much potassium and phosphorus for your body to handle. A single cup of brown rice contains about 154 mg of potassium and around 150 mg of phosphorus. Compare that to a cup of white rice. The difference is remarkable; you will find just 54 mg of potassium and around 68 mg of phosphorus in the white rice. That's less than half the amount that brown rice has!

If you do not want to include white rice into the diet, try alternatives to brown rice such as couscous, bulgur, buckwheat, and pearled barley. They are not only nutritious but delicious as well.

Dairy

Milk is often recommended for strong bones and muscles. But for those with kidney diseases, having milk increases the potassium and phosphorus content in the blood. It might be important for people to consume milk in many cases since it aids them with other medical conditions. If you require milk in your diet, ensure that you communicate your medical history, issues, current diet, and other vital information to your doctor. By doing so, you will get proper recommendations on including milk in your diet.

When you visit your doctor, make sure that you are completely honest about your medical history, habits, and diet. Of course, don't try to hide the fact that you occasionally sneak in a cup of that good, sweet, chilled soda pop in the middle of the night. But, on the other hand, don't be embarrassed to admit something if it concerns your kidneys or your health. Your doctors are not there to judge you. Trust me; there is nothing you can say that they haven't seen or heard before. And in some cases, what they might have experienced could be quite shocking to you.

Alkaline foods you should include in your daily diet

Alkaline foods help counter the potential risks of acidity and acidity refluxes, bringing some kind of relief. Most traditional Indian foods contain alkaline foods to make a balanced diet.

If you have indulged in excessive reddish meats and processed foods, isn't it about time you included some alkaline food in what you eat? Here is a list to truly get you started.

Green Leafy Vegetables

The majority of green leafy vegetables are thought to have an alkaline effect inside our system. So, without reason, our elders and wellness experts always recommend adding greens to our daily food diet. They contain important minerals essential for your body to handle various processes.

Citrus Fruits

Contrary to the fact that citric fruits are highly acidic and could have an acidic influence on your body, they will be the best way to obtain alkaline foods. Lime, lime, and oranges contain Vitamin C. They are recognized to assist in detoxifying the machine, including providing rest from acidity.

Seaweed and Ocean Salt

Did you know seaweed or ocean vegetables have 10-12 times more mineral content material than those grown on land? They are also regarded as highly alkaline meal sources and produce various advantages to the body program. You can suggest adding nori or kelp to the soup plate or making sushi at home. Or simply sprinkle some ocean salt into the salads, soups, omelets, etc.

Seasonal Fruits

Every nutritionist and wellness expert will let you know that adding seasonal fruits to your diet can benefit your well-being. They come filled with nutritional vitamins, nutrients, and antioxidants that look after various stomach functions. They may be good alkaline meal sources too.

Nuts

Don't you love to chew on nut products when food cravings activate? Besides being resources of great fats, also, they create an alkaline impact on the stomach. For this reason, add walnuts and Brazilian nuts to your daily meal strategy.

Chapter 9: Dr. Sebi Method to Heal Kidneys

Dr. Sebi's Official method for treating Chronic Kidney Disease, such as any other disease, is composed of 3 main steps. Please note that any of these parts can't be passed over to succeed in your healing journey.

The three steps I'm talking about are:

Cleansing → The body must be cleaned on an intra-cellular level through detoxification to purify each cell and remove the excess mucus.

Revitalizing → After cleansing, you need to nourish your body to regenerate your cells and strengthen the immune system.

Keeping the Body Healthy → Follow Dr. Sebi's nutrition guide and adopt healthy lifestyle habits every day to keep your mind and body in good shape.

CLEANSING

How to Prepare Cleansing Herbs?

Preparing your cleansing herbs would depend greatly on the form you purchased them. It's easier to prepare cleansing herbs that come in powder forms, as you can easily make herbal teas with them in the specified or recommended dosage. However, for other forms form herbs, especially roots or leaves, it is better to use a ratio of 1 teaspoon to 1 cup (8 oz) of spring water for each herb.

However, I recommend preparing herbs in batches of mixtures for easier batch preparation and storage. That would mean mixing them up according to function and benefit. Again, this will depend on the state of your health and what minerals are most important for you. You can combine similar herbs with similar functions into a batch. Like our healer, Dr. Sebi would say: *"If you want calcium, you know where to go to (sea moss), if you want Iron, you go to Burdock, and if you want a mix of both Iron and Fluorine, you go to Lily of the Valley".*

In all, try not to mix more than 2 or 3 herbs. Remember, these herbs are electric, and it's best to preserve their organic carbon, hydrogen, and oxygen nature as much as we can. But, again, if you mix more than that, you may not get their accurate concentrations per ml of water, so try to limit it to 3, possibly 2.

For a clearer understanding, you can use the following mix:

- Mix **Colon and gallbladder** cleansing herbs together

- Mix **liver and kidney** cleansing herbs

- Mix **respiratory and mucus cleansing** herbs

- Mix **lymphatic and heavy-metal** cleansing herbs.

Since these herbs perform a whole-body cleanse (not just colon), including the skin, eyes, colon, liver, lymphatic system, and gallbladder, you can decide to choose how to combine them. Also, note that when you make larger batches of these herbs for storage, try not to make batches that last more than 7 to 14 days.

For pre-purchase cleansing packages
Please follow the recommended dosage or instructions that are provided for that cleansing package

For fresh Green leafy herbs
- Place in spring water and boil on low heat for 5 to 7 min

- For dried leafy herbs, boil longer – 10 to 15 min

For Dried ground (or powder) herbs
For dried ground or powder leaves or roots, mix in recommended ratios for the herb. Powder herbs are the easiest to mix in dosage proportions, so you can simply follow the package instructions

For Chunks of Dried Root herbs
If you've purchased chunks of roots or stems, you can prepare them in the following way:

- Cut or break up chunks

- Place in spring water and boil for 15 minutes

- Let cool and serve

- Alternatively, prepare in larger batches and place in jars to store in the refrigerator.

For bulk purchase herbs
If you have purchased herbs in bulk and are making your teas, find out the recommended dosage for each herb. You should prepare each herbal tea ratio of 1 teaspoon to 8 ounces of spring water as a general rule.

For capsules
I recommend that you do research and find out what the recommended dosage is for each herbal capsule

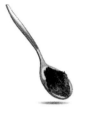 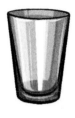

1 teaspoon **+** **1 Cup (8 oz)**
Herb **Spring water**

How To Take The Prepared Cleansing Herbs

If you are on medication, I recommend taking the herbs one hour before taking your meds; Dr. Sebi recommended this. Your colon cleansing herbs should not be consumed for longer than 30 days because your body may become dependent on them, and you want to start to reduce the dose during your last 3 to 5 days, depending on how long you've been taking them.

Routine:

- **Twice a day** - morning and night

- **Daily Consistency** - Try to stay consistent both in timing and duration. That is, try not to skew the duration. Make it consistent, and take the cleansing herb throughout the cleanse. For example, for a 14-day cleanse, the cleansing herbs can be taken twice daily, and you should take them around the same time you do take them on both mornings and evenings.

- **Gradual Wean Off** – Just like medications, it is not the best to go cold-turkey when it comes to herbal detox. Towards the end of the cleanse duration, wean off your herbs by gradually reducing the dosage and duration. The duration of the wean will depend on the length of the fast you choose. For example, I usually start weaning a week towards closure for a one-month fast. For a 14 day fast, I begin weaning on day 11 or 12. You can begin the wean by reducing it from twice a day to once a day. Or simply take half the dosages each for mornings and night.

You must do this because you need to signal to your body to start functioning independently without dependence on the cleansing herbs. And no other way to do this than to take it slow and gradual, without bringing too much "shock" to your body.

How to break a detox fast?

- Slowly reintroduce solids

If you are doing water or a liquid fast, you will need to reintroduce solid foods slowly. You can begin by introducing solids like high water-content fruits. These include watermelon, apples, and berries. After that, you can introduce softer fruit solids like bananas and avocados. Later, you can incorporate harder solids like veggies. All foods must be listed on the nutrition guide. However, if doing a fruit or raw veggie fast, you can break the fast right away on solid foods.

- Drink 1-gallon spring water daily

Drink spring water daily together with the revitalizing herbs and sea moss.

How long should you detox/cleanse?

How long you should detox depends on your state of health, that is, your body's toxification level (the less healthy you are, the more toxic your body is) and tolerance level. Typically, it is recommended to fast for 7-14 days, but Dr. Sebi recommends a minimum of at least a 12 day fast. Dr. Sebi himself fasted for 90 days to cure diabetes, asthma, and impotence. It is great to cleanse at least once a year for 7 days if you consume an alkaline diet. If you are not consuming an alkaline diet, then you should cleanse/detox every 3 months

I fasted for 14 days, and I recommend fasting for between 14 days and 1 month if you have high blood pressure. Again, your body's tolerance level will ultimately determine the length, so watch your body and study its reaction as you begin the fast. We are all different, and you may find that you cannot handle a basic liquid fast (water or juice). In that case, you can get started with fruit or raw vegetables fast. But make sure all foods and fruits are listed in the Dr. Sebi Nutrition Guide. Whether liquid, juice or raw food fast, the results are virtual all the same – the only major difference is when it takes to begin to see results. While raw food fasts take longer, liquid fasts are much faster. So do not worry; the most important thing is to stay committed and focused on whatever fasting method you choose.

Common Symptoms Expected During Detox Cleanse

- Cold and Flu symptoms
- Changes in Bowel movements
- Fatigue and Low Energy
- Difficulty sleeping
- Itching
- Headaches

- Muscle aches and pains
- Acne. Rashes and breakouts
- Mucus expels (catarrh, etc.)
- Lower blood pressure

Be happy if you relate to any of these symptoms during the cleansing stage. That's because your body is pushing out all the toxins and mucus you have been keeping inside for so long. In addition, these symptoms are only temporary and usually resolve after the first one to two weeks.

Herbs to Take During cleansing

PRODIGIOSA

Prodigiosa, also known as 'Prodijiosa or Hamula, is a perennial plant with large bushy leaves and flowers, and it's from the daisy family and native to Mexico and California. These plants have a grey-purple hue on the underside and dark green leaves on the upper side and grow up to 5 feet in height, with their flowers growing in clusters. This plant has a long history with the Mexicans. It has been used for centuries to treat diabetes, arthritis, diarrhea, and stomach disorder and relieve aching joints.

Because of the chemical and compound composition of Prodigiosa, research has shown that it is very effective for the treatment of diabetes II because it aids in stimulating the pancreatic gland to secret and reduces or lowers blood sugar level and burn down fat in the gallbladder. The irony is that Prodigiosa can cause more damage to people suffering from Type I diabetes. Furthermore, consuming Prodigiosa's tea/infusion helps boost the digestion of fat, improve bile synthesis in the liver, dissolve tiny gallstones, and treat chronic gastritis and other digestive systems disorders. Although there is no research to prove its effectiveness in treating cataracts, it is believed that it can cure cataracts.

Prodigiosa is used for several reasons, including:

- Treatment of diabetes (type II).
- Treatment of diarrhea.
- Treatment of stomach pain.
- Treatment of gallbladder disease.
- Enhancing the digestion of fat and boosting the digestive system's healthiness.

The note-full precautions to beware of before using or consuming Prodigiosa includes:

Pregnant and breastfeeding mothers should not use or consume Prodigiosa as there is no research to back it to whether it is safe or not.

It is a no-go area for people suffering from diabetes I. People with diabetes II should control their sugar levels while consuming

this herb.

How to prepare Prodigiosa tea/infusion:

- Dry the fresh leaves until it is dried.
- Once the fresh leaves are dried, or the one you ordered for is available, boil 8 or 16ounce of water and brew 1 or 2 tablespoons of Prodigiosa leaves in the warm water for 15minutes.
- After brewing it, strain the Prodigiosa leaves.
- Take a cup (8ounce) of Prodigiosa tea/infusion two times per day for the dosage.

BURDOCK ROOT

Burdock root is the root of a delicious plant called Burdock, which all its body or parts are useful as either food or medicine. This plant can be found all over the world. I called this plant the wonder plant because everything about it is important as we consume its root as food and use it for medicinal purposes. Both its leaf and seed are used for medicinal purposes.

People worldwide have been using burdock root orally to treat and prevent various health disorders for over five centuries.

Because of Burdock root's chemical composition, such as; quercetin and luteolin, research has shown that it can serve as a great effective antioxidant that can treat and prevent cancer by preventing cancerous cells from growing and mutating combating aging. A compound like 'Phytosterols' helps scalp and hair follicles grow healthy hair even from baldheads. The vitamins-C helps in boosting the immune system and combat bacterial. It also helps cleanse or detoxify the liver and lymphatic system, etc.

The potassium helps reduce blood sugar levels and filter the blood by removing impurities through the bloodstream and eradicating toxins through the skin and urine.

The benefits of using or consuming burdock root tea/infusion include:

- It cleanse/detox the liver and lymphatic system.
- Treat and prevent diabetes by reducing blood sugar levels in the body.
- Eliminate toxins from the body by inducing sweetness and urine.
- Purify the blood by removing heavy metals from the bloodstream.
- Treat various skin disorders and combat aging.
- Treat and prevent cancer by inhibiting the growth and mutation of cancerous cells.
- Boost the immune system and enhance circulation.

Until at the time of writing this book, there have been no side effects recorded by researchers or people who have used these herbs.

However, research has it that applying this root to your skin might cause rashes.

For the dosage and how to prepare Burdock root tea/infusion, kindly take the following steps:

- Scrub the uprooted root of burdock heartily under running water to remove all the dirt that accompanied it from the soil.
- You should chop the Burdock root into smaller pieces (less than 1 inch). Please note that it will come dried and already chopped if you order it online.
- Pour 2-3 cup of water into your saucepan and add ¼ cup of the chopped burdock root and boil it.
- Lower your gas once the water is boiling, re-boil it for 30-40 minutes, and put off your gas.
- Once it is cold, strain it and consume it.
- For the dosage, drink one glass cup daily

DANDELION

Dandelion is a flowering plant known as 'yellow gowan' or 'lion's tooth. This plant is native to Eurasia and today. It is common in over 60 countries worldwide in the mild climates of the northern hemisphere. For centuries, these flowering plants have been used for the treatment of swelling (inflammation) of the pancreas, relieve pains that are caused by inflammation, treat and prevent cancer, tonsils (tonsillitis), skin disorder, bladder or urethra disorder, digestive and liver problems and enhance the general health of the liver and digestive system.

Researchers proved that it is a very effective cleansing/detoxification herb because of the chemical compositions and nutrients.

The benefits of using or consuming Dandelion include:

- It helps to detoxify or cleanse the liver and the kidney.
- It helps to treat and prevent diabetes by regulating blood sugar levels.
- It helps to fight against and relieve pains that are caused by inflammation.
- It helps to deactivate and inhibit the negative effects of free radicals in the body because of its antioxidant properties.
- It reduces the level of cholesterol.
- It lowers blood pressure by getting rid of excess fluid in the body.
- It helps to naturally shed excess weight gain by improving the metabolism of carbohydrates.
- It helps in boosting the digestive system.
- It helps to boost the immune system.
- It helps to keep the skin healthy and treat and prevent skin diseases.

Till at the time of writing this book, Dandelion is 100% safe, but consuming an overdose of it can result in some side effects like:

Experiencing stomach upset or irritation

Allergic reactions

The special precautions before using/consuming dandelions are:

Pregnant and breastfeeding mothers should stay off dandelion as there is no research to know if it is harmful to them or not.

If you are suffering from Eczema, stay off dandelion as more than 85% of people with eczema suffer an allergic reaction to dandelion.

For the dosage and how to prepare Dandelion tea/infusion, kindly take the following steps:

- Get some fresh leaves of dandelion and wash them under running water to remove all the dirt.
- After washing it, pour ½ - 1 cup of the washed dandelion into your saucepan.
- You should boil 4-5 cups of water and pour the boiled water inside the saucepan. Next, you pour the dandelion and cover it for 12-15 hours or throughout the night (overnight).
- The next day, strain out the dandelion leaves, and you will be left with the dandelion tea/infusion.

- For the dosage, take ½ tablespoon of Dandelion per ¾ cup of water three times daily. And if you ordered your dandelion online, you can take 4-10 grams of dry leaf of dandelion three times daily.

ELDERBERRY

Elderberry is a dark purple berry from the elder tree, also known as European Black Elderberry or Sambucus Bacchae. This plant is a flowering plant from the family of Adoxaceae and native to Europe. Both the leaves and fruit (berries) of elderberry have been used for centuries to treat pain and swelling arising from inflammation. It also helps to stimulate urine production and induce sweat to detoxify the body system.

Because of how rich elderberry is with various compounds and nutrients like vitamin-C, dietary fiber, phenolic acids, which is a great and powerful antioxidant that helps to prevent and decrease the damage that is caused by oxidative stress in the body, it also contains some compounds like flavonols such as kaempferol, quercetin, isorhamnetin and anthocyanins which gives the fruit the black-purple color and makes it a strong antioxidant and anti-inflammation agent.

Elderberry also contains some nutrients, like:

- Calories

- Carbs

- Minute amounts of protein and fat

- And anthocyanins, making the plant a strong and effective antioxidant with anti-inflammatory properties.

The benefits of using/consuming elderberry include:

- It helps cleanse and detoxify the lungs and respiratory system by eliminating mucus from the upper respiratory system and the lungs.

- It helps to treat constipation.

- It helps to treat flu and cold in less than 24hours.

- It combats harmful bacteria in the body by preventing bacterial growth through its antibacterial properties.

- It boosts and supports the immune defense system by increasing white blood cell production.

- It protects and keeps the skin healthy.

- It helps to relieve chronic fatigue syndrome and depression.

Till at the time of writing this book, there is no record of any side effects from researchers and people who have used elderberry, but because of the compound that is present in elderberry, it will be wise to use it for not more than 12 weeks and take a break for at least a week before using it again.

The special precautions before using elderberry include:

- Ensure children below 12 years do not use/consume elderberries, and children above 12 and under 18 should not use them for more than 10days.

- Since there is no reliable information to know if elderberries are safe or not for pregnant and breastfeeding mothers, I strongly advise that they stay off elderberries.

- People who have a history of suffering from an autoimmune disease like; multiple sclerosis, lupus, rheumatoid arthritis, etc., should stay off elderberry as it has the potency to boost the immune system to become more active which could worsen their situation.

- Since elderberries have the potency to increase or boost the immune defense system, any medications designed to decrease the immune system's function will certainly interact with Elderberry.

For the dosage and how to prepare Elderberry tea/infusion, kindly take the steps below:

- Boil 8-12oz of water in your saucepan.
- Once the water is boiling, measure one tablespoon of dried elderberries and add it to the boiling water.
- Reduce your gas and allow it to boil for at least 15 minutes.
- After the 15 minutes timing, allow it to get cold and strain it using a filter.
- For the dosage, consume 3-4 cups daily.

SARSAPARILLA ROOT

Sarsaparilla root is the root of a tropical wood climbing vine that belongs to the genus Smilax family. Dr. Sebi recommends it as a revitalizing herb for many diseases, including cancer, because it is rich in iron, calcium, and phosphate.

The benefits of consuming Sarsaparilla roots are:

- It helps to destroy and prevent cancerous cells from mutating.
- It binds the endotoxins responsible for the lesions in psoriasis patients and eliminates them from the body system.
- It helps to fast-track healing and recovery.
- It treats and prevents health issues caused by inflammations like joint pain, swelling of any parts of the body, arthritis, rheumatoid, etc.
- It soothes and heals sexually transmitted diseases such as syphilis, herpes, gonorrhea etc.
- It helps to treat and prevent leprosy
- It helps protect and reverse damages done to the liver to function perfectly.
- It makes the body absorb nutrients and other herbs easily

There are no side effects attributed to this herb's consumption when writing this book. However, because of the 'saponins' that it contains, I advise you to consult your doctor before using this herb, as saponins can cause stomach irritation.

For the dosage and how to prepare sarsaparilla root tea, kindly take the following steps:

- Harvest some sarsaparilla plant roots and wash them under running water to remove all the dirt that accompanied it from the soil.
- After washing it, pill off the outer skin, chop it into smaller pieces and dry it in a well-ventilated place (indoors) for at least seven days (ensure you turn the drying root daily for the seven days until it is completely dried.) iii. Once it is dried, store it in a paper bag or cardboard box. (Ensure you don't store it in a plastic container as it will get mold).
- Measure 1teaspoon of the dried chopped Sarsaparilla root and add it to your saucepan and add 8 ounces of water. Boil it for 15-20minutes v. Strain it using a filter. You are done!
- For the dosage, consume 1cup (8ounce) 3 times daily.

GUACO

Guaco is a climbing plant with different names like Huaco, Guace, or Vejuco. This climbing plant belongs to the Asteraceae and cordifolia species' family and is rich in numerous minerals and compounds. Its leaves are very medicinal and nutritional. The people of Aztecs used them to clean the blood system and clear heavy metals from the bloodstream.

There are a lot of benefits that one can benefit from using or consuming Guaco. Some of them are:

- It lessens the effect or symptoms of snake poison.

- It is used to thin the blood through the coumarin activities it contains (anticoagulant and blood-thinning.)

- It helps to combat inflammation through its anti-inflammatory properties.

- It treats stomach irritation through the effect of its cleansing activities.

- It helps treat respiratory disorders like coughs, rheumatism, bronchitis, etc.

- It enhances quick recovery from the wound.

- It helps to cleanse or detoxify the blood and skin by clearing heavy metals from the blood.

- It boosts and builds the immune defense system.

- It can treat some infections diseases such as; candida yeast infection, herpes, etc.

There are no severe side effects that researchers or uses have recorded until writing this book.

Like I said earlier, Guaco is 100% safe for consumption by mouth, but if you are taking or using any Coumadin drugs, please consult with your doctor before using it.

And if you have any history of bleeding, do not use Guaco unless your doctor approves of it. Like I said earlier, Guaco helps to thin the blood, so any medications that can thin the blood or slow blood clotting do interact with Guaco.

For the dosage and how to prepare Guaco tea/infusion, kindly take the following steps:

- Get some handful of fresh Guaco and wash it under running water or 2 ounces of its dried leaves if you have the dried ones.
- Pour about 6cups of water in your saucepan together with the Guaco leaves. Boil it until it is reduced to 2 cups.
- You can add some brown sugar (optional) if you add the brown sugar; allow it to boil for another 20 minutes.
- Strain the syrup with a strainer.
- You should bottle it and store it in a refrigerator.
- For dosage, take 1 soupspoon 3-4 times daily.

EUCALYPTUS TREE

The eucalyptus tree is a fast-growing evergreen tree native of Australia. This plant's leaves and bark are used for medicinal purposes like joint and muscle pain, cold, cough, congestion, etc. However, the Chinese, Greek, and Indian Ayurvedic people have incorporated this amazing herb to treat various conditions for thousands of years before now.

This plant/tree has more than 400 different species. The most used is the Eucalyptus globulus or the Australian fever tree, also known as Blue Gum.

Eucalyptus leaves cineole that is also known as eucalyptol, in which the leaf's gland contains essential oil (eucalyptus oil) and also; flavonoids and tannins, which are plant-based antioxidants that aid in reducing inflammation, controlling blood sugar, fighting against the activities of bacteria and fungi and the oil can help in relieving pain and inflammation as well as blocking chemicals that usually cause asthma.

The benefits of using or consuming eucalyptus tea/infusion include:

- Cleansing the skin through steaming/sauna.
- Relieving common cold symptoms like cough lozenges and inhalants and also sore throat and sinusitis
- Relieving symptoms of bronchitis. Inhaling the vapor of eucalyptus tea helps serve as a decongestant by loosening phlegm and easing congestion.
- It aids in relieving asthma: research showed that eucalyptus has the potency to break up mucous in people who have asthma.
- It aids in dental plaque and improves gingivitis
- It helps in improving bad breath

Until writing this book, eucalyptus leaves are 100% safe for consumption.

However, eucalyptus oil is not as safe as the leaves. Applying the oil directly to the skin without diluting it can lead to serious nervous system problems.

For the dosage and how to prepare eucalyptus tea/infusion, kindly take the following steps:

- Boil water to 194-205 Fahrenheit. Alternatively, you can boil the water and drop it down for a minute or two to reduce the temperature.
- Pour a teaspoon of dried eucalyptus leaf into a teacup/mug.
- Pour 6 ounces of water inside the teacup/mug and allow the leaves to be steep for 10-15minutes.
- Get a filter to strain the loose leaves of the eucalyptus.
- You are a god. You can now enjoy the cup of eucalyptus tea/infusion at a go.
- For the dosage, take 3-4 cups per day.

REVITALIZING

Revitalization is restoring, rejuvenating, and recovering all the energy the body has lost due to the disease it has suffered from and during the cleansing period. According to Dr. Sebi, all the revitalizing herbs are rich in phosphate, calcium, iron, etc. Therefore, the body needs a speedy recovery.

The recommended revitalizing herbs for kidneys health include:

IRISH SEA MOSS

Irish Sea Moss is red algae that belong to the family of Florideophytes that grows on the rocky parts of the Atlantic coast of various countries, including the British Isles, Jamaica, Scotland, etc. Dr. Sebi recommends this herb for revitalizing the body after cleansing because it has over 92 out of 102 minerals that the body needs to be healthy. Some minerals are, for example:

- Phosphorus
- Iodine
- Selenium
- Calcium
- Bromine
- Iron
- Potassium

Some of the benefits of consuming Irish Sea Moss are:

- It heals and boosts the immune defense system.
- It treats and prevents hyperthyroidism and boosts the functionalities and health of the thyroid.
- It helps to soothe joint pain and swelling and treat arthritis.
- It helps to enrich the overall mood and reduce fussiness.
- It helps to combat infections caused by viruses and bacterial.
- It helps treat and prevent various skin disorders like acne, skin wrinkling, and alleviating inflammation.
- It helps to treat and prevent digestive and respiratory tract disorders.

The note-full precautions to beware of before consuming Irish Sea moss include:

Because of how rich Irish Sea moss is with iron can trigger hypothyroidism for people suffering from Hashimoto's disease.

Stop using the herb if you notice any allergies or reactions.

For the dosage and how to prepare Irish Sea Moss tea, kindly take the steps below:

- Measure and boil 1cups (8ounce) of water in a ceramic pot.
- Once the water is boiled, measure 2-3 tablespoons of Irish Sea moss gel (or 1teaspoon for the fine form) and add it to the boiling water.
- Allow the Irish Sea moss for 10-15 minutes to dissolve completely.
- You are done!
- For the dosage, take 1cup of Irish Sea moss tea daily in the morning.

PAO PEREIRA

Pao Pereira is a tree that belongs to the Apocynaceae family and is native to South America. This tree's bark is rich in various compounds that effectively destroy, eliminate, and inhibit cancerous cells. Because of and how effective the bark of this tree is, Dr. Sebi recommends this herb to revitalize the body system after cleansing.

The benefits of consuming Pao Pereira include:

- treating malaria and other infections caused by parasites.

- It helps treat and prevent cancer by destroying cancer and preventing cancerous cells from mutation.

- Soothing and relieving liver pain.

- It helps to treat and prevent stomach disorders like constipation and irritation.

- It helps to boost sexual arousal

Till at the time of writing this book, no side effect is attributed to the consumption of Pao Pereira; but since there is no vital information to show that this herb is 100% safe for pregnant and breastfeeding mothers, I advise that they avoid this herb's consumption.

For the dosage and how to prepare Pao Pereira tea, kindly take the steps below:

- Harvest some Pao Pereira by cutting some of its bark down the tree, chopping it, and drying it.

- Once it is dried, boil 1liter of water and pour two tablespoons of the dried Pao Pereira into the boiling water.

- Lower the heat of the fire to a medium-low and place the lid on the pot.

- Boil the mixture at medium temperature for 20 minutes.

- Allow it to get cold and train it using a strainer or filter.

You are done!

For the dosage, consume 1 cup of tea times daily.

SOURSOP

Soursop is the fruit of the "Annona Muricata" tree, a native of tropical regions in the Americas that belong to the Annonaceae family. Its leaves are widely used because they are rich in various nutrients like iron, calcium, phosphorus, magnesium, sodium, potassium, zinc, etc. That makes the tea very effective in fighting against the mutation of cancerous cells.

Other benefits of consuming soursops tea are:

- It helps to destroy and eliminate cancerous cells and inhibit the growth of cancer cells.
- It is a very strong and effective antioxidant that helps neutralize free radicals that damage the cells.
- It helps to soothe heart disorders.
- It helps lower blood sugar levels for people who have type 2 diabetes.
- It helps to fight against infectious diseases caused by bacterial. Such diseases like yeast infections, cholera, gingivitis, Staphylococcus, tooth decay etc.
- It helps to soothe and alleviate swelling (inflammation) etc.

The note-full precautions before consuming soursops tea include:

Since there is no information about this herb's harmful effects on pregnant and breastfeeding mothers, I advise that they stay off this herb.

Although this herb is tempting, please make sure you consume this herb under a medical practitioner's supervision.

For the dosage and how to prepare soursops tea, kindly take the following steps:

- Harvest some fresh Soursops leaves, dry them until it is dried, chop them, or pound them into smaller pieces. On the other hand, you can place an order online, and it will come dried and chopped.
- Measure 1 teaspoon of the chopped leaves of the Soursops and pour it into your teacup or mug.
- Boil 8 ounces of water and add it to the Soursop leaves in the teacup or mug and cover it.
- Allow the leaves to steep for 10-15 minutes and strain them.
- You are done!
- For the dosage, consume 2-3 cups of Soursops tea daily.

When Should I Consume the Revitalizing Herbs?

The best time to consume the revitalizing herbs is the next day after finishing your cleanse. For instance, if you fast for 14days, on the 15day, you should start consuming your revitalizing herbs.

What Are the Things That I Shouldn't Forget?

Drink at least a gallon of spring water daily.

Eat foods only on Dr. Sebi's nutritional guide once you are done with your detox /cleanse.

Consume the revitalizing herbs, including Irish Sea moss and sarsaparilla root.

Ensure you do an intra-cellular cleanse once per year for at least 7days if you consume only an alkaline diet from Dr. Sebi's nutritional guide. Still, you should always do an intra-cellular cleansing after every three months if you are not.

Please note that consuming acidic food can only put your body at the risk of relapsing.

KEEPING THE BODY HEALTHY

Maintaining a Healthy Weight

Maintaining a healthy weight is important for renal patients. Frequent weight changes may further damage your kidneys and harm your health. You need to make sure that you are not overeating to make up because you are missing out on certain types of meals. In addition, you are restricted from some food groups that may harm your condition and damage your renal functions. The best way of maintaining a healthy weight is to eat regularly and try having smaller meal portions with fewer calories while taking all the nutrients you need. Follow up with tips we have previously listed for healthier weight maintenance, which means that you should avoid extra fat, sugar, and processed foods for the best results. Eating regularly and establishing a routine with your meals are also recommended. As mentioned earlier in the book, when it comes to food preparation, use cooking techniques that originally required less oil and fat. Your diet may be diverse; however, you need to take care of portions, avoid responding to food cravings, and eat more than your body needs.

Watch Your Calorie Intake

Calories should be watched closely in terms of avoiding consuming empty calories. This kind can give you the energy your body needs, but that won't offer the essential nutrients that your body needs. Empty calories are usually found in sweets, sugary beverages, and snacks. Avoid munching on snacks and sweets and find healthier alternatives in fruit and vegetables. These food groups will provide you with essential nutrients and fewer calories than processed food with added sugar or sodium.

Don't Take Weight Supplements

Maintaining a healthy weight is important for your health and will help you live a normal life even when your renal system is giving you a hard time; however, you should never take an alternative in a shortcut, meaning that you shouldn't rely on weight supplements and weight loss products for helping you lose or maintain your weight. Weight supplements may impose more threat to your health by adding more toxins and waste to your organism.

No Over-the-Counter Pills and Medications

Common pain killers are usually taken and bought over the counter and without a prescription and used to diminish or relieve pain. Anti-inflammatory drugs raise the risk of getting kidney disease or worsening the kidney's condition when taken regularly. Avoid taking painkillers unless prescribed by your doctor otherwise. If in pain, talk to your physician or a doctor specialist about which medications are safe for you. Avoid taking any type of medicines and pills that are no9t specifically prescribed for you and your doctor. Your condition will most certainly worsen. In addition, you will be putting extra pressure on your kidneys due to these medications' consumption.

Avoid Sweets and Sugar-packed Goods

Patients with diabetes represent a risk group for getting chronic kidney diseases. In contrast, patients with kidney conditions may worsen with frequent sugar consumption and processed foods with added sugar. Just as we recommend cutting on your salt consumption to avoid having an increased sodium level in your body and further complications caused by redundant sodium, it is likewise recommended to cut on your sugar intake. Sugar may cause diabetes if taken regularly and in large quantities and should be avoided. You may use fruit as a healthier alternative but avoid high-potassium foods such as bananas.

Get Plenty of Sleep

Sleep deprivation may cause all kinds of health conditions that cause further damage to the body. That's because we use sleep to help our cells renew and our bodies recover. Whenever we don't get enough sleep, we get tired, feel fatigued, our blood pressure fluctuates, we lose focus, and we are often unable to perform the daily tasks we normally do. Not getting the sleep you need will also make your body more prone to all kinds of diseases and illnesses. In contrast, it will make your entire body feel alarmed and stressed, which should further have a devastating effect on your renal health. So make sure to address your body's needs and get as much sleep as you need.

Eat Healthily

Eating healthy should be the centerpiece of your new lifestyle. Healthy food improves health and has numerous benefits for our bodies and minds. However, when eating unhealthy food in the long run, we introduce our body to lots of waste that our organism doesn't need. The role of kidneys and our renal functions is crucial for our well-being. In cases where renal function is weak, slow, or failing in performance, waste introduced through an unhealthy diet causes various damage to the body.

Furthermore, it brings more damage to the kidneys and renal system, creating a vicious circle where your health condition is only getting worse. Make sure to cut on fast food and snacks, junk food, processed food, sweets, and food packed with salt and additives. Instead, focus on fresh groceries and healthily prepared food.

Check Your Blood Pressure

Blood pressure is the cause of many serious health conditions. It also represents one of the main causes and symptoms of renal diseases. High blood pressure causes kidney damage, harms cardiovascular health, and causes a heart attack. If you have high blood pressure, you should cut your sodium intake. At the same time, kidney patients are advised to lower their sodium intake at all costs to prevent increased blood pressure that is more likely to be triggered by salt intake and consumption of bad fat and highly processed foods.

Check Your Blood Sugar

As mentioned earlier, kidney disease can even be triggered by diabetes. In cases where patients develop diabetes due to an improper diet or/and genetic predispositions, kidney disease's overall condition is set to worsen. That is why we recommend cutting on sugary treats and beverages, added sugar, and processed foods. In addition, prepare your food by yourself to follow up on the amounts of sugar present in your everyday diet.

Quit Smoking!

Smoking may cause all kinds of cancer, stroke, heart attack, and cardiovascular diseases, increasing kidney cancer. Patients who have already been diagnosed with kidney disease should stop smoking as inhaling cigarette smoke may cause further damage to the kidneys because smoking slows down the flow of blood that runs through the kidneys, disabling these vital organs from performing crucial functions for your health.

Cut Your Meat Meals

Meat is packed with protein, and your kidneys are set to eject the leftover waste produced when our organism processes the protein. In addition, our muscles take what they need from nutrients introduced with meat. Meat is delicious and nutritious, yes; however, too much meat is surely set to mess with your health and will place more pressure on your kidneys. Processed protein creates waste that your body needs to eliminate; as mentioned before, this waste is called urea and creatinine. Our body ejects it with the help of kidneys and through urine, keeping us healthy and our body free of waste. To improve your renal health, you may seek meat substitution in salmon or start eating meat moderately and in smaller portions. The general recommendation would be twice to three times a week, once a day, for meat portions, while you should also make sure to cook your meat with less oil and no fat added. Make sure to choose meat pieces with less fat and more lean meat. Cook or slow cook your meat with herbs and spices instead of frying your meat and adding salt.

No Alcohol

Drinking is proven to have devastating effects on kidneys, even in people who haven't been diagnosed with a form of kidney disease, as frequently. Excess alcohol consumption increases the risk of chronic kidney disease and brings extended damage to an already damaged renal system. Stay away from alcohol, even if you feel tempted. Alcohol is another form of liquid that your kidneys need to process and take care of, alongside introducing toxins to your body that may cause inflammation. Sugary alcohol beverages also contribute to weight gain, which could bring more damage to your kidneys.

Dietary Choices for a Healthier Lifestyle

Carbohydrates and Fiber: Although carbohydrates may be difficult to process at later stages of kidney disease, they provide a vital energy source to combat lethargy feelings. As a low protein diet is recommended, carbohydrates can also help to replace calories. Some carbohydrates are also sources of fiber. It is recommended that you eat at least 25 grams of fiber per day, even when suffering from stage 5 kidney disease and undergoing dialysis. You may become frustrated when trying to count your fiber levels. Many high fibrous foods are also high in potassium, phosphorous, and fluid (all restricted). The food lists are a useful starting point for ingredients and various nutritional values.

Fats: Fats often get a bad reputation as we don't distinguish between healthy and unhealthy fats. Polyunsaturated and monounsaturated fats are healthy when consumed in moderation, whereas trans fats and saturated fats should be avoided.

Protein: Although bodybuilders usually come to mind when we think of protein, it is an essential component of our diets and vital for repairing tissues, keeping infections at bay, and, of course, building muscle, even in the most exercise-phobic of us! Suppose you have chronic kidney disease in the first few stages. In that case, it is usually advised to consume protein for up to 15% of your daily diet, with carbohydrates and fats making up 85%, the same amount recommended for an average adult's daily intake. At stage 4, this recommendation usually decreases to only 10% protein. During stage 5, if you are on dialysis, the dialysis will filter out the waste toxins from your body and protein; therefore, you must include protein as part of your diet. Please note that you must follow your doctor's advice on how much protein you consume at each stage. It depends on various factors such as your height, weight, and which stage of the disease you have. Always consult a professional for individual guidance before making any changes to your diet.

Phosphorus and Calcium: Phosphates are salt compounds that include salt and other minerals; they work, as it does calcium, to strengthen and keep our bones healthy. Our kidneys usually remove extra phosphorous from the blood. Still, kidney disease will prevent this process from functioning as it should. Unfortunately, it's not as simple as just removing all phosphates from your diet as they are pretty much in most foods, but we can look out for those high in phosphorous. A list of foods identifies low, medium, or high in phosphorous. You should typically stay away from processed foods as these often contain additives. Too much phosphorus can also lead to a calcium deficit, which can, in turn, lead to the extreme bouts of itchiness that many chronic kidney disease sufferers report. If low calcium levels persist, this can lead to further pain, a general weakening of the bones, and even bone disease. It might be that your doctor will recommend taking a calcium supplement if your phosphorus levels remain too high. After this, medicines known as phosphorous binders may be required but always consult a professional.

Fluids: As the kidneys start to decrease in functionality, waste toxins and excess liquids are not removed from the body as they should be. That may lead to your doctor recommending you limit the liquids you consume. This is more likely during the later stages of kidney disease, and you should consult a professional for specific advice.

Potassium: This is a mineral that has an essential role in keeping your heart healthy and regulating water levels in the body. Again, this is another mineral usually removed when in excess through the kidney filtration system. Too much of one particular mineral is problematic as the kidneys cannot remove it in the way they can when they are completely healthy. Still, extremely low levels are also harmful. Potassium is commonly found in many fruits and vegetables—stick with watermelon, berries, apples, cherries, pears, grapes, and peaches as low potassium fruits.

Iron: Anyone whose chronic kidney disease has resulted in anemia will need extra iron in their diet. As some iron-rich sources may conflict with other dietary considerations such as protein, ensure you find out from your doctor which sources of iron you can have.

7 Worst Foods for your Health

1) Alcohol

2) Soy

3) Eggs

4) Dairy

5) Sweetened Juices

6) Coffee

7) Any kind of Meat

10 Important Alkaline Fruits and Vegetables that Fit the Alkaline Diet

1) Cucumber

2) Onions

3) Zucchini

4) Avocado

5) Lettuce

6) Elderberries

7) Seeded grapes

8) Mango

9) Papaya

10) Tamarind

Manage your Stress During Kidney Failure

When you are suffering from kidney failure, it's normal to be stressed out all the time. However, it might lead you to skip meals or even forget your medication, which might affect your health even more.

But you need to understand that life is full of hurdles and setbacks, and you really can't let them hold you back.

In that light, here are six tips to help you keep your stress under control:

Make sure to take some time just to relax and unwind. Try to practice deep breathing, visualization, meditation, or even muscle relaxation. These will help you stay calm and keep your body healthy.

Try to accept the things that are not under your control, and you can't change. Trying to enforce a chance on something that is not within your reach will only make things worse. Better advice is to look for better ways of handling the situation instead of changing it.

Don't pressure yourself; try to be good and don't expect much. You are a human being, after all, right? You can make mistakes, so accept that. Just try your best.

And lastly, always try to maintain a positive attitude. Even when things go completely wrong, try to see the good instead of the bad and focus on that. Try to find things in all phases of your life that make you happy and that you appreciate, such as your friends, work, health, and family, for example. You have no idea how much help a simple change of perspective can bring.

Keep yourself hydrated

You should always ensure that you are sufficiently hydrated, but you shouldn't overdo this. No studies have shown that over-hydration is good for enhancing the performance of your kidneys. It is good to drink sufficient water, and you can drink around four to six glasses of water per day. Consuming more water than this wouldn't help your kidneys perform better. It would just increase the stress on your kidneys.

Read the labels carefully

The next time you go shopping for groceries, make sure you carefully read the labels on food products. Read the nutritional chart that's printed on the cover, and if you don't recognize anything on it, it's better if you don't pick it up. You need to be very careful about the food products you consume when on a renal failure diet.

Accept Practical and Emotional Support

If you have a network of encouraging you, it is advantageous for your health, mostly emotional encouragement or support. Research conducted has put side by side individuals who had the most and smallest amount of social support. It was recorded that those who had the most social support had a much better quality of healthy life and lived longer.

Below are some recommended ideas for building a support system:

Request for assistance or for someone who can listen. Individuals, in most cases, want to assist but do not know how to go about it. Therefore, you will have to be precise and state your request.

Enter into a support group. Sharing with other people who have related experiences might assist you to cope.

Encourage others; It will form a healthy cycle of giving and receiving.

Avoid Environmental Toxins

Reduce your exposure to environmental toxins that can raise your chances of having cancer and other deadly diseases, including asbestos, formaldehyde, tobacco smoke, styrene (seen in Styrofoam), and tetrachloroethylene (perchloroethylene).

Prepare Your Meals

The best way of knowing what you are consuming to the tiniest detail is to prepare your food by yourself; you may love take-outs and nights when you have your dinner out but try to prepare most of your food by yourself, including your snacks. When making your meals, make sure that the food you are using is mostly fresh and low in sodium, potassium, and low concentrations of other nutrients that can harm your renal health. Try to take your lunch from home when going to work instead of eating in a cafeteria or a restaurant. Focus on preparing meals by boiling, steaming, slow cooking, or baking instead of frying techniques.

No Added Salt and Processed Foods

Besides encouraging more fresh groceries with low-sodium and low-potassium concentrations, we also encourage you to avoid adding salt to your meals and follow up with food labels to ensure that you are not consuming food with high concentrations of sodium and potassium. Processed foods such as processed meat, boxed and packaged goods, snacks, junk food and fast food, sweets and cookies, candy, and similar sugary treats are bad for you in general, and with added salt may additionally harm our kidneys and slow down your renal functions, that way damaging your kidneys as these vital organs are not able to process and level all the sodium in your body with the presence of chronic kidney disease.

Watch for Your Potassium Intake

Follow up with the grocery list we have made on foods normally low in potassium concentrations so that your body may receive the quantity of this vital mineral it needs without struggling with excess waste. However, be aware that some low-sodium products may have increased potassium concentrations. Consult your doctor on potassium and discuss the average amount of potassium you may have weekly and daily with your condition.

Be Active and Exercise

Being active and exercising is important for everyone. Your body needs activity to burn calories that you introduce to your body with every meal. Physical activity also encourages serotonin production – the happiness hormone – which makes you feel motivated and refreshed once healthy physical activity becomes a part of your routine. Physical condition is great for your health and should help you battle issues with your renal health. However, ensure not to overestimate yourself or underestimate the effects of activity and exercising.

Common forms of exercise include:

- Stair climbing
- Tai Chi
- Stretching
- Yoga
- Cycling
- Walking
- Swimming

To perform these normal workouts, you don't have to join a gym or even buy any sort of expensive equipment! Instead, you can simply take a walk around your streets, do yoga at home, and so on.

Just make sure to consult with your doctor to determine which exercise is suitable for you and adjust it to your dialysis routine.   If you were already consuming healthy foods, it would also make sense if you were exercising regularly because regular physical activity will prevent weight gain and regulate your blood pressure. But you should be careful about the amount of time you exercise or how much you exercise, especially if you aren't acclimatized to exercising. Don't overexert yourself if you are just getting started. This would increase your kidneys' pressure and break down your muscles.

Seek treatment for hypertension

Pressure is now considered the leading cause of chronic renal failure. According to nephrologist Nestor Scho, professor at Unifesp, the increase in blood pressure damages the kidneys' blood vessels and may cause hypertensive nephropathy. "This way, the organ becomes overloaded, and little by little loses its filtering capacity," he explains. Taking care of hypertension is essential even when it is not the cause of chronic renal failure. It becomes even more important in the advanced stage of the disease.

Control of diabetes

"Diabetes is the second leading cause of chronic renal failure," says nephrologist Lucio Roberto Moura of Hospital Israelita Albert Einstein. That is because the disease triggers the so-called 'diabetic nephropathy, a change in kidney vessels that leads to a protein loss in the urine. Also, diabetes favors atherosclerosis, forming plaque fat in the arteries that hinder the kidneys' filtration work. Over time, more and more toxic substances are trapped in the body, leading to death. Therefore, one way to detect the problem is to do urine tests to determine if the protein is eliminated. Those already diagnosed with diabetes need to be more aware of their kidney health.

Chapter 10: Supplements

The very best approach to acquire the critical substances you desire (minerals, vitamins, essential fatty acids, fats -- the list continues on and on) is via a balanced, healthful, nutritional supplement (one which is 100 percent natural if possible). However, the truth is that several individuals have quite a difficult time eating enough of the ideal sorts of foods to acquire the materials they require in the right amounts. That is why it is highly suggested that you carefully think about using nutritional supplements to improve the quantities of important stuff your body needs to work at its best.

It might appear overwhelming to consider carrying ten (or more) distinct supplements daily but remember that doing this could be a true advantage to your body and head. Additionally, it might allow you to stay longer and much healthier. Nevertheless, suppose you are aware that you are getting a fantastic amount of a few of these chemicals in your diet plan. You are interested in maintaining the number of supplements you are taking comparatively low. In that case, you can correct your nutritional regimen so.

Here is one important note to remember while you're considering nutritional supplements: Your daily recommended allowances for vitamins, minerals, nutritional supplements, and other chemicals that you see on food labels do not indicate a great deal. These tips show you the minimum quantities necessary for the body to keep working properly. However, they do not let you know what amounts you will need for the body to go beyond that foundation level.

Multivitamin

Some people today choose a once-a-day multivitamin. While that is better than simply taking nothing in any way, the tablet likely does not include large enough dosages of all the vitamins you want. How can I know? Suppose a once-a-day vitamin comprised adequately substantial doses of 14 essential vitamins. In that case, it might need to be as large as a golf club. The majority of the multivitamins offering comprehensive vitamin policy ask that you take a few pills every day. Four capsules or tablets per day is a fairly typical number.

A variety of great brands and moderately priced options can be found. You would like to locate an organization that does third-party analysis. Most of their better products aren't offered across the counter. They have to be bought via an undercover doctor or a drugstore involved in natural wellbeing. Guarantee that the multivitamin you select includes a great calcium source, and be certain it functions as calcium hydroxylapatite rather than calcium carbonate. You do not automatically realize the differences between both; simply ensure your multivitamin involves the former rather than the latter.

Multimineral

In general, you will need to provide your system using 16 distinct nutritional supplements if you want it to perform at an optimum level.

Multimineral nutritional supplements are simple to discover. In several instances, you can discover multivitamin/multi-mineral combination nutritional supplements. However, these options can be challenging. First, you have to be certain if you decide to go that path; you purchase an option that comprises all 14 vitamins and 16 nutritional supplements. (That is rather a good deal!)

If you pick a multi-mineral supplement, go with one that features chelated minerals. I will spare you all of the full details of this procedure, which produces chelated minerals. But remember that you are likely paying for nutritional supplements that wind up in your bathroom rather than on your own body's major systems unless you are getting chelated minerals.

Do not choose a multi-mineral supplement that arrives out of a clay resource. These goods aren't chelated, plus they feature tin, silver, and nickel. Sometimes they even record lead as a component!

Omega-3 Fatty Acids

You have probably read or heard about omega-3 fatty acids in the news lately. The significance of this essential fatty acid was getting a great deal of press and great reason. It is one of these substances your body needs to endure and flourish. But unfortunately, despite all of the wonderfully intricate chemical processes your own body can perform, it cannot fabricate omega-3 fatty acids.

To avoid germs but get your omega-3 supplement, use liquid fish oil or some capsule or soft gel. Take 1 g twice per day to get what you want.

Resveratrol

Resveratrol is a highly effective antioxidant, and I recommend that everybody get a dose of this every day. Resveratrol has generated a higher profile as a Harvard Medical School case study. A couple of years back, a fairly dramatic gain in mice's health and lifespan was revealed after they were given resveratrol. Should you read up about this particular antioxidant, you're likely to see it is in red wine, which is the reality. However, suppose you wished to receive an important dose of resveratrol from red wine. In that case, you'd need to glug a couple of hundred bottles of the material daily, which will kill you before you have to enjoy the advantages of resveratrol.

The fantastic thing is you can purchase resveratrol supplements in many health food shops and any vitamin store, either in person or on the internet. You will find it labeled either as resveratrol or red wine extract. I suggest getting 30 mg every day, which ought to be somewhat simple, given the width of nutritional supplement options available in the industry.

Vitamin C

If you choose a fantastic multivitamin, you will likely get a fantastic amount of vitamin C every day. But do not believe for a moment you are getting all your body should truly have the ability to work on a full degree.

I suggest carrying a 1,000-milligram vitamin C supplement two times every day. I know that seems like a great deal, but if you've read about it, you understand why I believe very strongly that vitamin C is a massive blessing for your great health. Though it's within plenty of vegetables and fruits, it may continue to be hard to get enough of the things on your diet plan. Hundreds (maybe thousands) of vitamin C supplement options are available, so do some research and speak with your naturopathic physician to discover which ones are ideal for you.

If you are fighting a disease, take 8,000 mg of vitamin C daily rather than the normal 2,000 mg.

Vitamin B Complex

The term vitamin B complex describes B vitamins: B1, B2, B3, B5, B6, B7, B9, and B12. A number of the B vitamins also have several other widely used titles – riboflavin and niacin are just two great examples.

The assortment of important features the vitamin B complex performs on the human body is shocking. I would not even try to cover all of the details. Just know that if you want to be healthy and live a long, comfy lifestyle, you had better concentrate on getting lots of B vitamins.

It's a fantastic idea to have a vitamin B complex supplement and a multivitamin daily. You'll discover such a supplement that can provide you exactly what you need in just one dose every day.

Magnesium

Several strong studies performed over the past couple of years have demonstrated powerful connections between elevated levels of magnesium intake and cardiovascular disease avoidance. Individuals who get lots of calcium – within their diets and during supplementing – normally possess a reduced heart disease risk. Additionally, magnesium is also involved in approximately 300 different biochemical reactions that happen within your own body, which means that you may see why it is a fantastic idea to be certain that you're getting enough. To be sure, have a supplement that provides you 600 mg each day.

Sulforaphane

Not everybody has heard of sulforaphane, and that is too bad. But, on the other hand, it has been making headlines on a fairly regular basis recently, and everybody ought to be regularly carrying it as a nutritional supplement.

Recent studies have suggested that sulforaphane will help thwart some sorts of cancer and may slow tumor growth. Additional studies reveal that sulforaphane lessens the quantity of H. pylori bacteria from the gut, which triggers stomach lining inflammation and nausea. If those are not good reasons to choose sulforaphane every day, I do not understand what exactly they are.

Vitamin E

Along with vitamin C and vitamin B complex, vitamin E is something that will almost surely be included in your multivitamin routine but likely not in large enough quantities. However, you'll be able to see continuing health benefits of supplementing with vitamin E around 800 mg every day. Therefore, don't be reluctant to take that much.

What are a few of the health advantages of taking extra vitamin E? To begin with, vitamin E has strong antioxidant effects. But vitamin E does several other fantastic things for the body, too, from boosting your immune system to maintaining blood vessels at tiptop form.

Do yourself massive favor, and do not scrimp on the vitamin E.

Alpha-Lipoic Acid (ALA)

You will frequently see the lipoic acid known as ALA. It is a top-notch antioxidant that helps your body fight infection. In addition, it retains your cells working at a higher level.

Choose an ALA nutritional supplement and locate a capsule type that produces about 800 mg every day. That amount was demonstrated to provide many health benefits with no overpowering or side-effects within the human body. It's possible to locate ALA supplements in any fantastic health food shop and the regional vitamin retailer.

Conclusion

We encourage you to return to our guidebook any time you are in doubt or whenever you would like to get back to useful tips on how to live a healthier life with damaged renal functions and chronic kidney disease. The state of your renal function defines how well your organism and your body function; however, as explained in the book, your health should see crucial improvements with changing your everyday diet.

Make sure always to check your labels when shopping for groceries. Take care that the meals you are preparing are prepared following the low-potassium and low-sodium diet for best results. Remember that healthy habits make a healthy life.

Patients who struggle with kidney health issues, go through kidney dialysis and have renal impairments need to undergo medical treatment and change their eating habits and lifestyle to improve the situation. Much research has been done on this, and the conclusion is that food has a lot to do with how your kidney functions and its overall health.

The first thing to changing your lifestyle is knowing how your kidney functions and how different foods can trigger different kidney function reactions. Certain nutrients affect your kidney directly. Nutrients like sodium, protein, phosphate, and potassium are risky. You do not have to omit them altogether from your diet, but you need to limit or minimize their intake as much as possible. You cannot leave out essential nutrients like protein from your diet, but you need to count how much protein you have per day. It is essential to keep balance in your muscles and maintain a good functioning kidney.

At the point when you eat flippantly and fill your body with toxins, either from nourishment, drinks (liquor or alcohol, for instance) or even from the air you inhale (free radicals are in the sun and move through your skin, through dirty air, and numerous food sources contain them). In general, your body will convert numerous things that appear to be benign until your body's organs convert them into things like formaldehyde because of a synthetic response and transforming phase.

A profound change in kidney patients is measuring how much fluid they drink. Too much water or any other form of liquid can disrupt their function. How much fluid you can consume depends on your kidney's condition. Most people assign separate bottles to measure how much they have drunk and how much more they can drink throughout the day.

Human kidneys also need much care and attention to work effectively like all other body parts. It takes a few simple and consistent measures to keep them healthy. Remember that no medicine can guarantee good health, but only a better lifestyle can do so.

Since the early signs of kidney disease are hardly detectable, it is important to keep track of the changes you witness in your body. Even the frequency of urination and loss of appetite are good enough reasons to be cautious and concerning. Indeed, only a health expert can accurately diagnose the disease. Still, personal care and attention to minor changes are of key importance to CKD.

BOOK 6: <u>DR. SEBI ANXIETY SOLUTION</u>

THE ULTIMATE DR. SEBI GUIDE TO GET OUT OF YOUR HEAD AND FREE YOURSELF FROM ANXIETY AND DEPRESSION

Introduction

The following chapters will discuss some of the many issues with having anxiety disorder or simply worrying too much. Of course, it's normal for everyone to get scared or worry sometimes. Still, suppose this is a common occurrence for you, in addition to feeling panic regularly. In that case, you might have an anxiety disorder in some form. You will discover how important taking a new attitude toward anxiety is to heal yourself. This book explains the crippling impacts of anxiety, the various risk factors for anxiety, and the treatments, including counseling and psychotherapies, to treat and manage anxiety. Anxiety is a devastating power that must be analyzed and understood to ensure its proper and timely diagnosis and effective treatment. This book contains a plethora of tips and techniques that you can apply to your current lifestyle to limit the effects of anxiety, all without any professional training. Ultimately, it will ensure that you understand anxiety's core mechanism and workings to determine a better strategy for understanding and managing your anxiety.

Anxiety is something that can take over your life if you let it. While you're having an anxiety attack, your breathing will be rapid. You have crazy thoughts, you may not be able to sleep, you may be worried about money, work, or family, and you can't stop thinking about anything else but that. Anxiety is very real and can significantly affect your health. So taking action to reduce your anxiety is vital.

Anxiety is very bad for your health in so many different ways. Therefore, you must take control of your life and conquer the anxiety you might have.

Learn how to combat your fears.

Figure out who provides an anxiety diagnosis to get the help you need.

Discover what an anxiety attack is.

What anxiety disorder you have, the best treatment for your case's severity, and how much you are willing to work towards an effective solution.

Discover the what, who, where, when, and how of anxiety for yourself. You no longer have to live with the severe panic attacks, the fear, stress, and health issues arising from your disorder. Instead, you can gain the strength to fight through mindfulness, therapy, and, if necessary, medication.

You owe it to yourself and your family to live worry, stress, and fear-free. Stop hiding because of your fears and live instead.

Chapter 1: Anxiety

What is Anxiety?

The emotion of anxiety is simply a feeling of worry, fear, or general unease. As mentioned above, it's a perfectly natural response and a very human one. Without feelings of anxiety, it's likely that our ancestors would not have survived very long or that the human race would have been so successful. For our ancestors, anxiety at the sight of a prowling lion sent adrenaline through their systems, which prompted the "fight or flight" response and helped them to live another day.

Today, anxiety remains a common emotion, but the focus is often shifted to more abstract and usually more trivial issues than prowling predators. For example, bill payments worries over jobs, loss, or divorce stimulate feelings of uncertainty and anxiety. Even relatively mundane things such as going out, being late, and tests can cause anxiety to flare up. The emotion becomes a disorder when we fail to control our worries and concerns; some can do this more effectively than others. For those with normal anxiety responses, the emotion is quickly dispelled. Still, this is much harder for those with an anxiety disorder. The condition can affect every aspect of their daily lives – in some cases to a crippling extent.

Anxiety is not considered normal and healthy if it exceeds a certain limit. If it reaches that severe limit, it becomes a disorder that needs to be treated like any other. But first, we need to dig deeper to understand the problem we are treating. An anxiety disorder is defined as that level of anxiety that blows out of proportion compared to the original stressor. It is the kind that takes longer than normal and, in the process, starts interfering with normal body functions and, generally, the victim's life. An anxiety disorder can deal with high blood pressure, heart attack, hypertension, stroke, and nausea.

Anxiety becomes a disorder if it starts interfering with certain aspects of an individual's life like studying, social life, work, and general inability to execute daily tasks.

Sometimes abnormal anxiety goes away by itself, so you won't have to see a doctor or therapist about it. However, if the symptoms persist, you will have to see one as soon as possible. You know the symptoms are severe if you experience too much stress and cannot normally carry on your daily activities. Symptoms for an anxiety disorder must not be confused with anxiety as they are the same, only that those for the latter are short-lived.

Who is affected?

Anxiety disorder is relatively common, affecting an estimated 1 in 25 people. Like many depression and stress-related disorders, this estimate is only very rough – it's likely that anxiety disorders are underreported or not correctly identified. Anxiety disorder affects men and women – although the latter seems to have a slightly higher incidence. Again, this could be through underreporting. Women are more likely to raise concerns with doctors and clinicians than men, especially regarding what is perceived as "emotional" issues.

In reported cases, anxiety does seem to be more common between approximately 30 and 60. However, the condition can be found in people of any age group. Race, ethnicity, or religion seem to have little impact on the risk of developing anxiety-related illnesses. The conditions are found in every community and amongst people from every background – across the globe. Ultimately, anxiety disorder is a very human condition and can affect anybody.

Types of Anxiety Disorder

Generalized Anxiety Disorder (GAD)

GAD is a chronic anxiety disorder often characterized by excessive worry and long-lasting anxiety about specific situations, life events, and objects. GAD sufferers battle with fear and often worry about particulars like money, health, work, school, or family. They exhibit a certain fear but are often faced with the challenge of identifying the specific cause of tension and how to control the worries after that. This unexplained fear may cause them to be unrealistic about the situation. More often than not, their actions blow the situation out of proportion, contrary to what may be anticipated. Sufferers showcase a result, sufferers thoughts and expect disas

In many cases, this is a long-term condition, and sufferers feel anxious over a wide range of situations. Anxiety, in this case, is not normally a response to one single situation or event. Instead, patients with the condition will feel anxious daily and may not remember when they were last relaxed. Restlessness or constant worrying are two psychological symptoms of the condition. Poor concentration or poor sleep are physical symptoms often found with GAD.

Panic Disorder

This type of anxiety combines both physical and psychological elements. Your body reacts to panic naturally, and emotionally you may feel overwhelmed by emotions, including fear and apprehension. You may feel that you are about to die, go mad, or lose control. Physical symptoms include sweating, feeling sick, shaking, or the sensation that your heart is beating irregularly. A common side effect of panic disorder is the development of phobias, including complex phobias (agoraphobia or social phobias) and simple ones that include fear of certain animals, situations (the dentists, for example), or bodily fluids (blood, vomit, or injections being common examples). It is a type of anxiety that is often characterized by sudden or brief attacks of intense apprehension or terror, which automatically leads to confusion, shaking, nausea, dizziness, and sometimes sufferers experience some difficulty in breathing. Panic attacks rise abruptly, and they tend to peak after 10 to 15 minutes, after which they may last for hours without end. Any panic anxiety disorder may occur after a frightening experience or an event of prolonged stress, but it can also be spontaneous. A panic attack also makes the individual very alert; they tend to be aware of their changes. To some extent, the individual may interpret certain changes in normal body function as a life-threatening illness. This false interpretation may cause the individual to change behavior-wise to avoid the suspected illness and its resultant attacks.

Post-Traumatic Stress Disorder (PTSD)

Post-traumatic stress disorder or PTSD is anxiety that results from previous traumatic events or episodes such as rape, military combat, serious accident, hostage situations, abusive relationships, and abusive childhood. People living with PTSD are often aware of their environment; they inhibit a fear of repeating the traumatic event every time a situation triggers the flashback. Individuals with this anxiety disorder are often withdrawn and may showcase certain phobias and behavioral changes to avoid certain stimuli.

Real events in life usually trigger this condition; these are usually serious and very frightening. They include involvement in road accidents, violent assault (including sexual assault), witnessing violent events, military combat, witnessing or being involved in terrorist attacks or severe natural disasters. Of course, not everyone involved in traumatic events develops the condition. Still, estimates suggest that up to 30 % of those involved in traumatic situations will develop PTSD.

Social Anxiety Disorder (Social Phobias)

This type of anxiety disorder is characterized by a fear of being in public places, social gatherings, being negatively judged by others, or fear of public humiliation. Symptoms like stage fright, speech anxiety, fear of embarrassment, and fear of intimacy are common with individuals suffering from a social anxiety disorder. The disorder may also cause the sufferers to be withdrawn, self-conscious, and avoid contact with fellow humans or public situations. Sometimes people mistake this disorder with a simple notion of being "shy." Still, the truth is, if you are always shy. You get that feeling whereby you wish the ground could just open up and swallow you every time you are in a public situation, then you have a social anxiety disorder.

This disorder can be part of Panic Disorder or can occur independently. This condition is often seen as "shyness" but is a much more severe issue. Normal activities such as making a phone call, going to the store, or interacting with other people prompt strong anxiety. Social anxiety disorder has wide-ranging implications for those who experience it, affecting relationships, working lives, and education. Feelings that you will lose control, humiliate yourself, or be rejected by people are common symptoms of the condition.

Phobia

Phobia is an irrational fear that leads to avoidance of certain objects or situations. For example, we have heard people say that they are hydrophobic or claustrophobic; they are phobias that create an anxious feeling. Any phobia has a fear reaction identified with a particular cause. The fear may be seen or described as unnecessary or irrational.

Separation anxiety disorder

This type of anxiety disorder is caused by separation or panic attacks once a sufferer is separated from a place or person that provides that feeling of safety or security. A good example that best explains this disorder is when a stranger practically draws a baby from its mother and tries to take it to an estranged place where the mother will be out of sight. The baby's face will change automatically, and the anxiety that builds in them may cause them to cry or create a tantrum. In addition, it is a natural stimulus for them to panic because of the sudden separation, and even as the baby is taken away, it will stretch its arms towards its mother.

Is it All in Your Head?

Anxiety disorders can be mild or very severe. In the latter case, they can disrupt your ability to live a normal life. They can damage relationships and make it difficult for you to find or keep working. In addition, they can lead to depressive illnesses and isolation, which will often only make things worse.

In the past, anxiety disorders (and other psychological) illnesses were viewed by many people, including the medical profession, as signs of weakness. However, since the development of psychotherapy (and the advances in the discipline), the medical and psychological professions now fully recognize the range and implications of anxiety disorders. As a result, they have now considered conditions in their own right and (and here comes the good news) treatable ones.

Causes, treatments, and options for recovery vary depending on a range of factors. Addressing the underlying issues is important, and, in some cases, medication may be required. Where this is the case, you should always take the medication as prescribed. In many cases, however, a combination of self-help techniques and Cognitive Behavioral Therapy (CBT) – a form of counseling – will be all that is required.

Emotional and physical symptoms of anxiety

Have you ever felt like there are so many problems in your life that you don't know which way to turn?

Then the chances are that you are suffering from anxiety, but don't worry, you're not alone.

According to the Anxiety Disorders Association of America, over 40 million adults suffer from anxiety, America's most common mental illness. Anxiety can take many forms; the most common is called Generalized Anxiety Disorder (GAD). People who suffer from GAD have gone beyond the everyday worrying to suffering so much that the body feels distressed in many ways. It disrupts your daily functioning as the mixed-up emotions make the mind dysfunctional.

Here are a few examples of the symptoms which indicate that anxiety has become a serious condition:

Broken sleep pattern

Cannot get to sleep at night? When you do, do you often wake up in a panic, having had bad dreams?

Poor sleep can leave you exhausted during the day, destabilizing emotional levels.

Developing a phobia

Hate being in a crowd?

Scared to leave the house?

Have a fear of confined spaces?

These and many other phobias are symptoms of a high anxiety level.

Muscles aches

Do your shoulders, neck, back, and all suffer from a dull ache?

That is because you are probably constantly tensing your muscles throughout the day without even realizing it.

Digestive problems

Do you have Irritable Bowel Syndrome (IBS), indigestion, lack of appetite, or overeating the wrong things, such as sugary foods?

Again, common symptoms of anxiety.

Being over self-conscious

Do you have low self-esteem, such as?

A feeling that you are unattractive?

That people are staring or watching you and only you?

Blushing excessively?

All of which can be signs of a high anxiety level.

The onset of panic attacks for no reason

Do you suddenly get a feeling of fear?

Do you find yourself breathing fast with short breaths?

Do you get tingling fingers, nausea, headache regularly?

It can be a dominoes effect; one symptom can trigger another until you find that you are overwhelmed by extreme anxiety.

Living in the past

Do you often find yourself reminiscing and remembering bad things from your past?

Do you have Flashbacks of bad childhood memories?

Do you ponder overtimes that you suffered bullying?

Can you not forget times you suffered an embarrassing moment?

More signs that you are struggling emotionally and are overanxious.

Obsessive-Compulsive Disorder (OCD)

Do you have impulsive thoughts that you have no control over?

Maybe you feel compelled to repeat a certain behavior such as hand washing?

All of these can be symptoms of OCD, another effect of high anxiety levels.

These are but a few, the tip of the iceberg, but probably the most obvious signs that all is not well. Often, they come on slowly, as you are less and less able to cope with daily life. But, it could be a major change that brings any of these symptoms on:

Newlywed.

Becoming a parent.

New job.

Moving.

Suffering a tragic event.

Financial difficulties.

Many situations can major impact your life and throw your emotions into turmoil. Once it starts, it feels like a downward spiral with no escape.

Persons suffering from anxiety disorders showcase an array of physical and nonphysical symptoms.

Listed below are some of the symptoms that are associated with anxiety disorders:

I. Trembling	**VII.** Numbness
II. Nausea	**VIII.** Heart palpitations
III. Churning stomach	**IX.** Restlessness
IV. Headache	**X.** Sweating
V. Diarrhea	**XI.** Irritability
VI. Backache	**XII.** Easily tired

XIII. Muscle tension

XIV. Trouble concentrating

XV. Frequent urination

XVI. Often startled

XVII. Trouble sleeping (insomnia)

With post-traumatic stress disorder, the sufferer exhibits a range of symptoms such as:

I. Nightmares or flashbacks of reliving the traumatic experience

II. Avoidance of places, people, or anything associated with the traumatic event

III. Withdrawal or poor concentration

IV. Difficulty in sleeping

V. Hypervigilance (closely monitoring the surroundings)

VI. Irritability

VII. Diminished feelings

VIII. Keen eye o detail as if they are always looking out for particular places, people, or objects.

Causes of anxiety

Any negative factor that creates a stressful environment for an individual automatically triggers anxiety.

Medical factors are:

· Anemia, asthma, heart conditions and infections

· Stress from a serious medical condition like cancer, HIV, diabetes, or hepatitis.

· Anxiety may also be a side effect of medication

· Symptom of an illness

· Lack of sufficient oxygen supply in the lungs.

Environmental /external factors are:

· Trauma from certain life events

· Stress in marriage, personal relationship, or divorce

· Stress from work

· Stress at school

· Financial stress

Substance abuse:

In cases where one is intoxicated from an illicit drug such as morphine or cocaine, they may become more aware of what's happening around them. As a result, the anxiety levels build up. Anxiety is also common to recovering drug and alcohol addicts; the withdrawal method used to eliminate and detox the substances from an individual's system may cause numerous anxiety bouts.

Brain chemistry:

Brain chemical imbalance is a theory that seeks to explain the creation causes of anxiety disorders in some individuals. Whereas a theory remains challenged, I have still merited this factor as a cause of anxiety. The theory states that when serotonin, a neurotransmitter in the brain, is available at low levels, it causes depressive and anxiety disorders.

Genetic causes:

Genetic studies on genes as a cause of anxiety disorders are still ongoing; scientific researchers have identified certain genes that may predispose to anxiety disorders in individuals. In addition, majorly biological and environmental factors cause some disorders like (SAD) social anxiety disorder.

How to diagnose an anxiety disorder

Apart from observing a person's character, and identifying certain anxiety disorder symptoms, a proper medical diagnosis from a mental health provider must ascertain the condition. The symptoms mentioned above are common with other diseases like cancer, diabetes, and hepatitis. Therefore, do not self-conclude that you are suffering from an anxiety disorder unless you are sure.

Anxiety Affecting Daily Life

As you deal with stress regularly, whether it's because of financial pressures, schooling, relationship problems, worries about your job or finding work, or anything else, it can develop into anxiety over time.

What usually happens is that the worry starts to consume your thoughts. You begin thinking about the challenges you're regularly facing. For example, you could be thinking about the rent that's late while driving home from work, knowing you can't possibly pay it right now.

You could be worried about the company you work for downsizing. You might be concerned about your adult child's well-being because he's out partying every night, doesn't seem to be taking any responsibility for his life, is getting himself into debt, and nothing you say or do –aside from paying those bills for him-is making a difference.

When you try to fall asleep at night, when the TV is off and everything is quiet, you can't shut the worry and stress off. You keep turning those fears over and over in your mind.

At some point in the middle of the night, you might finally drift off to sleep, but the alarm blares just two or three hours later. So now you're tired and deal with another day like that.

Multiply that night after night, and the anxiety will continue to build even more because now you're trying to focus at work, impress the boss, or get impatient with people around you.

You might snap at somebody then feel bad about it right away, and that's going to make things worse in your mind. Eventually, you may feel tightness in your chest, shortness of breath at times, and have a difficult time getting anything done.

Over time you might withdraw from some of the activities you used to enjoy because you're spending all of your time worrying about everything, even though you're not able to do anything about them.

In time, you're living a completely different life with little to enjoy. That can lead to depression and a general state of worry about many other things, even those things that weren't a major concern for you in the past.

Your husband might be spending less time talking with you, mostly because he doesn't know what to say, and has become frustrated because you've been withdrawing from him. So now you start worrying about whether he's having an affair.

You see, your mind can begin creating more problems than exist, and the initial issues will still be there.

What Anxiety Does to the Body and Brain

Anxiety is a reaction to fear or stress with physical and psychological symptoms. Biologists and psychologists believe feelings arise from the amygdala. The amygdala decides on the emotional responses your brain will have in or to certain situations.

The brain functions with neurotransmitters that carry impulses to the sympathetic nervous system. These neurotransmitters tell your heart how to beat and your lungs how to breathe. If you feel fear, the neurotransmitters may send messages to increase your heart and breathing rates, tense your muscles for a flight or fight response, and divert blood flow from certain organs to your brain. By gaining more blood flow to your brain, your brain has more oxygen and energy to function at a higher capacity to confront the danger.

You can physically feel nausea, lightheadedness, diarrhea, or the need to urinate, often because your body is no longer balanced. Moreover, it asserts the requirement for adrenaline. When anxiety is a persistent state, your body and mind feel it. It shows through in physical and mental symptoms.

Anxiety becomes an illness with chronic symptoms, such as migraine headaches, irritable bowel syndrome, and abnormal heart rates. In addition, a person can feel muscle pain that radiates throughout the entire body due to stress brought about by anxiety.

Individuals with anxiety may show signs of heart disease, gastrointestinal conditions, and chronic respiratory disorders. In addition, untreated anxiety can lead to early death.

The long-term effects of stress on the body are difficult to see. Doctors only recently explained that chronic physical illness may result from anxiety, fear, or stress, making the cause a mental versus a physical one. Repeated increases in heart rate, shortness of breath, and fainting spells can overtax the heart.

To avoid what anxiety does to the body, you or your loved one will need treatment. However, before you seek medication as treatment, you need to learn about the different anxiety disorders the symptoms of these disorders and see a psychologist obtain a diagnosis.

Who Can Help?

Now that you know who is at risk and suffers from anxiety disorders, you need to know who you can trust to treat you or a loved one's disorder. Psychology training can lead to different specialties.

A psychiatrist is one person who you can see to get help. A psychiatrist is a medical doctor. They specialize in diagnosing, preventing, and treating mental disorders, including anxiety disorders. A psychiatrist goes through an undergraduate degree program, master's program, and four years of medical school with at least one internship year.

A psychologist passes an undergraduate and master's degree program before entering a doctoral degree program in psychology. Licensed psychologists can work in counseling, psychotherapy, psychological testing, and give treatment to patients. The difference is a lack of a medical degree, so psychologists cannot prescribe medications.

Licensed mental health counselors have a master's degree in psychology or counseling. Clinical social workers have also obtained a master's degree, typically in social work, specializing in evaluating and treating mental disorders.

Another possibility is to seek a psychiatric or mental health nurse. These nurses have specialized training to help in mental health services. Nurses can be patient advocates and work in case-management services. The supervision of a doctor may be necessary for some US states.

Who Should I Talk To?

You have plenty of licensed and educated professionals to choose from when seeking help for your anxiety troubles. However, who do you want to speak with to get help? Who can provide the most help when it comes to the effects of anxiety on your life?

You can eliminate a psychiatrist from the list of potential professionals if you are not seeking medication as a treatment. However, psychiatrists and many mental health nurses can prescribe anxiety medications.

A psychologist or licensed mental health counselor is enough to help you if you want treatment using cognitive behavior therapy or other therapy instead of medication. Both professionals are there to counsel you, listen to you, and assess your stress levels based on the fears or phobias you have. Then, they can help guide you to a better solution, such as being more mindful of your triggers, how to deal with your panic attacks as they happen, and how you can approach a situation differently.

Who you approach to help you with your anxiety disorder depends partly on who is readily available in your area and the affordability of treatment? More health insurance plans offer mental health treatment, but not enough companies assist this need. In addition, you may not have insurance for mental health visits. The fees can be $75 or more per hour for psychologists.

Chapter 2: Depression

What is depression

Depression is one of the most widespread mental health problems in the universe. Besides causing significant mortality and morbidity (suicide), it also contributes to or is associated with several other serious problems. Depression typically means a break from an individual normal style of life and position

Depression is a common disease with a large level of morbidity and mortality. About 5% of the population has major depression at any given time, with men experiencing a lifetime risk of 7-12%; and women 20-25%.

Mortality rates by suicide are estimated to be as high as 15% among patients hospitalized for severe depression. Most patients receive much or all of their care for major depression from their primary care physician.

However, depression is poorly diagnosed and poorly treated because of competing priorities in primary care with the care of other chronic medical conditions, patient stigma, and variability in physician skills and interest.

Depression affects individuals differently, even if it mostly occurs in women than men due to hormonal factors and lifestyles. In men, depression always occurs when tired and angry, making them drink more alcohol and take drugs without caution.

Depression may contribute to atherosclerosis, perhaps by impairing glucose tolerance. Depression has been repeatedly linked to depressed immune function.

It is estimated that 17% of individuals in the United States experience major depression at some point in their lifetime.

Depression can attack an individual at any age and is a particularly significant problem in sufferers who are elderly.

The surgeon general of the United States recently noted that the suicide rate increases with age. In addition, nearly 5 million of the 32 million Americans suffer from depression.

Nowadays, allopathic anti-depressant drugs are all-too-often prescribed and dispensed without a second thought. Therefore, the decision to begin or maintain sufferers on these drugs should be made carefully.

The profitable new antidepressant drugs (selective serotonin reuptake inhibitors) are more effective than older drugs, psychotherapy, or cognitive behavioral therapy.

New drugs may not even have fewer adverse effects than some older agents, and reports on unforeseen negative consequences of these drugs, such as gastrointestinal bleeding, are emerging.

Antidepressant drugs have strong placebo effects, and placebo is very effective for treating individuals who are depressed.

Depression also resolves on its own in up to 50% of patients. Therefore, it is critical to support the mind-body in mild cases instead of ruthlessly suppressing any signs of depression.

Ultimately, the antidepressant should be reserved for treating more serious, recalcitrant cases of depression. However, even in those cases, the practitioner should continue to look for and treat the cause of the depression. Natural medicine offers many options for coping with problems despite the enormity of depression at any age.

Diagnosing and treatment of depression in the primary care center have many hindrances. First, the physician-patient encounters time is short, making it difficult to fully assess the patient for depressive signs and symptoms.

Depressed primary care patients typically present with physical complaints, often not admitting to a depressed mood and are reluctant to discuss depression. In one study, about two-thirds of patients with depression presented only with somatic problems.

Essential Fatty Acids and Oxidation

Essential fatty acids, particularly in the omega-3 family, exert a multi-factorial influence on mood. Omega-3 fatty acids have been shown to have a regulatory influence on serotonin release and degradation.

It is reported that omega-3 fatty acid levels are reduced in the serum and cell membranes in a significant proportion of people with depression.

There is concern that the desaturation of omega-3 fatty acids from precursors and excessive dietary omega-6 intake may play a certain role in these deficiencies. In addition, impaired absorption that results from the compromised gut may also reduce essential fatty acid levels, suggesting that herbs may be necessary and helpful once again.

Types of depression

Bipolar Disorder

Bipolar disorder or bipolar depression is a depressive problem that changes mood, concentration, and daily activities.

Bipolar depression consists of the following forms:

- Bipolar I disorder.
- Bipolar II disorder.
- Cyclothymia.

Bipolar I disorder is an overexcited or agitated disorder that occurs within a week. It could be extremely serious in that the patient will need emergency care.

Bipolar II disorder is regarded as an increase in agitation similar to bipolar I disorder. However, it is not a full episode of a typical bipolar I disorder. Hence, the individual experience depressive symptoms and minor manic symptoms.

On the other hand, Cyclothymia is a type of bipolar disorder that occurs within two years. It is also regarded as a drastic increase in elated behavior. In addition, patients experience hypomanic symptoms and depressive symptoms.

When individuals experience symptoms of bipolar disorder that do not match the three categories listed above, it is known as "other specified and unspecified bipolar disorders.

The symptoms associated with bipolar depression are; changes in sleep pattern, extreme emotion, change in activities pattern, involvement in activities that can harm…and many more.

Perinatal Depression

Perinatal depression is regarded as the type of disorder that affects women during pregnancy or after delivery. This type of depression is one of the common medical problems most women encounter during pregnancy and childbearing.

A woman is emotionally, mentally, and physically disturbed during pregnancy and after birth because she feels happy, sad, nervous, and swings mood. This is very common among one out of seven women.

Some symptoms associated with this type of depression are: persistent sadness, loss of interest in activities they initially enjoyed, emptiness, hopelessness, continuous crying, thoughts of death or suicide, loss of interest in caring for self-and/or child, limited ability to think or concentrate, difficulty in sleeping, reduced energy, irritability, increased feelings of anxiety and worry, reduced affection with baby, changes in appetite and weight.

Seasonal Affective Disorder

This type of depression is a biochemical imbalance in the brain stimulated by shorter daylight hours and less sunlight in winter.

In other words, as seasons change, people experience a shift in their biological circadian rhythm that can cause them to be out of step with their daily schedule.

This depression manifests in season, especially in the late fall and early winter. It disappears in the spring and summer.

This type of depression can affect your sleep, mood, appetite, energy level and affect your social life. Most times, individuals affected by this depressive disorder feel hopeless, stressed, sad, and tense.

The most unappealing month for the individual suffering from seasonal depression in the United States is mostly the first two months of the year. It mostly affects women than men.

The symptoms associated with this disorder are; guilt, sadness, depressed mood, continuous sleep, constant food intake, reduction in energy, poor social lifestyle, poor concentration…and many more.

Minor Depression

Minor depression is a depressive disorder that is not as severe as major depressive illness. Minor depression is similar to dysthymia, which is less severe than major depression and has fewer symptoms.

Mild depression is often very difficult to diagnose as some of its symptoms are similar to emotional responses.

The symptoms of this type of depression are; irritability, bad thoughts, feeling abnormally tired, hopelessness, sadness, difficulty focusing, feeling unmotivated, wanting to be lonely, minor aches and pains, losing empathy with others…and many others more.

Premenstrual Dysphoric Disorder

This type of depressive disorder occurs in women. It interrupts the normal daily activities of a woman before and during menstruation.

The symptoms associated with this illness are more severe, commonly occurring during the second half of the menstrual cycle.

The premenstrual disorder symptoms are confusion, anxiety, anger, lack of control, agitation, depression, poor concentration, vomiting, nausea, backache, paranoia, crying, fatigue, difficulty sleeping…and many more.

Disruptive Mood Dysregulation Disorder

Disruptive mood dysregulation disorder is a childhood problem related to extreme irritability, anger, and frequent intense temper outbursts.

This disorder starts with an angry mood every day. The causes of this disorder are unknown, but some factors are believed to cause it. Such factors include hereditary, temperament, co-occurring mental conditions, childhood experiences, family conflicts, poor parental support, parental substance use...and many more.

Symptoms of Depression

Some symptoms are associated with depression that every individual suffering from the depressive disorder can experience. The symptoms could be experienced almost every day, once in a week or more.

The signs and symptoms that are related to all the above types of depression are:

- A consistent feeling of hopelessness.
- Feeling irritated.
- Headache.
- Guiltiness and worthlessness.
- Helplessness.
- Poor concentration and difficulty in making decisions.
- Loss of interest activities that formally interest you.
- Constant sadness and feeling anxious.
- Having an empty mood.

- Loss of energy.
- Walking or talking more slowly.
- Body pains.
- Unexplainable health issues.
- Feeling restless.
- Sleeping problems, early-morning awakening, or oversleeping.
- Increase in appetite.
- Sudden reduction or increase in weight.
- Suicidal attempts.

Causes of Depression

In the United States, depression is regarded as a major mental/psychological problem. Several factors could cause you to be vulnerable to depression.

Depression starts in adulthood most times and can also occur at any age because it affects adolescents and children. It could be accompanied by other health problems such as Parkinson's disease, heart disease, diabetes, cancer…and more when it affects adults. The major causes of depression are unknown, although some possible factors could be considered.

Therefore, the causes of depression are:

- Stress.
- Hereditary factors.
- Health problems, such as cancer.
- Intake of certain medications.
- Trauma.
- Dead of loved ones.

- Substance abuse.
- Other personal problems.
- Sexual abuse.
- Emotional abuse.
- Conflict with family members or friends.

Relationship of anxiety and Depression

Depression is a feeling of fatigue, sadness, and lethargy. Anxiety disorders keep you hyper when you fear, stress, worry, and fatigue once the adrenaline wears off. When you feel fatigued, you do not feel like doing anything. If you do something like move or work, you will be drained. The more you think about your negative feelings, the sadder you will feel. You sink into depression.

Worries and stress can naturally lead to a feeling that nothing will ever change. You are in a constant state of anxiety; therefore, nothing will get better, and no matter how hard you try, things remain the same. When these thoughts enter your mind, you start to believe them over time.

You have effectively created a cycle of bad habits and thinking that it is difficult to rise against and return to better habits and thinking ways.

Other people, even loved ones, do not want to be around someone who is always anxious, unable to sleep, and depressed. At first, they may want to help, but eventually, they feel as if they will be dragged down by the person who has anxiety. They can also feel tired of repeating the same things, trying to help the person cope, and being there whenever they have a panic attack.

It makes anxiety worse when one thinks they may lose someone they depend on in their life. It increases the feelings of depression. Moreover, you have the reason why anxiety ruins relationships.

Moving Beyond Depression and Anxiety

If you suffer from past trauma, learn to release it or find a practitioner to help you release it. You can learn to eliminate or control it to no longer rears its ugly head. It occurred in the past, and you lived through it. There is no need for it to be a part of your presence in a painful way. You may want to pay attention to the age you feel when suffering from the trauma. Then, talk with that imagined version of yourself and assure them that you are living proof that they will survive. Encourage them.

Nutrition is important. Be sure that you eat healthy alkaline foods and get all the vitamins, minerals, and supplements your body needs to be healthy. Your mind and body can serve you well if you take care of them and provide them with what they need to function effectively.

You may be feeling overwhelmed and saying to yourself: "There is no way I can do all that is suggested in this book." Don't try to do it all at once. Begin slowly. Do those activities that are the easiest and most enjoyable in the beginning. Be patient with yourself. If you fail one day, forgive yourself and begin the next day again. Over time, you will learn how to be a better friend to yourself, and you will come to enjoy being nice to that special person, which is you!

We are convinced that you can be healthy. We had witnessed many clients and researched hundreds of accounts of people overcoming difficulties in their lives that seemed impossible when they began the journey. Your mind/body is wonderfully created to function effectively. We pray that this book will help you perform the miracle of living a happy, healthy life.

Chapter 3: Risk Factors for Anxiety

Neuroanatomy

The neural structures involved in the functioning of anxiety include Amygdala (which is the center for emotions such as anxiety and fear and stimulates the Sympathetic nervous system), Hippocampus (which is the center for emotional memory). People experiencing high levels of anxiety have been seen to have highly stimulated Amygdala and hippocampus. In addition, many research pieces regarding This automatically conclude a relationship between the structures that control reward and fear responses in anxiety suffering people.

Genetics

A family history of anxiety and genetic material is a huge risk factor contributing to anxiety. It renders a person vulnerable to anxiety disorders. Still, this anxiety disorder comes into action when triggered by specific stimuli, usually external and environmental. This genetic factor has contributed to 3% of anxiety disorders and 28% of the cases suffering from a generalized anxiety disorder. No complete single gene has been found to cause anxiety by itself.

Several parts of certain genes have been proven to contribute to anxiety, such as:

- PLXNA2
- CRH
- BDNF
- COMT
- SERT.

The mode of action for these genes to cause anxiety is their action on the neurotransmitters, e.g., epinephrine and serotonin, and some stress hormones such as cortisol, which have been seen in anxiety disorders.

Medical conditions

There are a huge number of medical conditions that can result in anxiety. Some of these medical conditions include breathing problems such as Asthma and COPD and the breathing problems experienced when on a death bed. Abdominal pain and chest-causing medical conditions can also cause anxiety. These conditions are usually somatic representations of anxiety, the same as sexual disorders. In teenagers, any conditions that affect appearances, such as skin and face conditions, trigger social anxiety. One of the main causes of social anxiety is a developmental disability in children. Similarly, chronic and fatal diseases, such as cancer, can also cause severe anxiety. Even so, many organic medical conditions cause symptoms mimicking anxiety.

Some of these medical conditions include:

Endocrine diseases, such as hypo or hyperthyroidism

Metabolic syndromes, e.g., diabetes, deficiency conditions such as deficiency of vitamins B2, B12, D, etc.

Gastric diseases include celiac, gluten sensitivity, bowel diseases, etc.

Heart conditions and blood diseases, like anemia

Cerebral accidents, like strokes and tumors etc.

Degenerative diseases of the brain, like Parkinson's, Multiple Sclerosis, Alzheimer's, dementia, Huntington's Chorea, and many more.

Substance-induced

There are many drugs that their uses can precipitate or increase the levels of already existing anxiety. Whether the drug is being used for intoxication or a heavy user, or going through withdrawal does not matter. Some of these drugs include Tobacco, Cannabis, sedatives (Benzodiazepines), alcohol, opioids such as pain killers that have been prescribed or illegal drugs like heroin, CNS stimulants like caffeine, amphetamines, and cocaine, hallucinogens like LSD, and inhaled drugs like Crack. The ironic part is that some people use these drugs to self-medicate themselves for existing anxiety. Still, these drugs treat anxiety for a short period. After that, the person becomes tolerant to their effect, and his anxiety worsens.

Psychological

Insufficient coping skills such as inflexibility, rigidity, inability to solve problems, denial, defense mechanisms, impulsive behavior, avoiding problems, instability, and escaping from threatening situations instead of focusing on solving them, are all related to causing or worsening already existing anxiety. In addition, anxiety is also related to how a person has pessimistic views about his future outcomes and how effectively they deal with the negativity in their life.

Some psychological dispositions like catastrophizing about the future, over-generalizing everything, attempting to read minds, binocular tricks, reasoning about emotions, and mental filtering can cause anxiety.

The psychodynamic theory of psychology suggests that anxiety results from different unconscious conflicts between your fears and desires. These conflicts are between the three forces of our psyche called id, ego, and superego. These conflicts end in anxiety, and the ego employs defense mechanisms to overcome this anxiety.

<u>Some of these defense mechanisms are:</u>

- Suppression
- Anticipation
- Repression
- Somatization
- Sublimation
- Repression
- Dissociation

For example, a child taught that anger is a negative emotion and never allowed to be angry will learn to repress his anger to avoid the anxiety caused by disapproving parents on his anger. These types of conflicts causing anxiety can be managed with the help of psychodynamic therapy.

Evolutionary psychology

From the perspective of evolutionary psychology, anxiety is good for us because it helps us remain cautious against all possible threats we can face in our environment and help us devise ways to avoid that threat. That may be true to some extent. Still, to remember, a person who suffers from anxiety starts avoiding all environments and situations that may not be dangerous. This is why people suffering from anxiety don't usually die due to accidents, as they avoid every situation that can be potentially threatening or dangerous.

Social

The social risk factors of anxiety range from trauma history, such as:

Emotional or physical abuse in childhood or teenage

High discipline

Negative experiences in childhood

No maternal warmth

Bad parenting

Anxious household environment

Rejecting

Drug abuse

Hostile parents

Dysfunctional parents

Harsh treatment

And the neglect of children.

Gender socialization

Other factors based on the context that has been seen to contribute to anxiety causation are Gender socialization and learning experiences. Learning mastery is the extent to which people think they control their own lives and instrumentality, which means factors like confidence about self-independence control the relationship between gender and anxiety.

Chapter 4: Conventional treatments

Medication is one treatment option. Going for medication first may be right for who you are, but it is not the only option. Medication may be the best treatment; however, drugs have side effects. Medication can also stop working. When medication stops working—what can you do? You have other drugs to try, but wouldn't it be nice if you could rely on other treatments available?

Keep in mind that you do have alternatives. When medication is right for you—use it. Treatment can involve both therapy and drugs. You may be on medication for the long term or short-term. The choice is the psychiatrists, typically based on the severity of your anxiety disorder.

Medication takes time to be effective. After three months, you may see the actual results of the drug you have chosen to use. Medication does not completely cure anxiety disorders. Still, they are very helpful in treating and managing anxiety symptoms. A doctor or medical health professional should only give medication for anxiety, not by yourself. Some authentic psychologists with the license to practice can also prescribe medication. Medication can be used in two ways. It can be used as the sole treatment for anxiety or used after psychotherapy has already been applied. No improvements were observed with psychotherapy. But to achieve the best results and obtain a faster recovery, it is better to combine the use of psychotherapy and medication

The medication used for treating anxiety disorders is most commonly anti-depressants, anti-anxiety meds, and beta-blockers. Unfortunately, these medicines only work if used regularly, and if their use is stopped, the anxiety symptoms will reemerge.

Antidepressants

Antidepressants are the main meds used for treating depression, but they work just to treat anxiety disorders. Their working duration is several weeks, and they must be used regularly. Their side effects include nausea, headache, and insomnia. However, these side effects are not usually severe. Therefore, they are not a huge problem

Anti-Anxiety Medications

The anti-anxiety medication helps elevate the anxiety symptoms, and the panic attacks often experienced with them. The most commonly used anti-anxiety meds are benzodiazepines. Benzodiazepines are the only meds used for the treatment of generalized anxiety disorder. Panic disorders and social phobia are also treated using benzodiazepines, but Antidepressants best treat them.

Beta-Blockers

Beta-blockers like atenolol and propranolol are very useful when treating different anxiety symptoms, especially social anxiety disorder's physical symptoms. Doctors prescribe these medicines to overcome shaking, blushing, trembling, and increasing anxiety.

Selecting the right kind of medicine for you, the right dose of that medicine, and the exact treatment method should be carefully adjusted to a person's unique needs and symptoms. They should be managed by expert medical healthcare professionals. Only an expert can tell you about each treatment plan's pros and cons and help you decide which one is best for you. Your doctor may have to try different methods and medicines with you before arriving at the right one.

You should make a point of discussing the following things with your doctor:

- Is the medication working for you or not, or to the extent it has improved your symptoms?
- The pros and cons of each type of medicine, especially the side effects
- Depending upon your medical history, which side effect can harm you the most

- The different changes you will be required to make in your lifestyle for your medication
- How much does each medicine costs, and what are the other cheaper alternatives
- Other alternatives that you can explore regards to your anxiety such as vitamin intake, therapies, and supplements that may affect your meds

You should stop using medicines because some medicines cause serious side effects if their use is stopped suddenly. They should be discontinued slowly and gradually with the help of a doctor's advice.

Selective Serotonin Reuptake Inhibitors

SSRIs or 'Selective Serotonin Reuptake Inhibitors relieve symptoms by blocking serotonin's absorption in your nerve cells. The drug works on the nerve cells in your brain. Serotonin affects your mood; therefore, blocking the uptake of serotonin enhances your mood. SSRIs typically prscribed include:

- Citalopram
- Fluoxetine
- Sertraline
- Escitalopram
- Paroxetine

This category of drugs offers fewer side effects than other medications such as tricyclic antidepressants. However, common side effects of these drugs include sleepiness, insomnia, weight gain, and sexual dysfunction.

Tricyclic Antidepressants and Benzodiazepines

This classification of medicines replaced benzodiazepines due to concerns of long-term use by patients. Benzodiazepines help induce relaxation, reduce muscular tension, and alleviate many anxiety symptoms. However, long-term use of Benzodiazepines leads to dependence and tolerance. They become ineffective.

<u>Tricyclic antidepressants include:</u>

- Imipramine
- Amitriptyline
- Nortriptyline
- Benzodiazepines are:

- Diazepam
- Alprazolam
- Lorazepam
- Clonazepam

Patients on tricyclic antidepressants may drop blood pressure, urinary retention, constipation, blurry vision, or dry mouth.

Serotonin-Norepinephrine Reuptake Inhibitors

SNRIs like Duloxetine and Venlafaxine increase serotonin and norepinephrine by inhibiting their absorption in the brain cells. However, SNRIs can cause insomnia, stomachaches, headaches, increased blood pressure, or sexual dysfunction. Therefore, most doctors choose SSRIs or SNRIs before benzodiazepines or tricyclic antidepressants.

Ketamine

The recent clinical trials using Ketamine are favorable. Ketamine helps alleviate depression in a few hours, and some patients in minutes. The reaction time is faster than other medicines available. However, it is for depression—it will only relieve one symptom of your anxiety.

What You Should Know About Medications

If you take other medicines for other health conditions, anxiety meds may cause drug interactions. Therefore, you should let your mental health provider know about any prescriptions, over-the-counter medications, vitamins, or supplements that you take.

Speak with your doctor or psychiatrist about medications they may want to take. If it will help you, what the side effects are, avoid certain things or drug interactions.

Pharmacists recommend you drink or eat before taking your pills and suggest a time to take them. These recommendations prevent side effects and help your body absorb the substance correctly.

Before you decide to start medication for anxiety, discuss how long you may be on the meds with your doctor. Also, schedule a check-up to discuss how you feel about the medicine and if you need to extend the amount of time you will need to be on medication.

Due to dependency on drugs, you should carefully review the drug information and decide if it is right. You have other treatment options that may work better or conjunction with the meds to overcome your anxiety. If you find it necessary, obtain a second opinion. If you feel your doctor or psychiatrist is pushing medicine, speak with another mental health care worker.

Chapter 5: Anxiety and Alkaline Diet

Alkaline diets are completely free from acidic foods. They are also termed electric foods, which help the body heal naturally. They are naturally found in nature and are not modified, hybridized, or irradiated.

Alkaline foods increase iron, copper, and other essential vitamins and minerals that make the immune system immuno-competent.

Doctor Sebi Alkaline Food List

Spices and Seasonings

- Dill.
- Achiote.
- Habanero.
- Savory.
- Basil.
- Thyme.
- Pure Sea Salt.
- Bay Leaf.
- Cayenne.
- Sweet Basil.
- Cloves.
- Onion Powder.
- Sage.
- Oregano.
- Powdered Granulated Seaweed.
- Tarragon.

Fruits

- Cantaloupe.
- Prickly Pear.
- Cherries.
- Sour sups.
- Prunes.
- Bananas.
- Dates.
- Figs.
- Grapes.
- Apples.
- Pears.
- Limes.
- Orange.
- Soft Jelly Coconuts.
- Mango.
- Berries.
- Raisins.
- Papayas.
- Melons.
- Currants.
- Peaches.
- Plums.

Vegetables

- Izote flower and leaf.
- Kale.
- Mushrooms except for Shitake.
- Bell Pepper.
- Chayote.
- Cherry and Plum Tomato.
- Dulse.
- Garbanzo Beans.
- Arame.
- Wild Arugula.
- Avocado.
- Cucumber.
- Dandelion Greens.
- Amaranth.

- Watercress.
- Tomatillo.
- Turnip Greens.
- Wakame
- Lettuce except for the iceberg.
- Olives.
- Purslane Verdolaga.

- Squash.
- Okra.
- Hijiki.
- Nopales.
- Nori.
- Zucchini.
- Onions.

Alkaline Grains

- Quinoa.
- Rye.
- Kamut.
- Tef.

- Wild Rice.
- Spelt.
- Fonio.
- Amaranth.

Alkaline Sugars

- Date Sugar.
- Agave Syrup from cactus (100% Pure).

The Benefits of Dr. Sebi's Alkaline Diet

Dr. Sebi's alkaline diet is loaded with several benefits, such as:

- Absence of cholesterol in the diet.
- Absence of alcohol.
- Treats and prevents autoimmune diseases.
- Helps to prevent strokes.
- Treats and prevents high blood pressure.
- It contains very low saturated fats, which also prevent major heart-related diseases.
- It contains no processed sugar.
- Treats and prevents diabetes.
- Helps to lose weight quickly

Forbidden Foods

Doctor Sebi disregards all foods that are not alkaline. Most foods people eats are highly acidic, which prevents the fast healing process in the body.

The following foods are forbidden:

- Corn.
- Fish and Seafood.
- Colors and flavors.
- Poultry products.
- Alcoholic products.

- Soy and soy products.
- Meat of all kinds.
- Eggs.
- Processed foods.
- Canned fruits.

- Seedless fruits.
- Foods with yeast or another component such as baking powder.
- Sugar.
- Foods fortified with vitamins and minerals

- Genetically Modified Organism fruits.
- Wheat.
- Fast foods.
- Genetically Modified Organism vegetables.
- Dairy products.

Correct Nutrition can Help with Anxiety Disorder

The Mental Health Institute research shows that anxiety disorders are more common than any other mental illness in America. That means that 18 percent of United States citizens suffer from anxiety symptoms. Depression and anxiety go together frequently, and about 50 percent of depression sufferers experience anxiety regularly in their lives. Some medications and therapies can reduce anxiety, but only 30 percent of people (or less) seek out professional help for their condition. But there are chances that you can make it right at home to start helping your anxiety. With the techniques and mindset changes, we've already discussed, like meditation and floating through anxious thoughts, changing your diet can help you manage your nervousness and anxiety.

Can Antioxidants help with your anxiety?

Low levels of antioxidants in the body are related to a higher state of anxiety. This means that including more antioxidant-rich foods in your daily diet can help you experience fewer symptoms and feel calmer, in general. In the year 2010, looked at over 3,000 foods and their antioxidant levels, including drinks, supplements, herbs, and spices. Here are some foods that have high levels of antioxidants, according to USDA research:

FRUIT: Including plums, sweet cherries, prunes, and apples.

BERRIES: Blueberries, raspberries, cranberries, strawberries, and blackberries all have high levels of antioxidants and can help you manage symptoms of your disorder.

NUTS: Not only are nuts healthy for you in many ways, but they are also high in antioxidants. This is especially true of Brazilian nuts and walnuts.

SPICES: Ginger and turmeric have anti-anxiety and antioxidant properties and should be included in your diet.

VEGETABLES: Vegetables are great antioxidants, including kale and amaranth greens.

Chapter 6: Essential oils for anxiety relief

Essential oils are the pure derivative of the plants they are extracted from. The result is a highly concentrated oil. Essential oils are a healthy and natural way to calm your body, mentally and physically. The molecules in the aroma of the oils can affect your brain and control stress and anxiety feelings. They also can change heart rate, blood pressure, and the function of your immune system.

How do essential oils help with anxiety?

When essential oils enter your body, they have incredible healing effects. The fragrance molecules from the oils travel through your olfactory system (one of the sensory systems responsible for your sense of smell) and make it to your brain to combat those feelings of anxiety and stress. Your limbic system is connected to certain parts of your brain that also affect blood pressure, hormone balance, and stress levels. Essential oils can be used topically or inhaled using aromatherapy to soothe anxiety. As outstanding healers, your body can absorb and spread its healing powers through your body within five minutes of exposure.

Essential Oils for Anxiety and How to Use Them

Lavender Essential Oil
It is one of the most effective in treating anxiety. In addition, this oil can improve concentration, calm anger and irritability, and promote relaxation, combating insomnia.

In my experience, there are a couple of ways to use lavender oil:

Topically: Place two to three drops on your wrists and rub them together as if you were putting on perfume.

Use a diffuser: You can do this using an oil diffuser, which you can find at many stores and online.

In your bath: Run a hot bath and add a couple of drops of lavender to the water. While the steam from the warm bath will diffuse the oil and allow the soothing aroma to fill the room, your body will absorb some of it while relaxing in the bath.

On your pillowcase: Put a couple of drops on your pillowcase so that you can let the aroma help you fall asleep and stay asleep.

Cedarwood Essential Oil
An essential oil that promotes serotonin release is a neurotransmitter in your body that regulates mood. Also, this oil helps regulate appetite. That is beneficial because, in some cases, feelings of anxiety can cause loss of appetite. Cedarwood oil also helps if you have trouble falling or staying asleep. In my experience, this oil also brings me feelings of confidence. This oil gives me a sense of power to overcome my stress and anxiety.

A couple of ways to use cedarwood oil:

As a massage lotion: Mix ¼ cup of coconut oil with twelve drops of cedarwood oil and add six orange essential oil drops. Massage into your feet, arms, and neck before bed and drift effortlessly to sleep.

As a moisturizer: Add a few drops of cedarwood oil to your favorite unscented body lotion or mix some drops with coconut oil. Use these to moisturize your body and take advantage of its healing properties.

Eucalyptus Essential Oil

The strong aroma of this oil eliminates stress and gives you an energy boost. It is my favorite oil to use when I feel sluggish or mentally exhausted from stress and anxiety. It is the perfect pick-me-up to get rid of those feelings of sadness.

A couple of ways to use eucalyptus oil:

In your shower: Run a warm shower and plug the drain. Next, add three to five drops of eucalyptus oil to the water and let the warm water run over it. This will diffuse the oil and fill your shower with its refreshing aroma. Then, you'll be ready to tackle anything that comes your way!

As an air freshener: Free your space from negative energy and use this oil as an air freshener. Simply mix twenty drops of eucalyptus oil with eight tablespoons of water in a spray bottle. Use this to bring positivity to any space, whether your bedroom, car, or office.

Rose Essential Oil

This oil is one of my favorites when I need an extra positivity boost. Also, this oil amps up my confidence because the aroma, to me, is very feminine. Rose oil also boosts feelings of peace and well-being.

A couple of ways to use rose oil:

After shower body spray: As a cherry on top after a refreshing shower, mix a few drops of rose oil with water in a spray bottle. Then, spray it in your hair, on your body, and even on your clothes to leave yourself feeling cleansed of all of those negative energies and stresses.

As a perfume: Rub two to three drops of rose oil on your wrists and neck for a confidence-boosting aroma to follow you throughout the day.

Essential oils are a powerful and versatile way to free your body from anxiety. The aromas and the properties of these oils are essential in your self-care recipe. The next chapter will learn how meditation can rid your body and mind of anxiety. You will also learn to incorporate essential oils in your meditation practice for an extra soothing experience!

Chapter 7: Dr. Sebi's 3-Step Solution

Dr. Sebi's Official method for treating anxiety, such as any other disease, is composed of 3 main steps. Please note that any of these parts can't be passed over to succeed in your healing journey.

<u>The three steps I'm talking about are:</u>

Cleansing → The body must be cleaned on an intra-cellular level through detoxification to purify each cell and remove mucus excess.

Revitalizing → After cleansing, you need to nourish your body to regenerate your cells and strengthen the immune system.

Maintaining a Healthy Lifestyle→ Follow Dr. Sebi's nutrition guide and adopt healthy lifestyle habits every day to keep your mind and body in good shape.

CLEANSING

How to Prepare Cleansing Herbs?

Preparing your cleansing herbs would depend greatly on the form you purchased them. It's easier to prepare cleansing herbs in powder forms. You can easily make herbal teas with them in the specified or recommended dosage. However, for other forms form herbs, especially roots or leaves, it is better to use a ratio of 1 teaspoon to 1 cup (8 oz) of spring water for each herb.

However, I recommend preparing herbs in batches of mixtures for easier batch preparation and storage. That would mean mixing them up according to function and benefit. Again, this will depend on the state of your health and what minerals are most important for you. You can combine similar herbs with similar functions into a batch. Like our healer, Dr. Sebi would say: *"If you want calcium, you know where to go to (sea moss), if you want Iron, you go to Burdock, and if you want a mix of both Iron and Fluorine, you go to Lily of the Valley"*.

In all, try not to mix more than 2 or 3 herbs. Remember, these herbs are electric, and it's best to preserve their organic carbon, hydrogen, and oxygen nature as much as we can. But, again, if you mix more than that, you may not get their accurate concentrations per ml of water, so try to limit it to 3, possibly 2.

For a clearer understanding, you can use the following mix:

- Mix **Colon and gallbladder** cleansing herbs together

- Mix **liver and kidney** cleansing herbs

- Mix **respiratory and mucus cleansing** herbs

- Mix **lymphatic and heavy-metal** cleansing herbs.

Since these herbs perform a whole-body cleanse (not just colon), including the skin, eyes, colon, liver, lymphatic system, and gallbladder, you can decide to choose how to combine them. Also, note that when you make larger batches of these herbs for storage, try not to make batches that last more than 7 to 14 days.

For pre-purchase cleansing packages
Please follow the recommended dosage or instructions that are provided for that cleansing package

For fresh Green leafy herbs
- Place in spring water and boil on low heat for 5 to 7 min

- For dried leafy herbs, boil longer – 10 to 15 min

For Dried ground (or powder) herbs
For dried ground or powder leaves or roots, mix in recommended ratios for the herb. Powder herbs are the easiest to mix in dosage proportions, so you can simply follow the package instructions

For Chunks of Dried Root herbs
If you've purchased chunks of roots or stems, you can prepare them in the following way:

- Cut or break up chunks

- Place in spring water and boil for 15 minutes

- Let cool and serve

- Alternatively, prepare in larger batches and place in jars to store in the refrigerator.

For bulk purchase herbs

If you have purchased herbs in bulk and are making your teas, find out the recommended dosage for each herb. You should prepare each herbal tea ratio of 1 teaspoon to 8 ounces of spring water as a general rule.

For capsules

I recommend that you do research and find out what the recommended dosage is for each herbal capsule

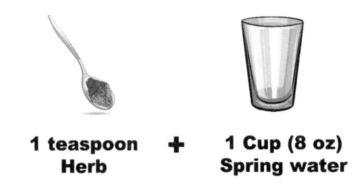

1 teaspoon Herb **+** **1 Cup (8 oz) Spring water**

How To Take The Prepared Cleansing Herbs

If you are on medication, I recommend taking the herbs one hour before taking your meds; Dr. Sebi recommended this. Your colon cleansing herbs should not be consumed for longer than 30 days because your body may become dependent on them, and you want to start to reduce the dose during your last 3 to 5 days, depending on how long you've been taking them.

Routine:

- **Twice a day** - morning and night

- **Daily Consistency** - Try to stay consistent both in timing and duration. That is, try not to skew the duration. Make it consistent, and take the cleansing herb throughout the cleanse. For example, for a 14-day cleanse, the cleansing herbs can be taken twice daily, and you should take them around the same time you do take them on both mornings and evenings.

- **Gradual Wean Off** – Just like medications, it is not the best to go cold-turkey when it comes to herbal detox. Towards the end of the cleanse duration, wean off your herbs by gradually reducing the dosage and duration. The duration of the wean will depend on the length of the fast you choose. For example, I usually start weaning a week towards closure for a one-month fast. For a 14 day fast, I begin weaning on day 11 or 12. You can begin the wean by reducing it from twice a day to once a day. Or simply take half the dosages each for mornings and night.

You must do this because you need to signal your body to prepare to start functioning independently without dependence on herbs' cleansing. And no other way to do this than to take it slow and gradual, without bringing too much "shock" to your body.

How to break a detox fast?

- Slowly reintroduce solids

If you are doing water or a liquid fast, you will need to reintroduce solid foods slowly. You can begin by introducing solids like high water-content fruits. These include watermelon, apples, and berries. After that, you can introduce softer fruit solids like bananas and avocados. Later, you can incorporate harder solids like veggies. All foods must be listed on the nutrition guide. However, if doing a fruit or raw veggie fast, you can break the fast right away on solid foods.

- Drink 1-gallon spring water daily

Drink spring water daily together with the revitalizing herbs and sea moss.

How long should you detox/cleanse?

How long you should detox depends on your state of health, that is, your body's toxification level (the less healthy you are, the more toxic your body is) and tolerance level. Typically, it is recommended to fast for 7-14 days, but Dr. Sebi recommends a minimum of at least a 12 day fast. Dr. Sebi himself fasted for 90 days to cure diabetes, asthma, and impotence. It is great to cleanse at least once a year for seven days if you consume an alkaline diet. If you are not consuming an alkaline diet, then you should cleanse/detox every three months

I fasted for 14 days, and I recommend fasting for between 14 days and one month if you have high blood pressure. Again, your body's tolerance level will ultimately determine the length, so watch your body and study its reaction as you begin the fast. We are all different, and you may find that you cannot handle a basic liquid fast (water or juice). In that case, you can get started with fruit or raw vegetables fast. But make sure all foods and fruits are listed in the Dr. Sebi Nutrition Guide. Whether liquid, juice or raw food fast, the results are virtual all the same – the only major difference is when it takes to begin to see results. While raw food fasts take longer, liquid fasts are much faster. So do not worry; the most important thing is to stay committed and focused on whatever fasting method you choose.

Common Symptoms Expected During Detox Cleanse

- Cold and Flu symptoms
- Changes in Bowel movements
- Fatigue and Low Energy
- Difficulty sleeping
- Itching
- Headaches

- Muscle aches and pains
- Acne. Rashes and breakouts
- Mucus expels (catarrh, etc.)
- Lower blood pressure

Be happy if you relate to any of these symptoms during the cleansing stage. That's because your body is pushing out all the toxins and mucus you have been keeping inside for so long. In addition, these symptoms are only temporary and usually resolve after the first one to two weeks.

CLEANSING HERBS

Below are listed the herbs Dr. Sebi recommended to use to cleanse your body and relieve anxiety symptoms:

CASCARA SAGRADA

It is a natural laxative, purgative shrub plant from Rhamnaceae's family that Dr. Sebi recommended because of its potency to cause muscle contractions in the intestine, detox/cleanse the colon, and stimulate the colon the colon the colon liver and pancreas secretion, and moves stool through the bowel. In addition, this herb is rich in glycosides, Vitamin-A, B, C, and D, emodin, and anthracoid, making it effective in cleansing and revitalizing herbs.

The benefits of Consuming Cascara Sagrada include:

- It helps to get rid of toxins from the colon.

- It serves as a laxative for constipation.

- It helps to soothe and dissolve gallstones.

- It helps to treat and prevent liver problems.

- It helps to destroy and inhibit cancerous cells from mutation.

- It helps to soothe and treat digestive problems.

- It relieves joint and muscle pain and other pains caused by inflammation.

- It treats transmitted diseases caused by viruses and bacterial

When writing this book, there are no side effects attributed to healthy adults who consume Cascara sagrada for a short period.

The note-full precautions before Consuming Cascara Sagrada are:

- Nursing mothers should avoid these herbs because they can inflict their babies with diarrhea.

- If you suffer from disease or health disorders like; stomach irritation or upset without knowing the cause, colitis, kidney disorders, intestinal blockage, or Crohn's disease, please do not use this herb without medical supervision.

For the dosage and how to prepare cascara sagrada tea, kindly take the steps below:

- Get Cascara Sagrada plants, remove some of the bark, and chop it.
- Once you have chopped it, dry it until it is dried, or you can order it online, and it will come chopped and dried.
- Pour 8-10 ounces of water into your saucepan and add 1-1½ teaspoon of cascara sagrada bark in the saucepan.

- Steams the mixture for 15-20 minutes on your cooker.
- After 15-20 minutes, steam, allow it to reduce its hotness and strain it to remove the chopped bark of cascara sagrada.
- You are done. For the dosage, consume1cup (8-10ounce) of Cascara Sagrada tea 2-3 times daily.

RHUBARB ROOT

Rhubarb Root is a very effective laxative that Dr. Sebi recommended because it boosts the digestive tract's health. However, Rhubarb roots are rich in various nutrients, making them a perfect herb for cleansing the body.

The benefits of Consuming Rhubarb Root are:

- It helps treat various types of sores like; canker sores, cold sores, etc.
- It helps to destroy various viruses like; herpes simplex virus, HIV, etc.
- It helps to enhance and relieve the symptoms of menopause.
- It helps to serve as a remedy for treating pancreatitis (swelling of the pancreas).
- It helps boost and enhance people's respiratory system suffering from ARDS to breathe healthier.
- It helps to soothe and cure menstrual pain (dysmenorrhea).
- It helps to treat and stop blood bleeding in the stomach.
- It helps to treat and prevent gastrointestinal (GI) bleeding.
- It helps to shed excess body weight (cholesterol) naturally.

When writing this book, there are no side effects attributed to consuming Rhubarb root and its rhizome for over two years, except it leaves that contain oxalic acid, which is unsafe.

For the dosage and how to prepare Rhubarb root tea, kindly take the steps below:

- Uproot some roots of the Rhubarb plant (make sure that the plants uprooted are above four years, in autumn).
- Wash the uprooted roots under running water to remove all dirt from the soil, remove the external fibers, and dry it on a plane surface.
- Once it is dried, chop it into smaller pieces. (Not more than 0.5 inches) or pound it and store it in a tightly closed container. Alternatively, you can order it online, and it will come dried and chopped.
- Pour 8 ounces of water in a saucepan, add 1tablespoon of the pounded or chopped rhubarb root, and boil the mixture for 15-20minutes v. After the timing, reduce the heat of the gas for about 10 minutes and put off the fire.
- Allow it to get cold for at least 10-15minute and strain out the root.

You are done. Take 1 cup (8ounce) of the infusion three times per day for the dosage.

ASHWAGANDHA

The benefits of using or consuming Ashwagandha also include:

- It helps to reduce stress fast by regulating chemicals in your brain
- It is widely used to fight anxiety in herbal medicine
- Being an energy booster, it helps not to feel fatigued
- It may help improve heart health by reducing cholesterol and triglyceride levels
- It may help to reduce sugar levels in people suffering from diabetes
- It acts as a pain reliever, preventing pain signals from traveling along with the central nervous system.
- May increase muscle mass and muscle strength
-

Dosage and administration:

Take 250mg to 3000mg daily with abundant water in the morning.

MULLEIN

Mullein is a flavorful beverage flowering plant that has been used for centuries to treat various ailments. Research shows that this herb is an effective anti-microbial, anti-inflammatory, anti-cancer, anti-hepatotoxic, antioxidant, and anti-viral herb with potency to prevent many health disorders. In addition, it helps to cleanse and detoxify the lungs and lymph system and destroy cancer.

The benefits of consuming Mullein include:

- It helps treat and prevent various types of cancer by destroying cancerous cells and preventing them from mutating.
- It helps to eliminate mucus from the small intestine
- It helps to activate healthy lymph circulation in the chest and neck
- It helps neutralize the negative effects of free radicals by protecting the cells from damages caused by free radicals.
- It helps treat and prevent various bacterial and virus infections like herpes viruses, HIV etc.
- It helps to treat and prevent respiratory tract infections.
- It helps to treat and prevent tuberculosis.
- It helps to treat earaches.
- It helps treat various health disorders like bronchitis, stroke, heart diseases etc.
- It helps prevent some chronic brain diseases like Alzheimer's, Parkinson's etc.
- It helps to treat atherosclerosis and others in the biological systems.
- It helps treat and relieve pain caused by inflammation and tumor.
- It also helps treat various ailments like asthma, bronchitis, migraine, congestion etc.

There are no negative side effects attributed to mullein consumption by mouth when writing this book. However, since there is no information

When writing this book, there are no medications that interact with mullein. Therefore, it can be combined with other herbs and drugs without issues.

For the dosage and how to prepare Mullein tea, kindly take the steps below:

- Harvest some fresh mullein leaves, dry them until they are dried, and chop them into smaller pieces. Alternatively, you can place an order online, and it will come dried and chopped.
- Once the fresh leaves are dried, measure 1-2 teaspoons and pour them into your teacup or mug.
- Measure 8-10 ounces of water and boil it.
- Once the water is boiling, pour it inside your teacup or mug where the mullein leaves are and allow it to steep for 15-20 minutes.
- Strain it, and you are done!
- Take 1 cup (8-10ounce) 2-3 times daily for the dosage.

GERMAN CHAMOMILE

German chamomile is a natural laxative and anti-inflammation herb native to southern and eastern Europe. The herb smells slightly like an apple and is popular throughout the world. The name "chamomile" is Greek for "Earth Apple".

The benefits of consuming German Chamomile include:

- It helps to treat and calm the central nervous system.
- It helps to treat and prevent swelling (inflammation)
- It helps to boost the functionalities of the brain and heal the brain.
- It helps serve as a laxative that helps to enhance healthy sleep and relieve depression.
- It helps relieve and soothe stomach and intestine cramps and soothe indigestion (dyspepsia).
- It helps to shed excess body fat by reducing cholesterol in the body.
- It helps treat and prevent skin disorders like eczema, etc., and cold and flu.

The note-full precautions before consuming German Chamomile are:

Because there is not much information regarding whether German Chamomile is harmful to pregnant and breastfeeding mothers or not, I advise that they stay off this herb completely.

People allergic to plants from the Asteraceae/Compositae family should stay off German Chamomile.

Because German Chamomile increases estrogen, people suffering from; hormone-sensitive disorders like; breast, uterine and ovarian cancer, uterine fibroid, endometriosis, etc., should stay off this herb.

For the dosage and how to prepare German Chamomile, kindly take the steps below:

- Get some fresh flowers of German chamomile and dry them on a plane surface
- Once it is dried, pound it into smaller pieces, or you can order it online, and it will come dried and chopped.
- Boil 10 ounces of water.
- Measure 1-2 teaspoons of the dried flower of German chamomile and pour it into your teacup/mug.
- Pour the boiled water into the teacup/mug, cover it and allow it to steep for 10-15 minutes.

- Filter it using a filter and press the marc to get the new active principle inside the cell.
- You are done. Take 1 cup (10ounce) of the tea/infusion 1 time per day before eating anything for the dosage.

VALERIAN ROOT

The benefits of consuming valerian roots include:

- It helps treat and calm the central nervous system relieving anxiety, stress, depression, and chronic fatigue syndrome (CFS).
- It helps to treat and prevent sleeplessness (Insomnia).
- It helps relieve and reduces the severity and frequency of hot flashes in postmenopausal women and relief premenstrual disorders (PMS).
- It helps soothe dysmenorrhea (menstrual cramps) and relieve pains during menstruation.
- It may help to lower blood pressure and the rate of heartbeat.
- It is used to remedy Attention-deficit hyperactivity disorder (ADHD).
- It is used to treat and relieve some health issues like headaches, convulsions, epilepsy, mild tremor, joint pains, stomach irritation, etc.

Valerian root has no side effects if used for less than 28 days, but if you consume too much of it, you might suffer some side effects like:

- Stomach irritation.
- Headache
- Swing mood
- Sleeplessness
- Sluggishness

The note-full precautions before consuming valerian root include:

Since much is unknown about this herb's safety for pregnant and breastfeeding mothers, I advise them to stay off this herb.

Because of this herb's drowsiness effect, I strongly advise you not to drive or operate any machinery after consuming valerian root.

For the dosage and how to prepare Valerian root tea, kindly take the following steps:

- Harvest some valerian plants' roots, wash them, chop them into smaller pieces, and dry them.
- Alternatively, you can order it online, and it will come dried and chopped.
- Boil 8-10 ounces of water and add 1teaspoon of the valerian root and allow it to boil for 15-20 minutes.
- Allow it to get cool and strain.
- You are done! For the dosage, take 1 cup (8-10ounce) of valerian tea 30-60minutes before going to bed daily.

DANDELION

Dandelion is a flowering plant known as 'yellow gowan' or 'lion's tooth. This plant is native to Eurasia and today. It is common in over 60 countries worldwide in the mild climates of the northern hemisphere. For centuries, these flowering plants have been used for the treatment of swelling (inflammation) of the pancreas, relieve pains that are caused by inflammation, treat and prevent cancer, tonsils (tonsillitis), skin disorder, bladder or urethra disorder, digestive and liver problems and enhance the general health of the liver and digestive system.

Researchers proved that it is a very effective cleansing/detoxification herb because of the chemical compositions and nutrients.

The benefits of using or consuming Dandelion include:

- It helps to detoxify or cleanse the liver and the kidney.
- It helps to treat and prevent diabetes by regulating blood sugar levels.
- It helps to fight against and relieve pains that are caused by inflammation.
- It helps to deactivate and inhibit the negative effects of free radicals in the body because of its antioxidant properties.
- It reduces the level of cholesterol.
- It lowers blood pressure by getting rid of excess fluid in the body.
- It helps to naturally shed excess weight gain by improving the metabolism of carbohydrates.
- It helps in boosting the digestive system.
- It helps to boost the immune system.
- It helps to keep the skin healthy and treat and prevent skin diseases.

Till at the time of writing this book, Dandelion is 100% safe, but consuming an overdose of it can result in some side effects like:

- Experiencing stomach upset or irritation
- Allergic reactions

The special precautions before using/consuming dandelions are:

Pregnant and breastfeeding mothers should stay off dandelion as there is no research to know if it is harmful to them or not.

If you are suffering from Eczema, stay off dandelion as more than 85% of people with eczema suffer an allergic reaction to dandelion.

For the dosage and how to prepare Dandelion tea/infusion, kindly take the following steps:

- Get some fresh leaves of dandelion and wash them under running water to remove all the dirt.
- After washing it, pour ½ - 1 cup of the washed dandelion into your saucepan.
- You should boil 4-5 cups of water and pour the boiled water inside the saucepan. Next, you pour the dandelion and cover it for 12-15 hours or throughout the night (overnight).
- The next day, strain out the dandelion leaves, and you will be left with the dandelion tea/infusion.
- For the dosage, take ½ tablespoon of Dandelion per ¾ cup of water three times daily. And if you ordered your dandelion online, you can take 4-10 grams of dry leaf of dandelion three times daily.

PRODIGIOSA

Prodigiosa, also known as 'Prodijiosa or Hamula, is a perennial plant with large bushy leaves and flowers, and it's from the daisy family and native to Mexico and California. These plants have a grey-purple hue on the underside and dark green leaves on the upper side and grow up to 5 feet in height, with their flowers growing in clusters. This plant has a long history with the Mexicans. It has been used for centuries to treat diabetes, arthritis, diarrhea, and stomach disorder and relieve aching joints.

Because of the chemical and compound composition of Prodigiosa, research has shown that it is very effective for the treatment of diabetes II because it aids in stimulating the pancreatic gland to secret and reduces or lowers blood sugar level and burn down fat in the gallbladder. The irony is that Prodigiosa can cause more damage to people suffering from Type I diabetes. Furthermore, consuming Prodigiosa's tea/infusion helps boost the digestion of fat, improve bile synthesis in the liver, dissolve tiny gallstones, and treat chronic gastritis and other digestive systems disorders. Although there is no research to prove its effectiveness in treating cataracts, it is believed that it can cure cataracts.

Prodigiosa is used for several reasons, including:

- Treatment of diabetes (type II).
- Treatment of diarrhea.
- Treatment of stomach pain.
- Treatment of gallbladder disease.
- Enhancing the digestion of fat and boosting the digestive system's healthiness.

The note-full precautions to beware of before using or consuming Prodigiosa includes:

Pregnant and breastfeeding mothers should not use or consume Prodigiosa as there is no research to back it to whether it is safe or not.

It is a no-go area for people suffering from diabetes I. People with diabetes II should control their sugar levels while consuming this herb.

How to prepare Prodigiosa tea/infusion:

- Dry the fresh leaves until it is dried.
- Once the fresh leaves are dried, or the one you ordered for is available, boil eight or 16ounce of water and brew 1 or 2 tablespoons of Prodigiosa leaves in the warm water for 15minutes.
- After brewing it, strain the Prodigiosa leaves.
- Take a cup (8ounce) of Prodigiosa tea/infusion two times per day for the dosage.

BURDOCK ROOT

Burdock root is the root of a delicious plant called Burdock, which all its body or parts are useful as either food or medicine. This plant can be found all over the world. I called this plant the wonder plant because everything about it is important as we consume its root as food and use it for medicinal purposes. Both its leaf and seed are used for medicinal purposes.

People worldwide have been using burdock root orally to treat and prevent various health disorders for over five centuries.

Because of Burdock root's chemical composition, quercetin and luteolin, research has shown that it can serve as a great effective antioxidant. A compound like 'Phytosterols' helps scalp and hair follicles grow healthy hair even from baldheads. In addition, vitamins-C helps in boosting the immune system and combat bacterial. It also helps cleanse or detoxify the liver and lymphatic system, etc.

The potassium helps reduce blood sugar levels and filter the blood by removing impurities through the bloodstream and eradicating toxins through the skin and urine.

The benefits of using or consuming burdock root tea/infusion include:

- It cleanse/detox the liver and lymphatic system.
- Treat and prevent diabetes by reducing blood sugar levels in the body.
- Eliminate toxins from the body by inducing sweetness and urine.
- Purify the blood by removing heavy metals from the bloodstream.
- Treat various skin disorders and combat aging.
- Treat and prevent cancer by inhibiting the growth and mutation of cancerous cells.
- Boost the immune system and enhance circulation.

Until at the time of writing this book, there have been no side effects recorded by researchers or people who have used these herbs.

However, research has it that applying this root to your skin might cause rashes.

For the dosage and how to prepare Burdock root tea/infusion, kindly take the following steps:

- Scrub the uprooted root of burdock heartily under running water to remove all the dirt that accompanied it from the soil.
- You should chop the Burdock root into smaller pieces (less than 1 inch). Please note that it will come dried and already chopped if you order it online.
- Pour 2-3 cup of water into your saucepan and add ¼ cup of the chopped burdock root and boil it.
- Lower your gas once the water is boiling, re-boil it for 30-40 minutes, and put off your gas.
- Once it is cold, strain it and consume it.
- For the dosage, drink one glass cup daily

REVITALIZING

Below are listed the herbs Dr. Sebi recommended to use for revitalizing your body's cells and fighting anxiety:

IRISH SEA MOSS

Irish Sea Moss is red algae that belong to the family of Florideophytes that grows on the rocky parts of the Atlantic coast of various countries, including the British Isles, Jamaica, Scotland, etc. Dr. Sebi recommends this herb for revitalizing the body after cleansing because it has over 92 out of 102 minerals that the body needs to be healthy. Some minerals are, for example:

- Phosphorus
- Iodine
- Selenium
- Calcium

- Bromine
- Iron
- Potassium

Some of the benefits of consuming Irish Sea Moss are:

- It heals and boosts the immune defense system.
- It treats and prevents hyperthyroidism and boosts the functionalities and health of the thyroid.
- It helps to soothe joint pain and swelling and treat arthritis.
- It helps to enrich the overall mood and reduce fussiness.
- It helps to combat infections caused by viruses and bacterial.
- It helps treat and prevent various skin disorders like acne, skin wrinkling, and alleviating inflammation.
- It helps to treat and prevent digestive and respiratory tract disorders.

The note-full precautions to beware of before consuming Irish Sea moss include:

Because of how rich Irish Sea moss is with iron can trigger hypothyroidism for people suffering from Hashimoto's disease.

Stop using the herb if you notice any allergies or reactions.

For the dosage and how to prepare Irish Sea Moss tea, kindly take the steps below:

- Measure and boil 1cups (8ounce) of water in a ceramic pot.
- Once the water is boiled, measure 2-3 tablespoons of Irish Sea moss gel (or 1teaspoon for the fine form) and add it to the boiling water.
- Allow the Irish Sea moss for 10-15 minutes to dissolve completely.
- You are done!
- For the dosage, take 1cup of Irish Sea moss tea daily in the morning.

SENSITIVA

Also known as 'Mimosa pudica', which is of the Fabaceae family, is a species that is native to Central and South America. However, it is currently spread in other tropical regions. In addition, it is gaining popularity worldwide as a medicinal herb.

Besides being a fun, intriguing element of nature, Sensitive plant is also filled with many health benefits.

The health benefits of consuming Sensitiva herb are:

- It helps cure joint pain and arthritis
- It treats insomnia and sleeplessness
- It treats Asthma
- It helps to cure gum problems and toothaches
- It fights hair loss
- It lowers blood sugar levels and helps those who suffer from diabetes
- It lowers high blood pressure
- It helps to treat stomachaches

Dosage and administration:

Liquid: Dose about 3 to 6 ml of 1:2 mimosa liquid extract daily is advisable

Capsule: 1 tablet, three times daily with meals is advisable.

However, capsule and liquid extract formulations are proprietary herbal blends and are available in several strengths; besides this powder, teas are also available.

SOURSOP

Soursop is the fruit of the "Annona Muricata" tree, a native of tropical regions in the Americas that belong to the Annonaceae family. Its leaves are widely used because they are rich in various nutrients like iron, calcium, phosphorus, magnesium, sodium, potassium, zinc, etc. That makes the tea very effective in fighting against the mutation of cancerous cells.

Other benefits of consuming soursops tea are:

- It helps to destroy and eliminate cancerous cells and inhibit the growth of cancer cells.
- It is a very strong and effective antioxidant that helps neutralize free radicals that damage the cells.
- It helps to soothe heart disorders.
- It helps lower blood sugar levels for people who have type 2 diabetes.
- It helps to fight against infectious diseases caused by bacterial. Such diseases like yeast infections, cholera, gingivitis, Staphylococcus, tooth decay etc.
- It helps to soothe and alleviate swelling (inflammation) etc.

The note-full precautions before consuming soursops tea include:

Since there is no information about this herb's harmful effects on pregnant and breastfeeding mothers, I advise that they stay off this herb.

Although this herb is tempting, please make sure you consume this herb under a medical practitioner's supervision.

For the dosage and how to prepare soursops tea, kindly take the following steps:

- Harvest some fresh Soursops leaves, dry them until it is dried, chop them, or pound them into smaller pieces. On the other hand, you can place an order online, and it will come dried and chopped.
- Measure one teaspoon of the chopped leaves of the Soursops and pour it into your teacup or mug.
- Boil 8 ounces of water and add it to the Soursop leaves in the teacup or mug and cover it.
- Allow the leaves to steep for 10-15 minutes and strain them.
- You are done!
- For the dosage, consume 2-3 cups of Soursops tea daily.

CORDONCILLO NEGRO

The cordincillo negro is a shrub whose leaves give off a spicy smell when squeezed and a bitter taste when chewed.

Cordoncillo negro has many important medical uses.

For example:

It can be used as a painkiller. Chewing on the leaves of cordoncillo anesthetizes the mouth. So if you squeeze and rub these leaves over a cut or wound, it can serve as an anesthetic.

It can treat digestion problems like vomiting, nausea, stomach ache, dyspepsia, dysentery, etc.

It can also prevent blood loss from internal bleeding

It can treat respiratory problems like colds, flu, coughs, bronchitis, and pneumonia.

Helps to keep the kidney healthy and prevent kidney stones

Dosage and administration:

Infusion: 1 cup 2-3 times daily

BLUE VERVAIN

Blue Vervain is a perennial flowering plant that belongs to the family of Verbenaceae. It is rich in nutrients like iron fluorine, which purifies the blood, phosphorus, phosphate, zinc, potassium, magnesium, etc. Because of this potency, Dr. Sebi recommends this herb for revitalizing your body after cleansing.

The benefits of using or consuming Blue Vervain include:

- It helps to treat and prevent anxiety and sleeplessness and enhance mood.
- It helps to treat and calm the central nervous system.
- It helps soothe the nerves and relaxes the mind, thereby treating migraine headaches.
- It helps boost and protect the heart's health treat and prevent myocardial ischemia, chest pain, and heart failure.
- It helps to fight against both internal and external inflammation.
- It helps to treat menstrual cramps or pain and stomach pain.
- It improves digestive health and protects the livers and kidneys by cleansing/detoxifying the kidney and liver.

The note-full precautions before consuming soursops tea include:

Because there is no information to show if these herbs are good for breastfeeding mothers or pregnant women, I advise avoiding these herbs' consumption.

Till at the time of writing this book, there were no medications that interacted with blue Vervain.

For the dosage and how to prepare Blue Vervain tea, kindly take the following steps:

- Get some fresh leaves and flowers of blue Vervain and dry them.
- Once it is dried, pound or chops it, or you can order it online, and it will come dried and chopped.
- Boil a cup of water (8ounce) in a saucepan.
- Once the water is boiled, pour it into a cup, measure 1 teaspoon of the Blue Vervain, and add it to the water.
- Allow it to steep for 10-15 minutes and strain it.
- You are done! For the dosage, take 2-4 cups daily.

When Should I Consume the Revitalizing Herbs?

The best time to consume the revitalizing herbs is the next day after finishing your cleanse. For instance, if you fast for 14days, on the 15day, you should start consuming your revitalizing herbs.

What Are the Things That I Shouldn't Forget?

- Drink at least a gallon of spring water daily.
- Eat foods only on Dr. Sebi's nutritional guide once you are done with your detox /cleanse.
- Never forget to use sea moss
- Ensure you do an intra-cellular cleanse once per year for at least seven days if you follow only the alkaline diet from Dr. Sebi's nutritional guide. Still, if you are not, you should always do an intra-cellular cleansing after every three months to cleanse your body from mucus and toxins.

Please note that consuming acidic food can only put your body at the risk of relapsing.

MAINTAINING A HEALTHY LIFESTYLE

Dieting

Nope, this isn't the latest fad diet to help you lose weight! Instead, dieting for anxiety is about eating healthily. As mentioned above, the food we eat directly (often fast-acting) impacts our mood and emotional state. Therefore, a balanced, healthy diet is essential for good physical health, a stable, healthy weight, and mental health.

Healthy diets should include a balance of low-fat protein sources and lots of fruits and vegetables.

There are several food types that you may need to avoid if you suffer from anxiety:

High sugar foods boost our energy levels quickly but may promote adrenaline production, which causes feelings of anxiety.

Processed foods often contain high levels of sugar and a range of other additives, which will potentially imbalance the chemicals in your brain, leading to more or more severe manic episodes.

As mentioned above, **caffeine** boosts and one cup is usually OK. However, in excess, it will promote imbalances in your brain chemistry, over-stimulating adrenaline production and leading to high anxiety levels.

Alcohol: long term misuse of alcohol can lead to developing anxiety disorders. It's also often a symptom of the conditions and those suffering from depression-related illnesses. Cutting alcohol consumption is strongly recommended but seeking help is also wise.

Some foods are better for us than others, and certain types of food can profoundly affect our mood when it comes to brain food. The following food types have been identified as having positive effects on our brain's functions and chemistry.

For those with anxiety-related disorders, incorporating them into your diet is a must:

Vitamin B is essential for good physical health, and it also helps to regulate mood. Sources include vitamin supplements, citrus fruits and leafy green vegetables,

Another essential is Omega-3; as with vitamin B, it helps regulate mood and has several positive physical effects. It's found mostly in oily fish, but you can find them in dried fruits too. As part of a healthy balanced diet, you should aim to consume at least two to three portions per week.

Exercise

While exercise has been clinically proven to reduce anxiety and improve mood, it can also treat many other health problems. Health issues can be a major anxiety trigger, and easing the symptoms of those ailments can further reduce anxiety symptoms.

Also, exercising can help people relax. When a person exercises, their body releases hormones that produce a calming effect. Exercise also increases body temperature, which can be very relaxing. Working up a sweat is tiring, but it's a great way to calm down.

When some people hear the word "exercise," they picture a gym full of lifting weights. However, many fitness activities can provide the exercise someone with anxiety needs. Even everyday activities like gardening or washing a car can elevate the mood.

Many people think they don't have time for exercise, but exercise doesn't take hours. Instead, people can find little ways to increase physical activity throughout the day. For example, they might stretch at their desk at work or take a quick walk during their lunch break.

Studies suggest that 30 minutes of exercise a day, three days a week, can dramatically reduce anxiety symptoms. However, those same studies show that even small amounts of activity can positively affect. So if someone doesn't have time for lengthy workouts, they should still find ways to exercise their body needs.

While increased physical activity provides several health benefits, they aren't lasting. For exercise to improve anxiety, it must be done consistently. That makes it all the more important for people to find exercise routines they can stick with and physical activities that they enjoy.

Beginning an exercise routine is the hardest part for many people who suffer from anxiety. However, once they get started, they find these physical activity periods one of the most enjoyable parts of the day. Sticking with an exercise routine can be very easy if planned out well.

Anyone beginning an exercise routine should think about the physical activities they enjoy most. Do they enjoy playing with their children? Riding a bicycle? Gardening in their backyard? When it comes to reducing anxiety symptoms, any activity that gets the body moving counts as exercise.

No one should feel like they have to decide on a workout plan and stick to it forever. Sampling a variety of different activities can help keep motivation levels high. Different kinds of exercises have different benefits, and switching between them gives people the chance to experience them all.

If the thought of joining a gym is enough to bring on a panic attack – you're probably not alone. You don't need to have a social phobia (or any other kind of anxiety disorder) to have an aversion to the gym! However, healthy exercise has surprising implications for anxiety disorders and other psychological conditions, including depression. The mechanisms by which exercise and mental health are related are not fully understood. Many medical experts worldwide now acknowledge that exercise has a major impact on many psychological conditions. For example, it is believed that exercise can effectively combat depression as many commonly prescribed drugs.

There is no need to join a gym for the good news. If you want to, then there is certainly no harm in signing up. However, "exercise", in this context, means simple, easy exercises that anybody should be able to manage. A few times a day, short bursts of activity are the type of exercise that experts recommend. For example, a brisk walk lasting only ten minutes is believed to be enough to raise your emotional state for a couple of hours. It can be hard for those with anxiety disorders to get out and about occasionally. For some, with severe conditions, it can seem impossible. However, exercise will help improve your emotional state and take your mind off the anxiety. Use the following tips to increase your chances of successfully incorporating exercise into your life.

Don't start with the intention of completing a 10K run. Instead, simply use small bursts of activity – the type that gets you a little out of breath and sweating – into the day. Ten minutes every so often is better than half an hour in one go.

Moderate level intensity exercise is recommended as perfect for improving physical and mental health. That includes walking briskly, cycling, jogging, or swimming. Walking and jogging should not need any investment, and if you're uncomfortable alone, partner up with a friend or relative. Ideally, buddy up with someone who addresses the same issues or has a good understanding of them for extra support.

Psychologists recommend that the exercises you choose should be rhythmic and repetitive. That helps to clear the mind and focus it on the task at hand. Walking, again, is the simplest of these and should be easy to achieve for many people.

If you begin to experience anxiety during a period of exercise, simply focus your mind on your breathing. Use a meditation technique like "mindfulness meditation" (described briefly in the next chapter) to become aware of your body, breathe simply, and limit the impact of negative or nervous thoughts. Experience the moment you are in, not the fears in your mind. Alternatively, simply count each step (out-loud if necessary) to distract your mind from the feelings of anxiety.

Good Sleep Does the Trick

When you don't get good sleep, you drain your entire body and brain of vital functioning energy. In response, your body and brain are reduced to anxiety; it may be hard for you to focus and make logical thoughts. On the other hand, anyone experiencing an anxiety episode is advised to get a maximum of 8 hours of uninterrupted sleep. I know I say 8 hours, and it may be hard even to make them fall asleep. You can try and prepare the environment in which they will sleep, make it cozy, warm, and secure; you can even sleep by their side so that they know you are there. When you do all these, the person's brain starts adjusting from anxiety mode to relief mode, and thoughts like, 'I think I am safe in this room, I think she will make me safe' is what will be crossing their minds.

Teas

Tea has the power to relieve anxiety on some levels. The very act of drinking tea is relaxing, particularly when that tea is hot. It also requires people to take a few minutes to sit and relax, which anxiety sufferers need badly.

It creates a positive routine, which is relaxing in and of itself. Studies have shown that following calming routines can play a role in reducing anxiety symptoms. Also, tea provides the body with the hydration it needs to fight back against anxiety symptoms.

However, the real benefit of teas comes from the herbs they contain. Many herbs found in tea can provide long-term anxiety relief. Drinking tea made from fresh herbs can have a particularly beneficial effect, but even packaged tea can be quite helpful.

Valerian root is one type of tea that is particularly good at easing tension. This herb is a natural sedative and can help the body process emotions more effectively. It works particularly well for people who cannot get enough sleep because of their anxiety. However, it should be noted that this tea could cause some people to feel lethargic.

Research has shown that blue vervain can calm the nervous system and effectively treat many nervous conditions. It can also help people get a more restful night's sleep. However, even though this tea works very well, experts recommend against drinking it regularly. It's better for occasional relief.

You can also use Chamomile Tea. Chamomile tea is famous for its ability to aid in relaxation. It soothes many anxiety symptoms and can also calm a nervous stomach. People who have experienced a reduction in appetite because of their stress should give chamomile a try. It may provide them with anxiety relief while restoring their appetite.

One of the advantages of chamomile is that children can safely consume this tea. Many children suffer from anxiety, and this natural relief method can help them cope with their symptoms. However, when it comes to people under the age of twelve, it's recommended that chamomile not be taken for an extended period.

Another type of tea that you can also use is Lime Balm Tea. Lime balm tea works to soothe the nervous system, reducing feelings of anxiety and stress. It also has the power to relieve headaches, which are commonly experienced by people with anxiety disorders. Those who don't enjoy hot tea can experience soothing lime balm tea by drinking it iced.

Green tea is also another type of tea that you can use to help treat your anxiety as long as you drink decaffeinated tea. Most green tea contains caffeine, which means that many anxiety sufferers often avoid it. However, it also contains theanine, promoting alpha waves in the brain. This can provide a significant amount of relaxation. Decaffeinated green tea allows people to reap theanine benefits while avoiding the negative side effects of caffeine.

Tea can ease the symptoms of anxiety on some levels. It's a good idea for anxiety sufferers to experiment with different teas. This allows them to see which types provide them with the most relief. Some teas are more effective when taken daily, while others should only occasionally.

Tea is healthy, calming, and can benefit the mind and body in several ways. It's more than a beverage; it's a potent way to treat health problems and reduce stress. Tea should be a part of any anxiety sufferer's life.

Acupuncture

For years, Western people have approached acupuncture with skepticism. They didn't understand how sticking needles into the body could relieve anxiety symptoms. Many people think that acupuncture should cause people to experience more anxiety.

It's easy to see why people have such a hard time wrapping their heads around the concept of acupuncture. Acupuncture is based on the ancient Chinese principle of qi. Proponents of acupuncture believe that balancing qi in the body can cure several ailments. While qi's concept hasn't been sufficiently studied, recent research has helped prove that acupuncture can relieve anxiety. More importantly, it has been discovered why it's so effective.

When the body is stressed, some hormones are secreted. These hormones affect the pituitary and adrenal glands and cause many symptoms most commonly associated with anxiety. Unfortunately, these hormones can also trigger the " fight or flight" response, leading to panic attacks.

However, acupuncture can block these stress-induced hormone elevations. In addition, it can change the way blood circulates in the body and improve overall nerve function. Study after study has demonstrated that acupuncture works.

Although acupuncture was once considered alternative medicine, its increased legitimacy has led to acupuncture treatments being covered by several insurance companies. This allows many people to take advantage of one of the most effective anxiety treatments available.

It is important to note that acupuncture simply isn't for everyone. Some people may not be comfortable with the unusual nature of the treatment. Others may not have a reliable acupuncturist in their area. However, those willing to give acupuncture a try can experience many powerful benefits.

Limit Alcohol

Alcohol is not a terrible thing. It is normal to enjoy a couple of drinks when hanging out with friends or out for a celebration. It makes you feel more confident and less worried because alcohol depresses your central nervous system. However, alcohol becomes an issue when used as an escape if you find yourself reaching for a drink when you feel upset or hopeless.

Alcohol temporarily increases the serotonin levels that your brain produces and then drops off as the alcohol leaves your body. Serotonin is a neurotransmitter in your brain that affects mood. When the alcohol wears off, you may feel even more anxious and depressed as your body recovers. Feelings of sickness and worry induced by being hungover can cause you to feel more unsettled. When you drink alcohol often, your brain rewires and tries to counteract the inhibition (being drunk) by building up your alcohol tolerance. What happens from there is that you can drink even more alcohol without feeling the effects, which will lead you to drink even more quantities.

Limit Caffeine

If you have trouble with anxiety, consider cutting down on your caffeine intake. Coffee, and sometimes strong teas, can cause your blood pressure to increase, along with your heart rate. If you struggle with anxiety, you most likely already feel unsettled and jittery. Caffeine can increase these feelings. Also, caffeine blocks the neurotransmitter in your brain that makes you tired, so it can affect your sleep and keep you awake. Try substituting your morning cup of coffee for a cup of tea instead.

Take Advantage of Sunshine

It is important to be outside. The sun provides vitamin D to your body, essential for your health. When the sun is shining bright on your shoulders or face, you feel more active. In addition, it can help boost your mood, as the sun actually increases your serotonin levels. So next time you feel down, t Enjoy it and feel the warmth hugging your skin and letting it rejuvenate you.

Take a Deep Breath

Sometimes, the blood pressure levels go up; it is just natural stimuli to worry and experience nervousness. The person may experience increased or heavy breathing as the adrenaline levels increase. It is always wise to take a deep breath and systematically breathe in and out whenever anxious. Deep diaphragmatic breaths are a powerful technique to reduce anxiety levels; the process activates the body's relaxation response and eases the nerves. Deep breaths also help the body move from fight or flight mode to a controlled and calm nervous system.

Start by slowly breathing into a maximum of four while filling the belly first, then the chest. Next, exercise your cardiac muscles by trying to hold your breath into a similar count of four gently. Finally, slowly breathe out to our count and repeat this procedure several times until you feel your body relaxed.

Accept That You Are Anxious

Anxiety is just a feeling like any other; let's say love, sympathy, and empathy; it only becomes a problem when it becomes a disorder, as I discussed earlier on. It is not a crime to be anxious, so do not judge yourself every time the feeling engulfs your system. Reminding yourself that anxiety is nothing more than a feeling and that you have the power to control it prepares you psychologically to confront the particular stimulus that causes your fear positively.

Acknowledge That Your Brain is Playing Tricks on You

Thoughts are a powerful tool; they may positively or negatively influence your daily operations. When an object, person, or situation causes high levels of fear to build up in you, your brain may, through the thoughts, emphasize the details to the point that you develop certain worries, fears, and phobias. During any panic attack, the brain quickly tries to get possible ways out of the situation, which is just in response to the cause of panic. Acting on an immediate impulse to your thoughts may not be the best decision; however, try out possible ways to calm your nerves and take time to debate on the range of remedies that your brain presents you with. Once you can calm yourself and think of the many possible remedies, you have mentally overpowered your fear; anxiety leaves you helpless and always gives that feeling of defeat.

Use a Calming Mental Picture or Visualization

Take stage fright. For example, fear may engulf you to the point that you may feel dizzy on stage. A mental picture distracts you and pulls part of your attention to other things that you best enjoy.

Focus on the Moment

Anxiety knows no boundaries. It makes individuals focus on illogical occurrences of future events should the fear factor confront them. Therefore, every time you are anxious, do not bother about the future; rather, focus on what is happening to you at that particular time.

Busy Yourself with Meaningful Activities

When the feeling of anxiety sets in, do not fret, immediate relief can be achieved through focusing your attention on meaningful and goal-oriented activities. The anxiety interrupted a chain of activities that you were undertaking. If you were going shopping, still go and if you were planning to cook a nice meal, still cook. The brain is always hungry for an idea; that's why we have numerous thoughts by the minute. Even when our bodies shut down and we fall asleep, thoughts in the form of dreams still rampage our minds. The worst thing to do is just sit down and do nothing when anxious. Focusing on nothing means focusing on thoughts that will do you no good but intensify your worries.

Self-Reward

Reward is positive reinforcement. Whenever you overcome your fears, you can reward yourself with something that leaves a mark of assurance and emphasizes that inner voice that keeps telling you 'you can do it every time you are anxious.

That was so much on achieving immediate anxiety relief; these steps can work for all anxiety disorders. You are advised to combine any three or more remedies when reduced to an anxious fit.

Meditation

There are so many types of meditation. They are all aimed at fine-tuning your thoughts into positive energy that will reflect most of your physical life. Meditation allows you ample time with yourself away from listening to what everyone is telling you about your condition. Every time you are anxious, take a deep breath and create a unique world of your own in your thoughts. Maintain a steady relationship with the air in the surroundings, the natural sounds, and your body's response to the stimuli introduced through meditation.

Decompress

Anxiety activates the nerves to quickly react to your fears by relaying messages to your brain and back to your body. Decompression keeps the nervous system in check to not run wild whenever you get anxious. Take a warm heat cloth, wrap it around your neck and shoulders for ten minutes, close your eyes and relax your muscles, face, upper chest, back muscles, and neck.

Massage Your Worries Away

Massage has been used as a natural anxiety remedy for ages; it may be as simple as rubbing your neck gently, but whichever the case, you are massaging your way to calm nerves. The benefits of any massage therapy are many. Stress relief relaxation, lower blood pressure, lower tension build in the muscles and improved deeper breathing. As the book unfolds, I will discuss therapeutic massage as a natural remedy for anxiety disorders. In this case, it will be much deeper and more precise.

Having a Little Fun Killed Nobody

Laughing is a great relaxation technique and stress reliever. It increases lots of good feelings and serves to discharge tension. One major problem with people prone to anxiety is that they tend to take life so seriously that they appear to be melancholy all the time, and they eventually stop creating fun moments in their life. Fun and play are essential for the brain's proper functioning; it is a technique that stimulates the brain to come up with creative ideas rather than concentrating on little worries and fears. Within the fun and play, you may develop various ways to apply in situations when you are rendered anxious and helpless. Remember that rigidity limits you to a certain scope of ideas that will directly influence your take on the world.

Tackle That Inner Voice (and Develop Your Positivity)

For many of us, the inner voice that provides the commentary to our every move isn't exactly kind. It can pull us up on our mistakes, criticize and whisper things that cut us the right to the core. But if you can foster the support and encouragement of this inner voice, you can get through even the toughest times. So who better to love you than yourself, right?
What might come as a surprise is that you don't have to listen to this voice. You have the power to challenge it and make it dance to the beat of your drum, not its own. So next time it whispers hurtful things inside your ear turn around and challenge it. Ask what it is hoping to achieve and tell it you will only listen if it speaks to you with kindness.
Switch that negative inner voice to positive affirmations. Practice positive affirmations daily to calm your anxieties and transform your mindset into a positive and peaceful one. These affirmations can be anything that resonates with you.

Here are some simple yet powerful examples you can try:

• I feel cool, calm, and collected.

• Every part of the body is relaxed and light.

- With every breath, I let go of anxiety and feel calmer.

- I am confident that I will successfully tackle life's challenges.

- I feel at peace and can escape stress.

- I love myself deeply and unconditionally.

- All is well in my world, and I am safe.

- I look forward to my future with hope and happiness.

- I can overcome my fears and live life courageously.

Taking Care of Your Body

There is a strong relationship between mind, emotion, and body. It will be easier to relax if you know that you are taking care of your body. Try to develop healthy eating and fitness eating habits. Exercise and a clean diet can do wonders for your anxiety.

Also, try to sleep well and on time. If you have a healthy routine, you will have more energy to face and handle life's ups and downs. Make wise food choices, develop a good sleeping habit, and exercise regularly. It sounds far too simple, but this has been one of the biggest factors in overcoming anxiety.

Talk About Your Problems with Other People

It helps if you have a trusted friend or relative willing to listen to your worries. Trying to contain your feelings can be very challenging. It will just allow your panic to snowball. When a person is willing to listen to your problems and vulnerabilities, you will be more at ease and realize that you are not alone. Secondly, things aren't as bad as they seem.

Do not always expect that the other person will comfort you completely. It is highly unlikely that the other person will be able to erase all your worries. However, talking about worries will prevent them from becoming bigger and bigger. It will prevent you from snapping in an unexpected situation. Talking about your problems will prevent you from exploding and may assist you in maintaining perspective.

Try Connecting with Nature

There is something about the harmony of nature that is incredibly calming and relaxing. Allow yourself to be comforted by the beauty of the universe. Find solace in parks or gardens. Choose a place that will make you feel safe and grounded. If you want, you can even ask a friend to accompany you as you enjoy nature's wonders. I love sitting on a bench in a park on a quiet Sunday morning and just watching the world go by. I may choose to read a book or simply sit and contemplate life and my surroundings. This has an amazing calming effect and ensures I see the world in all its beauty and splendor.

You can also engage in a hobby involving nature. For example, gardening or mountain climbing is a good way to improve your relationship with the wonders around you. You'll be surprised by what a little sunshine can do in your life. You will feel lighter, better, and maybe even happier.

Try to Be Grateful

To be honest, there are a million and one ways that things can go wrong at every moment. Your situation could be much worse than it is. Try to focus on the good things that are happening in your life. Look for things that you can be grateful for. Do you have a roof above your head? Are there people in your life that make you smile? If you focus on the good things that happen in your life, you will likely feel less anxious about what the future holds.

Try to Learn To Calm Yourself Down

People sometimes become slaves to their feelings. If you are anxious, you need to learn to find peace of mind. First, find your own "calm" place. That means knowing how to take charge when it seems like your emotions are taking over. There are many various ways to calm yourself down.

Learn to Keep Yourself Busy

If you are an anxiety sufferer, you will likely spend your free time worrying about unimportant things. Try to minimize your idle time so that you won't spend too much time worrying about things that don't matter. It is best to try and get a hobby to fill up your free time. Find something that interests you. For example, it is good to get into art or sports. Besides keeping you busy, it will also help you use your energy, so you won't have excess energy to worry about silly things that don't matter.

Practice Mindfulness

At times, we become so caught up in our minds that we forget to be present in the world around us and miss out on much of the beauty of life. Instead, we see the looming deadlines and stressful obligations instead of breathing in the joy. So slow down, open your eyes to the things that are right there around you and find things to be grateful for.

Meditation

Mediation is fast becoming one of the most popular self-help and wellness techniques of all time and is no longer a preserve of the 'green' crowds. Regularly practicing will help lower your heart rate, rebalance your hormones, help you to become more mindful, and stop your stress response right in its tracks. So why not give it a try; challenge yourself to meditate for just 30 days and see how better you will feel.

Here's a great exercise to get started with:

Sit down somewhere comfortable where you will not be disturbed for the duration of your practice and set your timer for an allotted time. Just 10 minutes can be effective, especially when you begin.

Adopt a comfortable position with your feet flat on the floor and your hands resting lightly in your lap.

Now focus your attention on the movement of your breath as it enters and leaves your body. Do not attempt to change it. Simply observe.

Begin to count your inhalations starting at one, up to a count of 10, and then repeat for as long as you wish.

Next, count your exhalations up to a count of 10 again until you feel the desire to switch to a different technique.

While focusing your attention in this manner, try to relax your mind as much as possible. You don't need to try to make your mind go blank, but instead, simply acknowledge your thoughts and allow them to float past you. That might be difficult for you at first, but you will improve as you continue to practice.

After the allotted period, simply open your eyes and gently return to reality.

Use Positive Visualization

Positive visualization is the super-effective technique that most top athletes, business people, and high achievers utilize to get them the results they want. By picturing the outcome that you dream of, you can move towards your biggest goals, overcome any obstacles that might come across your path, and fall in love with the journey itself.

Work with a Therapist

Don't be afraid of working with a therapist if your stress or anxiety severely interferes with your quality of life. Holistic help is only taking the edge off the problem. Therapists are experienced individuals trained to understand what you are going through and provide unconditional support to prevent you from descending into more serious anxiety disorders, depression, or stress-related disorders.

Tai Chi and Yoga

Being another stress and anxiety-killing activity, yoga involves stretching and deep breathing. Variations of yoga pose bring awareness to muscles that you may not use daily. For example, I carry my stress in my neck and my shoulders. Yoga helps stretch those muscles and relieve the tension from my body. Another important aspect of yoga is inward focus as well. Focusing on your breath is also an important yoga practice. That ensures that you deliver enough oxygen to your muscles as you stretch them. Finally, yoga and meditation can be used together for the ultimate anxiety-relieving experience.

Both yoga and tai chi are also effective relaxation exercises. Yoga can improve the body's relaxation response in day-to-day life. These exercises are slow-paced and not strenuous, making them a good fit for people of all ages.

Those unfamiliar with yoga and tai chi may want to begin taking a class. Some moves are hard to imitate without seeing them in motion. Video footage is also an option.

From deep breathing to full body stretches, relaxation exercises can provide long-term and short-term relationships. Once these techniques become a regular part of a person's life, they'll find that they feel far calmer and experience far less anxiety.

Relaxation exercises can provide people with much control over their anxiety symptoms. These techniques can help people experience fewer symptoms and far fewer panic attacks when regularly practiced. They're something anxiety sufferers should familiarize themselves with.

Psychotherapy

Psychotherapy is also called talk therapy. It has been seen as effective in helping people suffering from anxiety disorders cope with their anxiety. Psychotherapy needs to be given at the specific level of a person's anxiety to work effectively. Engaging in psychotherapy may be difficult for the person suffering from an anxiety disorder. He finds it extremely difficult to discuss his anxiety-provoking triggers and situations. He feels extremely uncomfortable at first when discussing facing his fears.

Cognitive Behavioral Therapy (CBT)

CBT is a very popular modern psychotherapy that has helped people deal with their anxiety disorders. CBT, a person's way of thinking, behavior, and reactions to situations that cause anxiety or make him fearful, can be altered productively. In addition, CBT helps people learn and apply social skills, which is the core of social Anxiety.

Conclusion

For millions of people worldwide, anxiety is a serious problem. It affects their daily life, interferes with their ability to get things done, and can even begin impacting their physical health and well-being.

The basic principle is that you can use the knowledge and tools to change your everyday life that does not work the way you want.

The knowledge or tools will not solve your problems; it is important to understand that you stand for change while we guide your work to change what you want to change.

The methods outlined in this book will help you take charge again so, if you ever feel another attack coming on, you have everything you need to regain control again, quickly.

You've now got the tools to work towards lessening the frequency of the attacks until they're just a distant memory.

You can do it. It's not even that difficult. But, if you truly want to change and rid yourself of panic attacks, the steps outlined in this book will get you there.

The next step is to decide on a treatment plan by seeking help. Mild anxiety cases specific to your life right now, without chronic symptoms, can be corrected and overcome using an alkaline diet, meditation, journaling, and mindfulness practices. You can live a life free of anxiety attacks and abnormal levels of worry, stress, and fear. You can develop techniques to retrain your brain to deal with mild upsetting situations that once brought on panic attacks. Use your stress and worry about pushing yourself to do better because some anxiety levels are healthy.

Just because your doctor might be telling you a prescription is the best remedy to help treat anxiety, there **are** extremely effective natural remedies.

This book laid out some of the most potent. If you ***truly*** want to overcome your anxiety and feel great every day into the future, combine the supplements with a healthier diet, exercise, **and** meditation techniques.

Before you realize it, you'll be feeling much better, more relaxed, and healthier than you have in a long, long time.

Now go out there and live your life on your terms.

BOOK 7: <u>DR. SEBI COOKBOOK</u>

MONEY-SAVING ALKALINE RECIPES TO SUPERCHARGE YOUR HEALTH

Chapter 1: Breakfast

• Alkaline Blueberry Spelt Pancakes

Preparation Time: 6 minutes

Cooking Time: 20 minutes

Servings: 3

Ingredients:

- 2 cups spelt flour
- 1 cup coconut milk
- 1/2 cup alkaline water
- 2 tbsps. grapeseed oil
- 1/2 cup agave
- 1/2 cup blueberries
- 1/4 tsp. sea moss

Directions:

1. Mix the spelled flour, agave, grapeseed oil, hemp seeds, and sea moss together in a bowl.

2. Add 1 cup of hemp milk and alkaline water to the mixture until you get the consistent mixture you like.

3. Crimp the blueberries into the batter.

4. Heat the skillet to moderate heat, then lightly coat it with the grapeseed oil.

5. Pour the batter into the skillet and let them cook for approximately 5 minutes on every side.

6. Serve and Enjoy.

Nutrition:

- Calories: 203 kcal.
- Fat: 1.4g.
- Carbs: 41.6g.
- Proteins: 4.8g.

• Alkaline Blueberry Muffins

Preparation Time: 5 minutes

Cooking Time: 20 minutes

Servings: 3

Ingredients:

- 1 cup coconut milk
- 3/4 cup spelt flour
- 3/4 tef flour
- 1/2 cup blueberries
- 1/3 cup agave
- 1/4 cup sea moss gel
- 1/2 tsp. sea salt
- Grapeseed oil

Directions:

1. Adjust the temperature of the oven to 365 degrees.

2. Grease 6 regular-size muffin cups with muffin liners.

3. In a bowl, mix together sea salt, sea moss, agave, coconut milk, and flour gel until properly blended.

4. You then crimp in blueberries.

5. Coat the muffin pan lightly with the grapeseed oil.

6. Pour in the muffin batter.

7. Bake for at least 30 minutes until it turns golden brown.

8. Serve.

Nutrition:

- Calories: 160 kcal.

- Fat: 5g.

- Carbs: 25g.

- Proteins: 2g.

• Crunchy Quinoa Meal

Preparation Time: 5 minutes

Cooking Time: 25 minutes

Servings: 2

Ingredients:

- 3 cups coconut milk

- 1 cup rinsed quinoa

- 1 cup raspberry

- 1/2 cup chopped coconut

Directions:

1. In a saucepan, pour milk and boil over moderate heat.

2. Add the quinoa to the milk, and then bring it to a boil once more.

3. You then let it simmer for at least 15 minutes on medium heat until the milk is reduced.

4. Cover it and cook for 8 minutes until the milk is completely absorbed.

5. Add the raspberry and cook the meal for 30 seconds.

6. Serve and enjoy.

Nutrition:

- Calories: 271 kcal.

- Fat: 3.7g.

- Carbs: 54g.

- Proteins: 6.5g.

• Coconut Pancakes

Preparation Time: 5 minutes

Cooking Time: 15 minutes

Servings: 4

Ingredients:

- 1 cup coconut flour

- 2 tbsps. arrowroot powder

- 1 tsp. baking powder

- 1 cup coconut milk

- 3 tbsps. coconut oil

Directions:

1. In a medium container, mix in all the dry ingredients.

2. Add the coconut milk and 2 tbsps. Of the coconut oil, then mix properly.

3. In a skillet, melt 1 tsp of coconut oil.

4. Pour a ladle of the batter into the skillet, then swirl the pan to spread the batter evenly into a smooth pancake.

5. Cook it for at least 3 minutes on medium heat until it becomes firm.

6. Turn the pancake to the other side and cook it for another 2 minutes until it turns golden brown.

7. Cook the remaining pancakes in the same process.

8. Serve.

Nutrition:

- Calories: 377 kcal.

- Fat: 14.9g.

- Carbs: 60.7g.

- Protein: 6.4g.

• Banana Barley Porridge

Preparation Time: 15 minutes

Cooking Time: 5 minutes

Servings: 2

Ingredients:

- 1 cup divided unsweetened coconut milk

- 1 small peeled and sliced banana

- 1/2 cup barley

- 1/4 cup chopped coconuts

Directions:

1. In a bowl, properly mix barley with half of the coconut milk.

2. Cover the bowl, then refrigerate for about 6 hours.

3. In a saucepan, mix the barley mixture with coconut milk.

4. Cook for about 5 minutes on moderate heat.

5. Then top it with the chopped coconuts and the banana slices.

6. Serve.

Nutrition:

- Calories: 159kcal.

- Fat: 8.4g.

- Carbs: 19.8g.

- Proteins: 4.6g.

• Zucchini Muffins

Preparation Time: 10 minutes

Cooking Time: 25 minutes

Servings: 16

Ingredients:

- 1 tbsp. ground flaxseed

- 3 tbsps. spring water

- 1/4 cup walnut butter

- 3 medium over-ripe bananas

- 2 small grated zucchinis

- 1/2 cup coconut milk

- 2 cups coconut flour

- 1/4 tsp. sea salt

Directions:

1. Adjust the temperature of your oven to 375°F.

2. Grease the muffin tray with the cooking spray.

3. In a bowl, mix the flaxseed with water.

4. In a glass bowl, mash the bananas, then stir in the remaining ingredients.

5. Properly mix and then divide the mixture into the muffin tray.

6. Bake it for 25 minutes.

7. Serve.

Nutrition:

- Calories: 127 kcal.

- Fat: 6.6g.

- Carbs: 13g.

- Protein: 0.7g.

-

Hemp Seed Porridge

Preparation Time: 5 minutes

Cooking Time: 5 minutes

Servings: 6

Ingredients:

- 3 cups cooked hemp seed
- 1 cup coconut milk

Directions:

1. In a saucepan, mix the rice and the coconut milk over moderate heat for about 5 minutes as you stir it constantly.
2. Remove the pan from the heat, then stir.
3. Serve in 6 bowls.
4. Enjoy.

Nutrition:

- Calories: 236 kcal.
- Fat: 1.8g.
- Carbs: 48.3g.
- Protein: 7g.

Alkaline Blueberry and Strawberry Muffins

Preparation Time: 15 minutes

Cooking Time: 5 hours

Servings: 6

Ingredients:

- 3/4 cup quinoa flour
- 3/4 cup tef flour
- 1/2 teaspoon salt
- 1/3 cup agave
- 1 cup fresh coconut milk
- 1/4 cup strawberries, chopped
- 1/4 cup blueberries

Directions:

- Place the quinoa flour, tef flour, and salt in a bowl.
- In another bowl, combine the agave and coconut milk. Slowly pour the wet ingredients into the dry ingredients.
- Mix until well-combined.
- Stir in the berries and mix until well-combined.
- Pour the batter into muffin pans.
- Place the muffin pans with the batter in the Instant Pot.
- Close the lid but do not set the vent to the Sealing position.
- Press the Slow Cook button and adjust the cooking time to 4 to 5 hours.

Nutrition:

- Calories: 271 kcal.
- Protein: 7.2g.
- Carbs: 36.6g.
- Sugar: 4.3g.
- Fat: 11.5 g.

Blueberry Spelt Flat Cakes

Preparation Time: 15 minutes

Cooking Time: 4 hours

Servings: 4

Ingredients:

- 2 cups spelt flour

- 1/4 teaspoon sea salt

- 1/4 cup hemp seeds

- 1 cup fresh coconut milk

- 1/2 cup spring water

- 2 tablespoons grapeseed oil

- 1/2 cup agave

- 1/2 cup blueberries

Directions:

1. Mix the spelt flour, sea salt, and hemp seeds in a bowl.

2. Pour in the coconut milk, water, grapeseed oil, and agave.

3. Stir until well-combined. Pour in the blueberries.

4. Line the Instant Pot with parchment paper.

5. Pour the batter into the Instant Pot.

6. Close the lid but do not set the vent to the Sealing position.

7. Press the Slow Cook button and adjust the cooking time to 4 hours.

Nutrition:

- Calories: 574 kcal.

- Protein: 16.1g.

- Carbs: 74.8g.

- Sugar: 14.8g.

- Fat: 27.8g.

▪ <u>Breakfast Quinoa Cereal</u>

Preparation Time: 15 minutes

Cooking Time: 15 minutes

Servings: 2

Ingredients:

- 1 cup quinoa

- 2 cups spring water

- A dash of cayenne pepper

- A dash of sea salt

- A dash of oregano

Directions:

1. Place the quinoa and spring water in the Instant Pot. Give a good stir.

2. Close the lid and set the vent to the Sealing position.

3. Press the Multigrain button and adjust the cooking time to 15 minutes.

4. Do natural pressures release.

5. Once the lid is open, ladle the porridge in bowls and top with cayenne pepper, salt, and oregano.

Nutrition:

- Calories: 322 kcal.

- Protein: 12.45g.

- Carbs: 56.7g.

- Sugar: 1.2g.

Chapter 2: Lunch

- ## Alkaline Macaroni and 'Cheese'

Preparation Time: 20 minutes

Cooking Time: 50 minutes

Servings: 8-10

Ingredients:

- 12 ounces of any alkaline pasta
- 1/4 cup chickpea flour
- 1 cup raw Brazil nuts
- 1/2 teaspoon ground achiote
- 2 teaspoons onion powder
- 1 teaspoon pure sea salt
- 2 teaspoons grapeseed oil
- 1 cup homemade hemp seed milk
- 1 cup spring water + extra for soaking
- Juice from 1/2 key lime

Directions:

1. Put the Brazil nuts in a medium bowl and cover them with spring water. Soak overnight.
2. Cook your favorite alkaline pasta.
3. Preheat your oven to 350 degrees Fahrenheit.
4. Place the cooked pasta in a baking dish and drizzle extra grapeseed oil to prevent it from sticking to the bottom.
5. Add all ingredients to a blender and blend for 2 to 4 minutes until smooth.
6. Pour the Brazil nut sauce over the macaroni and mix well.
7. Put the baking dish in the oven and bake for about 30 minutes.
8. Serve and enjoy your Macaroni and 'Cheese'!

Nutrition:

- Calories: 360 kcal.
- Fat: 6g.
- Carbs: 13.4g.
- Protein: 22.5g.

- ## Kamut Patties

Preparation Time: 15 minutes

Cooking Time: 30 minutes

Servings: 3-4

Ingredients:

- 3 cups cooked kamut cereal
- 1 cup minced red onions
- 1 cup chopped yellow & red peppers
- 1 cup spelt flour
- ½ cup homemade hemp seed milk (see recipe)
- 1 tablespoon basil
- ½ teaspoon cayenne powder
- 1 tablespoon oregano
- 1 tablespoon onion powder
- 1 teaspoon pure sea salt
- 2 tablespoons grade seed oil

Directions:

1. Combine vegetables, hempseed milk, seasonings, and kamut cereal in a large bowl.

2. Put 1/2 cup of spelt flour in the bowl and mix it well. Continue adding more flour until it can be formed into patties.

3. Warm the grapeseed oil in a skillet on medium heat. Form patties from the mixture and place them on the pan.

4. Cook patties for about 4 to 5 minutes on each side.

5. Serve and enjoy your Kamut Patties!

Nutrition:

- Calories: 412kcal.

- Fat: 7g.

- Carbs: 12g.

- Protein: 15g.

▪ Portobello Mushroom Burgers

Preparation Time: 25 minutes

Cooking Time: 50 minutes

Servings: 2

Ingredients:

- 2 cups portobello mushroom caps

- 1 sliced avocado

- 1 sliced plum tomatoes

- 1 cup torn lettuce

- 1 cup purslane

- 1/2 teaspoon cayenne

- 1 teaspoon oregano

- 2 teaspoons basil

- 3 tablespoons olive oil

Directions:

1. Preheat your oven to 425 degrees Fahrenheit.

2. Remove the mushroom stems and cut off ½ inch slice from the top slice, as if slicing a bun.

3. Mix onion powder, cayenne, oregano, olive oil, and basil thoroughly in a medium bowl.

4. Cover a baking sheet with foil and brush with grapeseed oil to avoid sticking.

5. Put mushroom caps on the baking sheet and brush them with the prepared marinade. Marinate for 10 minutes before cooking.

6. Bake for 10 minutes until golden brown, then flip. Continue baking for 10 more minutes.

7. Lay out the mushroom cap on a serving dish. This will serve as the bottom for the mushroom burger.

8. Layer the sliced avocado, tomatoes, lettuce, and purslane.

9. Cover the burger with another mushroom cap. Repeat steps 7 and 8 with the remaining mushrooms and vegetables.

10. Serve and enjoy your Portobello Mushroom Burgers!

Nutrition:

- Calories: 178kcal.

- Fat: 2g.

- Carbs: 3g.

- Protein: 16g.

▪ Veg-Meatballs

Preparation Time: 10 minutes

Cooking Time: 30 minutes

Servings: 7-9

Ingredients:

- 1 1/2 cups cooked garbanzo beans

- 1 cup garbanzo bean flour

- 2 cups mushrooms

- 1/4 cup diced red peppers

- 1/2 cup diced onions

- 2 teaspoons oregano

- 1 tablespoon onion powder

- 2 teaspoons basil

- 1 teaspoon fennel powder

- 1 teaspoon dill

- 1 teaspoon savory

- 1 teaspoon sage

- 1/2 teaspoon ginger powder

- 1/2 teaspoon ground cloves

- 1 teaspoon pure sea salt

- 1/2 teaspoon cayenne powder

- 6 cups fragrant tomato sauce (see recipe)

- 2 tablespoons grapeseed oil

Directions:

1. Place Mushrooms cooked garbanzo beans, onions, red peppers, and seasonings into a food processor. Blend them well for 1 minute.

2. Add blended mixture to a large bowl and mix in garbanzo bean Flour. Try to make balls. If balls do not form, add more flour.

3. Shape the meatballs and let them rest for a couple minutes.

4. Add grapeseed oil to a skillet and warm it on medium heat.

5. Place a couple of meatballs on the skillet. Cook for 2 minutes on each side.

6. Add fragrant tomato sauce to the meatballs and simmer for additional 5 minutes.

7. Serve and enjoy your Meatballs!

Nutrition:

- Calories: 321 kcal.

- Fat: 4g.

- Carbs: 6g.

- Protein: 7g.

▪ <u>Tomato & Greens Salad</u>

Preparation Time: 10 minutes

Cooking Time: 0 minutes

Servings: 4

Ingredients:

- 6 cups fresh baby greens

- 3 cups cherry tomatoes

- 2 tablespoons extra-virgin olive oil

- 1 tablespoon fresh lime juice

Directions:

1. In a large bowl, add all ingredients and toss to coat well.

2. Serve immediately.

Nutrition:

- Calories: 90 kcal.

- Total Fat: 7.3g.

- Saturated Fat: 1.1g.

- Cholesterol: 0mg.

- Sodium: 12mg.

- Total Carbs: 6.3g.

- Fiber: 2.2g.

- Sugar: 4.2g.

- Protein: 1.7g.

▪ Cucumber & Onion Salad

Preparation Time: 10 minutes

Cooking Time: 0 minutes

Servings: 5

Ingredients:

- 3 large cucumbers, sliced thinly
- ½ cup onion, sliced
- 2 tablespoons olive oil
- Sea salt, to taste
- ¼ cup fresh cilantro, chopped

Directions:

1. In a large bowl, add all ingredients and toss to coat well.
2. Serve immediately.

Nutrition:

- Calories: 81 kcal.
- Total Fat: 5.8g.
- Saturated Fat: 0.9g.
- Cholesterol: 0mg.
- Sodium: 49mg.
- Total Carbs: 7.7g.
- Fiber: 1.2g.
- Sugar: 3.5g.
- Protein: 1.3g.

▪ Apple Salad

Preparation Time: 10 minutes

Cooking Time: 0 minutes

Servings: 4

Ingredients:

- 4 large apples, cored and sliced
- 3 tablespoons extra-virgin olive oil
- 2 tablespoons hemp seeds
- Sea salt, to taste

Directions:

1. Add all the ingredients and toss to coat well in a large bowl.
2. Serve immediately.

Nutrition:

- Calories: 218 kcal.
- Total Fat: 11.1g.
- Saturated Fat: 1.5g.
- Cholesterol: 0mg.
- Sodium: 38mg.
- Total Carbs: 32.5g.
- Fiber: 6.4g.
- Sugar: 23.4g.
- Protein: 1.9g.

• Okra Curry

Preparation Time: 15 minutes

Cooking Time: 13 minutes

Servings: 2

Ingredients:

- 1 tablespoon olive oil

- ½ teaspoon cumin seeds

- ¾ pound okra pods, trimmed and cut into 2-inch pieces

- ½ teaspoon red chili powder

- 1 teaspoon ground coriander

- Sea salt and freshly ground black pepper, to taste

Directions:

1. Heat the oil over medium heat in a large skillet and sauté the cumin seeds for 30 seconds.

2. Add the okra and stir fry for 1-1½ minutes.

3. Reduce the heat to low and cook, cover for 6-8 minutes, stirring occasionally.

4. Uncover and increase the heat to medium.

5. Stir in the red chili powder, and coriander and cook for 2-3 more minutes.

6. Season with salt and remove from heat.

7. Serve hot.

Nutrition:

- Calories: 134 kcal.

- Total Fat: 7.6g.

- Saturated Fat: 1.1g.

- Cholesterol: 0mg.

- Sodium: 137mg.

- Total Carbs: 13.6g.

- Fiber: 5.9g.

- Sugar: 2.6g.

- Protein: 3.5g.

• Vegetable Party

Preparation Time: 15 minutes

Cooking Time: 35 minutes

Servings: 3

Ingredients:

- 1 tablespoon coconut oil

- 1 medium onion, chopped finely

- ½ tablespoon fresh ginger, minced

- 1 Serrano pepper, seeded and minced

- ¼ teaspoon cayenne pepper

- Sea salt, to taste

- 1 medium tomato, finely chopped

- 2 large zucchini, cubed

- 1 cup unsweetened coconut milk

- 2 tablespoons fresh cilantro, chopped

Directions:

1. In a large skillet, melt the coconut oil over medium heat and sauté the onion for 8-9 minutes.

2. Add the serrano pepper, cayenne pepper, salt, and sauté for 1 minute.

3. Add the tomato and cook for 3-4 minutes, crushing with the back of a spoon.

4. Add the zucchini and salt and cook for 1 minute, stirring occasionally.

5. Stir in the coconut milk and bring to a gentle boil.

6. Reduce the heat to medium-low and simmer, covered for 15-20 minutes or until done completely.

7. Serve with a garnish of cilantro.

Nutrition:

- Calories: 124 kcal.

- Total Fat: 6.4g.

- Saturated Fat: 5.3g.

- Cholesterol: 0mg.

- Sodium: 86mg.

- Total Carbs: 16.6g.

- Fiber: 7.5g.

- Sugar: 7.4g.

- Protein: 2.6g.

▪ Thick Alkaline Minestrone

Preparation Time: 10 minutes

Cooking Time: 15 minutes

Servings: 2

Ingredients:

- 1 tablespoon coconut oil

- ¼ onion, rinsed and diced

- ½ cup zucchini, rinsed and cubed

- ½ cup red bell peppers, rinsed and cubed

- ½ cup canned beans, such as white, navy, or kidney beans, rinsed and drained

- 1 cup tomato juice

- ½ cup vegetable stock

- Handful fresh basil leaves, rinsed

- Himalayan pink salt

- Freshly ground black pepper

Directions:

1. In a large pot over medium-high heat, heat the coconut oil. Add the onion, zucchini, and bell peppers. Sauté for 3 minutes.

2. Stir in the beans, tomato juice, and vegetable stock. Bring to a boil. Reduce the heat to simmer and cook for 10 minutes.

3. Stir in the basil, season with salt and pepper, and serve.

Nutrition:

- Calories: 168 kcal.

- Total Fat: 7g.

- Total carbohydrates: 25g.

- Fiber: 6g.

- Sugar: 11g.

- Protein: 4g.

▪ Sautéed Kale

Preparation Time: 10 minutes

Cooking Time: 20 minutes

Servings: 4

Ingredients:

- 1 tablespoon extra-virgin olive oil

- 1 lime, seeded and sliced thinly

- 1 onion, sliced thinly

- 2 pounds fresh kale, trimmed and chopped

- ½ cup scallions, chopped

- Sea salt and freshly ground black pepper, to taste

Directions:

1. Heat the oil over medium heat in a large skillet and cook the lime slices for 5 minutes.

2. Remove the lime slices from the skillet with a slotted spoon and set them aside.

3. Add the onion and sauté for about 5 minutes in the same skillet.

4. Add the kale, scallions, honey, salt, and pepper and cook for 8-10 minutes.

5. Add the lime slices and mix until well combined.

6. Serve hot.

Nutrition:

- Calories: 161 kcal.
- Total Fat: 3.6g.
- Saturated Fat: 0.5g.
- Cholesterol: 0mg.
- Sodium: 160mg.
- Total Carbs: 28.3g.
- Fiber: 4.6g.
- Sugar: 1.6g.
- Protein: 7.5g.

- ## Parsley Mushrooms

Preparation Time: 15 minutes

Cooking Time: 14 minutes

Servings: 2

Ingredients:

- 2 tablespoons olive oil
- 2-3 tablespoons onion, minced
- 12 ounces fresh mushrooms, sliced
- 1 tablespoon fresh parsley
- Sea salt and freshly ground black pepper, to taste

Directions:

1. Heat the oil over medium heat in a skillet and sauté the onion for 2-3 minutes.

2. Add the mushrooms and cook for 8-10 minutes or until desired doneness.

3. Stir in the parsley, salt and black pepper and remove from the heat.

4. Serve hot.

Nutrition:

- Calories: 162 kcal.
- Total Fat: 14.5g.
- Saturated Fat: 2g.
- Cholesterol: 0mg.
- Sodium: 128mg.
- Total Carbs: 6.9g.
- Fiber: 2g.
- Sugar: 3.4g.
- Protein: 5.6g.

Chapter 3: Dinner

• Easy Cilantro Lime Quinoa

Preparation Time: 5 minutes

Cooking Time: 15 minutes

Servings: 6

Ingredients:

- 1 cup quinoa, rinsed and drained
- ½ cup fresh cilantro, chopped
- 1 lime zest, grated
- 2 tbsp. fresh lime juice
- 1 ¼ cups filtered alkaline water
- Sea salt

Directions:

1. Add quinoa and water to the instant pot and stir well.
2. Seal pot with a lid, select manual mode and set the timer for 5 minutes.
3. When finished, allow releasing pressure naturally, then open the lid.
4. Stir in cilantro, lime zest, and lime juice.
5. Season with salt and serve.

Nutrition:

- Calories: 105 kcal.
- Fat: 1.7g.
- Carbohydrates: 18.3g.
- Sugar: 0g.
- Protein: 4g.

• Gingery Quinoa

Preparation Time: 10 minutes

Cooking Time: 25 minutes

Servings: 4

Ingredients:

- 1 cup quinoa
- 1 ½ cups filtered alkaline water
- 1 tsp. coriander powder
- 1 tsp. turmeric
- 1 tsp. cumin seeds
- 1 tsp. fresh ginger, grated
- 1 cup onion, chopped
- 2 tbsp. olive oil
- 1 fresh lime juice
- Pepper
- Salt

Directions:

1. Add oil to the instant pot and set the pot on sauté mode.
2. Add the onion in olive oil and sauté for 2 minutes or until it is softened.
3. Add ginger, spices, and quinoa and cook for 3—4 minutes.
4. Add water.
5. Seal pot with lid and cook on manual high pressure for 2 minutes.
6. When finished, allow releasing pressure naturally, then open the lid.

7. Add lime juice and stir well.

8. Serve and enjoy.

Nutrition:

- Calories: 268 kcal.

- Fat: 9.9g.

- Carbohydrates: 38.8g.

- Sugar: 3.4g.

- Protein: 7.6g.

• Spicy Zucchini

Preparation Time: 15 minutes

Cooking Time: 5 minutes

Servings: 4

Ingredients:

- 2 zucchini, cut into 1-inch cubes

- ½ cup filtered alkaline water

- 1 cup tomato, chopped

- ½ tsp. red pepper

- 2 tbsp. extra virgin olive oil

- ¼ tsp. sea salt

Directions:

1. Add zucchini and water into the instant pot.

2. Seal the pot with the lid and cook on manual high pressure for 5 minutes.

3. When finished, release pressure using the quick-release method, then open the lid. Drain zucchini well.

4. Add oil to the instant pot and set it on sauté mode.

5. Return the zucchini in the pot, tomato, red pepper and salt, and stir until combined.

6. Cook in sauté mode for 5 minutes. Stir occasionally.

7. Serve and enjoy.

Nutrition:

- Calories: 107 kcal.

- Fat: 7.6g.

- Carbohydrates: 10.5g.

- Sugar: 5.6g.

- Protein: 1.9g.

- Cholesterol: 0mg.

• Cajun Seasoned Zucchini

Preparation Time: 8 minutes

Cooking Time: 2 minutes

Servings: 2

Ingredients:

- 4 zucchinis, sliced

- 1 tsp. paprika

- 2 tbsp. Cajun seasoning

- ½ cup filtered alkaline water

- 1 tbsp. olive oil

Directions:

1. Add all ingredients into the instant pot and stir well.

2. Seal the pot with the lid and cook on low pressure for 1 minute.

3. When finished, release pressure using the quick-release method, then open the lid.

4. Stir well and serve.

Nutrition:

- Calories: 130 kcal.

- Fat: 7.9g.

- Carbohydrates: 14.7g.

- Sugar: 7.2g.

- Protein: 5.3g.

- Cholesterol: 0mg.

- ## Fried Cabbage

Preparation Time: 10 minutes

Cooking Time: 3 minutes

Servings: 6

Ingredients:

- 1 head cabbage, chopped

- ½ tsp. chili powder

- ½ onion, diced

- ½ tsp. paprika

- 1 onion, chopped

- 1 cup filtered alkaline water

- 2 tbsp. olive oil

- ½ tsp. sea salt

Directions:

1. Add olive oil into the instant pot and set the pot on sauté mode.

2. Add the onion in olive oil and sauté until softened.

3. Add the remaining ingredients and stir to combine.

4. Seal the pot with the lid and cook on high pressure for 3 minutes.

5. When finished, release pressure using the quick-release method, then open the lid.

6. Stir well and serve.

Nutrition:

- Calories: 75 kcal.

- Fat: 4.9g.

- Carbohydrates: 8g.

- Sugar: 4.2g.

- Protein: 1.7g.

- Cholesterol: 0mg.

- ## Zucchini Noodles

Preparation Time: 8 minutes

Cooking Time: 2 minutes

Servings: 2

Ingredients:

- 2 large zucchinis, spiralized

- 1 tbsp. fresh mint leaves, sliced

- 1/3 lime juice

- ½ lime zest

- 2 tbsp. olive oil

- ¼ tsp. pepper

- ½ tsp. sea salt

Directions:

1. Add oil into the instant pot and set the pot on sauté mode.

2. Add lime zest and salt in olive oil and stir for 30 seconds.

3. Add zucchini noodles and drizzled with lime juice and stir for 30 seconds.

4. Season with pepper and salt to taste. Top with mint.

5. Serve and enjoy.

Nutrition:

- Calories: 178 kcal.

- Fat: 14.6g.

- Carbohydrates: 12.2g.

- Sugar: 5.6g.

- Protein: 4.2g.

- Cholesterol: 0mg.

• Buckwheat Porridge

Preparation Time: 20 minutes

Cooking Time: 10 minutes

Servings: 4

Ingredients:

- 1 cup buckwheat groats, rinsed

- 2 tbsp. walnuts, chopped

- 3 cups coconut milk

Directions:

1. Add buckwheat, and milk in the instant pot and stir well.

2. Seal pot with lid and cook on manual high pressure for 6 minutes.

3. When finished, allow releasing pressure naturally, then open the lid.

4. Top with chopped walnuts and serve.

Nutrition:

- Calories: 151 kcal.

- Fat: 5.1g.

- Carbohydrates: 23.9g.

- Sugar: 1g.

- Protein: 5.2g.

- Cholesterol: 0mg

• Wild Mushroom Soup

Preparation Time: 10 minutes

Cooking Time: 15 minutes

Servings: 4

Ingredients:

- 4 oz. walnut butter

- 1 chopped shallot

- 5 oz. chopped portabella mushrooms

- 10 oz. chopped oyster mushrooms

- 1 minced chive clove

- 1/2 tsp. dried thyme

- 3 cups alkaline water

- 1 vegetable bouillon cube

- 1 cup coconut cream

- 1/2 lb. chopped celery root

- Fresh cilantro

Directions:

1. In a cooking pan, melt the butter over medium heat.

2. Add the vegetables into the pan, then sauté until golden brown.

3. Add the remaining ingredients to the pan, then properly mix it.

4. Boil the mixture.

5. Simmer it for 15 minutes on low heat.

6. Add the cream to the soup, then pour it using a hand-held blender.

7. Serve warm with the chopped cilantro as toppings.

Nutrition:

- Calories: 243 kcal.

- Fat: 7.5g.

- Carbs: 14.4g.

- Protein: 10.1g.

• <u>Grilled Vegetable Stack</u>

Preparation Time: 10 minutes

Cooking Time: 20 minutes

Servings: 2

Ingredients:

- 1/2 zucchini, sliced into slices about 1/4-inch thick

- 2 stemmed portobello mushrooms with the gills removed

- 1 tsp. divided sea salt

- 1/2 cup divided hummus

- 1 peeled and sliced red onion

- 1 seeded red bell pepper, sliced lengthwise

- 1 seeded yellow bell pepper, sliced lengthwise

Directions:

1. Adjust the temperature of your broiler or grill.

2. Grill the mushroom caps over coal or gas flame.

3. Add the yellow and red bell peppers, onion, and zucchini for about 20 minutes as you turn it occasionally.

4. Fill the mushroom cap with 1/4 cup of hummus.

5. Top it with some onion, yellow peppers, red, and zucchini.

6. Add salt to the season, then set it aside.

7. Repeat the process with the second mushroom cap and the remaining ingredients.

8. Serve.

Nutrition:

- Calories: 179 kcal.

- Fat: 3.1g.

- Carbs: 15.7g.

- Protein: 3.9g.

• <u>Stuffed Peppers</u>

Preparation Time: 5 minutes

Cooking Time: 20 minutes

Servings: 2

Ingredients:

- 1/2 cup chopped vegetables, zucchinis

- 1 cup cooked quinoa

- 1 tsp. coconut oil

- 2 seedless, cored bell peppers with reserved tops

- 1 tsp. sea salt

- 1 tsp. onion powder

Directions:

1. Adjust the temperature of the oven to 350°F.

2. Coat a baking pan with a little cooking spray, then set aside.

3. In a saucepan over moderate heat, sauté the vegetables in the coconut oil for 5 minutes until it becomes softened.

4. Add the onion powder, salt, and quinoa, then stir to mix them.

5. In the baking pan, place the bell peppers in an upright position.

6. Fill every pepper with half of the quinoa-vegetable mix.

7. Top every bell pepper with its reserved topping.

8. Cover the baking pan with a piece of aluminum foil, then bake it for about 15 minutes until the peppers become soft.

9. Serve.

Nutrition:

- Calories: 213 kcal.

- Fat: 5.1g.

- Carbs: 34.8g.

- Protein: 7.2g.

• Slow-Cooked Garbanzo Beans

Preparation Time: 10 minutes

Cooking Time: 4 hours

Servings: 4

Ingredients:

- 2 tablespoons avocado oil
- 2 pounds garbanzo beans, trimmed and halved
- 1 tablespoon cilantro, chopped
- 1 teaspoon turmeric powder
- 1 teaspoon curry powder
- Juice of ½ lime
- ¼ cup green onions, chopped
- 1 tablespoon sweet paprika
- A pinch of black pepper

Directions:

1. In the slow cooker, mix the garbanzo beans with the oil, cilantro, and the other ingredients, cover, and cook high for 4 hours.

2. Divide between plates and serve as a side dish.

Nutrition:

- Calories: 200 kcal.
- Fat: 7.5g.
- Fiber: 6g.
- Carbs: 12g.
- Protein: 7.5g.

• Lime Kale Mix

Preparation Time: 10 minutes

Cooking Time: 0 minutes

Servings: 4

Ingredients:

- 3 tablespoons olive oil
- 5 tablespoons lime juice
- 1 cup radishes, halved
- 1 cup cucumber, sliced
- 7 cups kale, torn
- A pinch of black pepper

Directions:

1. Mix the kale with radishes, and other ingredients in a bowl.

2. Toss and serve.

Nutrition:

- Calories: 180 kcal.
- Fat: 4.4g.
- Fiber: 5g.
- Carbs: 14g.
- Protein: 8g.

• Herbed Zucchini

Preparation Time: 10 minutes

Cooking Time: 20 minutes

Servings: 4

Ingredients:

- 4 zucchinis, quartered lengthwise
- ½ teaspoon thyme, dried
- ½ teaspoon coriander, ground

- ½ teaspoon oregano, dried

- ½ teaspoon basil, dried

- 2 tablespoons avocado oil

- 1 tablespoon chives, chopped

- 2 tablespoons parsley, chopped

- A pinch of black pepper

Directions:

1. Arrange zucchini pieces on a lined baking sheet, add all the other ingredients and toss.

2. Introduce in the oven and bake at 350 degrees F for 20 minutes.

3. Divide between plates and serve as a side dish.

Nutrition:

- Calories: 198 kcal.

- Fat: 4g.

- Fiber: 4g.

- Carbs: 14g.

- Protein: 5g.

Chapter 4: Smoothies

- ## Avocado Blueberry Smoothie

Preparation Time: 5 minutes

Cooking Time: 5 minutes

Servings: 1

Ingredients:

- 1 tsp. chia seeds
- ½ cup unsweetened coconut milk
- 1 avocado
- ½ cup blueberries

Directions:

1. Add all ingredients to the blender and blend until smooth and creamy.
2. Serve immediately and enjoy.

Nutrition:

- Calories: 389 kcal.
- Fat: 34.6g.
- Carbs: 20.7g.
- Protein: 4.8g.
- Fiber: 0g.

- ## Vegan Blueberry Smoothie

Preparation Time: 5 minutes

Cooking Time: 5 minutes

Servings: 2

Ingredients:

- 2 cups blueberries

- 1 tbsp. hemp seeds
- 1 tbsp. chia seeds
- 1/8 tsp. orange zest, grated
- 1 cup fresh orange juice
- 1 cup unsweetened coconut milk

Directions:

1. Toss all your ingredients into your blender, then process till smooth and creamy.
2. Serve immediately and enjoy.

Nutrition:

- Calories: 212 kcal.
- Fat: 6.6g.
- Carbs: 36.9g.
- Protein: 5.2g.
- Fiber: 0g.

- ## Berry Peach Smoothie

Preparation Time: 5 minutes

Cooking Time: 5 minutes

Servings: 2

Ingredients:

- 1 cup coconut water
- 1 tbsp. hemp seeds
- 1 tbsp. agave
- ½ cup strawberries
- ½ cup blueberries

- ½ cup cherries

- ½ cup peaches

Directions:

1. Toss all your ingredients into your blender, then process till smooth and creamy.

2. Serve immediately and enjoy.

Nutrition:

- Calories: 117 kcal.

- Fat: 2.5g.

- Carbs: 22.5g.

- Protein: 3.5g.

- Fiber: 0g.

- ## Avocado Kale Smoothie

Preparation Time: 5 minutes

Cooking Time: 5 minutes

Servings: 3

Ingredients:

- 1 cup water

- ½ Seville orange, peeled

- 1 avocado

- 1 cucumber, peeled

- 1 cup kale

- 1 cup ice cubes

Directions:

1. Toss all your ingredients into your blender, then process till smooth and creamy.

2. Serve immediately and enjoy.

Nutrition:

- Calories: 160 kcal.

- Fat: 13.3g.

- Carbs: 11.6g.

- Protein: 2.4g.

- Fiber: 0g.

- ## Apple Kale Cucumber Smoothie

Preparation Time: 5 minutes

Cooking Time: 5 minutes

Servings: 1

Ingredients:

- ¾ cup water

- ½ green apple, diced

- ¾ cup kale

- ½ cucumber

Directions:

1. Toss all your ingredients into your blender, then process till smooth and creamy.

2. Serve immediately and enjoy.

Nutrition:

- Calories: 86 kcal.

- Fat: 0.5g.

- Carbs: 21.7g.

- Protein: 1.9g.

- Fiber: 0g.

Cucumber-Ginger Water

Preparation Time: 5 minutes

Cooking Time: 5 minutes + night for infusion

Servings: 2

Ingredients:

- 1 sliced cucumber

- 1 smashed thumb of ginger root

- 2 cups of spring water

Directions:

1. Prepare and put all ingredients in a jar with a lid.

2. Let the water infuse overnight. Then, store it in the refrigerator.

3. Serve and enjoy your Cucumber-Ginger Water throughout the day!

Nutrition:

- Calories: 117 kcal.

- Fat: 2g.

- Carbs: 6g.

- Protein: 9.7g.

- Fiber: 2g.

Strawberry Milkshake

Preparation Time: 5 minutes

Cooking Time: 5 minutes

Servings: 2

Ingredients:

- 2 cups of homemade hemp seed milk

- 1 cup of frozen strawberries

- Agave syrup, to taste

Directions:

1. Prepare and put all ingredients in a blender or a food processor.

2. Blend it well until you reach a smooth consistency.

3. Serve and enjoy your Strawberry Milkshake!

Nutrition:

- Calories: 222 kcal.

- Fat: 4g.

- Carbs: 3g.

- Protein: 6g.

- Fiber: 1g.

Cactus Smoothie

Preparation Time: 5 minutes

Cooking Time: 10 minutes

Servings: 2

Ingredients:

- 1 medium cactus

- 2 cups of homemade coconut milk

- 2 frozen baby bananas

- 1/2 cup of walnuts

- 1 date

- 2 teaspoons of hemp seeds

Directions:

1. Take the Cactus, remove all pricks, wash it, and cut it into medium pieces.

2. Put all ingredients in a blender or a food processor.

3. Blend it well until you reach a smooth consistency.

4. Serve and enjoy your Cactus Smoothie!

Nutrition:

- Calories: 123 kcal.

- Fat: 3g.

- Carbs: 6g.

- Protein: 2.5g.

- Fiber: 0g.

- ## <u>Prickly Pear Juice</u>

Preparation Time: 5 minutes

Cooking Time: 10 minutes

Servings: 2

Ingredients:

- 6 prickly pears

- 1/3 cup lime juice

- 1/3 cup agave

- 1-1/2 cups spring water

Directions:

1. Take Prickly Pear, cut off the ends, slice off the skin, and put in a blender. Do the same with the other pears.

2. Add Lime Juice with Agave to the blender and blend well for 30-40 seconds.

3. Strain the prepared mixture through a nut milk bag or cheesecloth and pour it back into the blender.

4. Pour Spring Water in and blend it repeatedly.

5. Serve and enjoy your Prickly Pear Juice!

Nutrition:

- Calories: 312 kcal.

- Fat: 6g.

- Carbs: 11g.

- Protein: 8g.

- Fiber: 2g.

Chapter 5: Soups

• Fresh Garden Vegetable Soup

Preparation Time: 7 minutes

Cooking Time: 20 minutes

Servings: 1-2

Ingredients:

- 1 little zucchini
- 1 celery stem
- 1 yellow onion
- 1 quart (antacid) water
- 4-5 tsps. sans yeast vegetable stock
- 1 tsp. new basil
- 2 tsps. sea salt to taste

Directions:

1. Put water in a pot, include the vegetable stock just as the onion, and boil it.

2. When the water is bubbling, it would be ideal to turn off the oven as we would prefer not to heat up the vegetables. Instead, put them all in the high-temperature water and hold up until the vegetables arrive at the desired delicacy.

3. Permit to cool somewhat; at that point, all fixings into a blender and blend until you get a thick, smooth consistency.

Nutrition:

- Calories: 43 kcal.
- Carbohydrates: 7g.
- Fat: 1g.

• Rawsome Gazpacho Soup

Preparation Time: 7 minutes

Cooking Time: 3 hours

Servings: 3-4

Ingredients:

- 2 cups tomatoes
- 1 small cucumber
- 1 red pepper
- 1 onion
- 1 small chili
- 1 quart of water (preferably alkaline water)
- 4 tbsp. cold-pressed olive oil
- Juice of one fresh lime
- 1 dash of cayenne pepper
- Sea salt to taste

Directions:

1. Remove the skin of the cucumber and cut all vegetables into large pieces.

2. Put all ingredients except the olive oil in a blender and mix until smooth.

3. Add the olive oil and mix again until the oil is emulsified.

4. Put the soup in the fridge and chill for at least 2 hours (soup should be served ice cold).

5. Add some salt and pepper to taste, mix, place the soup in bowls, garnish with chopped scallions, cucumbers, tomatoes, and peppers and enjoy!

Nutrition:

- Calories: 39 kcal.

- Carbohydrates: 8g.

- Fat: 0.5g.

- Protein: 0.2g.

• Alkaline Pumpkin Tomato Soup

Preparation Time: 15 minutes

Cooking Time: 30 minutes

Servings: 3-4

Ingredients:

- 1 quart of water (if accessible: soluble water)

- 2 cups tomatoes, stripped and diced

- 1 medium-sized sweet pumpkin

- 5 yellow onions

- 1 tbsp. cold squeezed additional virgin olive oil

- 2 tsp. ocean salt or natural salt

- Touch of cayenne pepper

- Your preferred spices (discretionary)

- Bunch of new parsley

Directions:

1. Cut onions in little pieces and sauté with some oil in a significant pot.

2. Cut the pumpkin down the middle; at that point, remove the stem and scoop out the seeds.

3. Finally, scoop out the fragile living creature and put it in the pot.

4. Include the tomatoes and the water likewise and cook for around 20 minutes.

5. At that point, empty the soup into a food processor and blend well for a couple of

moments. Then, sprinkle with salt, pepper, and other spices.

6. Fill bowls and trim with fresh parsley. Then, make the most of your alkalizing soup!

Nutrition:

- Calories: 78 kcal.

- Carbohydrates: 20g.

- Fat: 0.5g.

- Protein: 1.5g.

• Turnip Green Soup

Preparation Time: 5 minutes

Cooking Time: 22 minutes

Servings: 2

Ingredients:

- 2 tbsps. Coconut oil

- 1 large chopped onion

- 3 minced cloves chive

- 2 in piece peeled and minced ginger

- 3 cups bone broth

- 1 medium cubed white turnip

- 1 large chopped head radish

- 1 bunch chopped kale

- 1 Seville orange, 1/2 zested and juice reserved

- 1/2 tsp. sea salt

- 1 bunch cilantro

Directions:

1. In a skillet, add oil, then heat it.

2. Add in the onions as you stir.

3. Sauté for about 7 minutes, then add chive and ginger.

4. Cook for about 1 minute.

5. Add in the turnip, broth, and radish, then stir.

6. Bring the soup to a boil, then reduce the heat to allow it to simmer.

7. Cook for an extra 15 minutes, then turn off the heat.

8. Pour in the remaining ingredients.

9. Using a handheld blender, pour the mixture.

10. Garnish with cilantro.

11. Serve warm.

Nutrition:

- Calories: 249 kcal.

- Fat: 11.9g.

- Carbs: 1.8g.

- Protein: 35g.

- ## Tangy Lentil Soup

Preparation Time: 5 minutes

Cooking Time: 15 minutes

Servings: 4

Ingredients:

- 2 cups picked over and rinsed red lentils

- 1 chopped serrano Chile pepper

- 1 large chopped and roughly tomato

- 1-1/2 inch peeled and grated piece ginger

- 3 finely chopped cloves chive

- 1/4 tsp. ground turmeric

- Sea salt

Topping

- 1/4 cup coconut yogurt

Directions:

1. Add the lentils with enough water to cover the lentils in a pot.

2. Boil the lentils, then reduce the heat.

3. Cook for about 10 minutes on low heat to simmer.

4. Add the remaining ingredients, then stir.

5. Cook until lentils become soft and properly mixed.

6. Garnish a dollop of coconut yogurt.

7. Serve.

Nutrition:

- Calories: 248 kcal.

- Fat: 2.4g.

- Carbs: 12.2g.

- Protein: 44.3g.

- ## Mushroom Leek Soup

Preparation Time: 5 minutes

Cooking Time: 8 minutes

Servings: 4

Ingredients:

- 3 tbsps. divided vegetable oil

- 2-3/4 cups finely chopped leeks

- 3 finely minced chive stalks

- 7 cups cleaned and sliced assorted mushrooms

- 5 tbsps. coconut flour

- 3/4 tsp. sea salt

- 1/2 tsp. ground black pepper

- 1 tbsp. finely minced fresh dill

- 3 cups vegetable broth

- 2/3 cup coconut cream

- 1/2 cup coconut milk

Directions:

1. Preheat oil in a dutch oven, then sauté the leeks and chive until they become soft.

2. Add in the mushrooms, then stir.

3. Sauté for about 10 minutes.

4. Add pepper, dill, flour, and salt.

5. Mix properly, then cook for about 2 minutes.

6. Pour in the broth, then cook to boil.

7. Reduce the heat in the oven, then add the remaining ingredients.

8. Serve warm with coconut flour bread.

Nutrition:

- Calories: 127 kcal.

- Fat: 3.5g.

- Carbs: 3.6g.

- Protein: 21.5g.

• <u>Grilled Vegetable Stack</u>

Preparation Time: 10 minutes

Cooking Time: 20 minutes

Servings: 2

Ingredients:

- 1/2 zucchini, sliced into slices about 1/4—inch thick

- 2 stemmed Portobello mushrooms with the gills removed

- 1 tsp. divided sea salt

- 1/2 cup divided hummus

- 1 peeled and sliced red onion

- 1 seeded red bell pepper, sliced lengthwise

- 1 seeded yellow bell pepper, sliced lengthwise

Directions:

1. Adjust the temperature of your broiler or grill.

2. Grill the mushroom caps over coal or gas flame.

3. Add the yellow and red bell peppers, onion, and zucchini for about 20 minutes as you turn it occasionally.

4. Fill the mushroom cap with 1/4 cup of hummus.

5. Top it with some onion, yellow peppers, red, and zucchini.

6. Add salt to the season, then set it aside.

7. Redo the process with the second mushroom cap and the remaining ingredients.

8. Serve.

Nutrition:

- Calories: 179 kcal.

- Fat: 3.1g.

- Carbs: 15.7g.

- Protein: 3.9g.

• <u>Date Night Chive Bake</u>

Preparation Time: 10 minutes

Cooking Time: 30 minutes

Servings: 2

Ingredients:

- 4 peeled and sliced lengthwise zucchinis

- 1 lb. radish chopped into bite-size pieces

- 2 tsps. Seville orange zest

- 3 peeled and chopped chive heads cloves

- 2 tbsps. coconut oil

- 1 cup vegetable broth

- 1/4 tsps. mustard powder

- 1 tsp. sea salt

Directions:

1. Adjust the temperature of the oven to 400°F.

2. In a separate bowl, mix all the ingredients.

3. Spread the mixture in a baking pan evenly.

4. Cover the mixture with a piece of aluminum foil, then place it in the oven.

5. Bake the mixture for about 30 minutes as you stir it once halfway through the cooking time.

6. Serve.

Nutrition:

- Calories: 270 kcal.

- Fat: 15.2g.

- Carbs: 28.1g.

- Protein: 11.6g.

• <u>Champions Chili</u>

Preparation Time: 5 minutes

Cooking Time: 25 minutes

Servings: 4

Ingredients:

- 1 cup diced red bell pepper

- 1 chopped onion

- 2 finely chopped chive stalks

- 2 cups sprouted garbanzo beans

- 1/4 cup fresh organic cilantro

- 1/4 cup organic salsa

- 8 oz. jar organic pasta sauce

- Dash of chili powder

Directions:

1. Apply some non-stick cooking spray to a pot.

2. Place the pot over moderate heat, then sauté the onion for about 5 minutes.

3. Add in the ingredients and stir.

4. Simmer for about 20 minutes.

5. Serve.

Nutrition:

- Calories: 101 kcal.

- Fat: 2.7g.

- Carbs: 18.5g.

- Protein: 3.9g.

Chapter 6: Salad

• Cherry Tomato & Kale Salad

Preparation Time: 10 minutes

Cooking Time: 0 minutes

Servings: 2

Ingredients:

- 2 tbsps. ranch dressing
- 2 cups organic baby tomatoes
- 1 bunch kale, stemmed, leaves washed and chopped

Directions:

1. Mix all the ingredients in a bowl.
2. Divide the salad equally into two serving dishes.
3. Serve.

Nutrition:

- Calories: 58 kcal.
- Fat: 6.9g.
- Carbs: 1.6g.
- Protein: 1.1g.

• Caprese Salad

Preparation Time: 5 minutes

Cooking Time: 0 minutes

Servings: 2

Ingredients:

- 1 sliced avocado
- 2 large sliced tomatoes

- 1 bunch basil leaves
- 1 tsp. sea salt
- 1 cup cubed jackfruit

Directions:

1. In a bowl, toss all the salad ingredients to mix.
2. Add the sea salt to the season.
3. Serve.

Nutrition:

- Calories: 125 kcal.
- Fat: 10.1g.
- Carbs: 9.1g.
- Protein: 2g.

• Avocado Power Salad

Preparation Time: 10 minutes

Cooking Time: 0 minutes

Servings: 2

Ingredients:

- 1 cubed avocado
- 1 cup cooled cooked quinoa
- 1 tbsp. freshly squeezed Seville orange juice
- 1 tsp. sea salt
- 1 tbsp. onion powder
- 1 tbsp. onion powder
- 1/4 cup chopped cilantro

- 1 cup peeled and diced cucumber

- 1 cup halved cherry tomatoes

- 5oz. fresh and roughly chopped kale

Directions:

1. Mix all the ingredients.

2. Keep the mixture in the fridge to chill for about 15 minutes.

3. Serve.

Nutrition:

- Calories: 433 kcal.

- Fat: 14.8g.

- Carbs: 63.6g.

- Protein: 13.7g.

• <u>Roasted Vegetables</u>

Preparation Time: 10 minutes

Cooking Time: 15 minutes

Servings: 2

Ingredients:

- 1—pint cherry tomatoes

- 1/2 cup halved mushrooms

- 1 tsp. sea salt

- 1 tbsp. onion powder

- 1 tbsp. coconut oil

- 1 seeded and chopped red bell pepper

- 1 peeled zucchini, cut into small bite-size pieces

Directions:

1. Adjust the temperature of your oven to 425° F.

2. In a bowl, mix all the ingredients and evenly coat the vegetables.

3. Transfer the vegetables into a baking pan.

4. Roast the vegetables for about 15 minutes until the vegetables are tender.

5. Serve.

Nutrition:

- Calories: 132 kcal.

- Fat: 7.3g.

- Carbs: 15.4g.

- Protein: 2.9g.

• <u>Summer Lettuce Salad</u>

Preparation Time: 5 minutes

Cooking Time: 0 minutes

Servings: 4

Ingredients:

- 2 cups halved cherry tomatoes

- 4 cups romaine lettuce or iceberg

- 1 peeled and sliced cucumber

- 2 thinly sliced radishes

- 1 sliced scallion

- 1/2 cup shredded zucchini

- 14 oz. garbanzo beans

Directions:

1. Add all of the salad ingredients in a large bowl, then toss 2 tbsps. of the dressing.

2. Serve.

Nutrition:

- Calories: 39 kcal.

- Fat: 0.3g.

- Carbs: 9g.

- Protein: 1.6g.

• Green Quinoa Salad

Preparation Time: 5 minutes

Cooking Time: 0 minutes

Servings: 4

Ingredients:

- 1 cup roughly chopped radish florets

- 1/2 tsp. sea salt

- 2 tbsps. Coconut oil

- 2 tbsps. Freshly squeezed Seville orange juice

- 1/2 cup water

- 2 cups cooled cooked quinoa

Directions:

1. In a bowl, mix the radish and quinoa, then stir.

2. Mix the water, coconut oil, salt, and Seville orange juice using a blender.

3. Blend until the ingredients emulsify.

4. Pour the mixture over the salad, then stir to mix.

5. Keep the salad in the fridge for about 15 minutes to chill.

6. Serve cold.

Nutrition:

- Calories: 364 kcal.

- Fat: 11.8g.

- Carbs: 53g.

- Protein: 12.2g.

• Salad Pop

Preparation Time: 5 minutes

Cooking Time: 0 minutes

Servings: 4

Ingredients:

- 1 yellow squash, sliced into pieces

- 1 zucchini, sliced into pieces

- 1 cucumber, sliced into pieces

- 8 steamed radish florets

- 8 cherry tomatoes

Directions:

1. Thread 1 zucchini slice onto a wooden skewer, followed by the yellow squash, cucumber, cherry tomato, and radish floret

2. Redo the process with the remaining ingredients and vegetable pieces.

3. Serve.

Nutrition:

- Calories: 142 kcal.

- Fat: 1.5g.

- Carbs: 31.2g.

- Proteins: 7.8g.

• Warm Kale Salad

Preparation Time: 5 minutes

Cooking Time: 2 minutes

Servings: 2

Ingredients:

- 1 tbsp. sesame oil

- 1/2 cup toasted and chopped coconuts

- 6 oz. package baby Kale leaves

- 1 cup chopped shiitake mushrooms

- 1 tsp. sea salt

- Water

Directions:

1. In a bowl, mix the coconuts and kale.

2. Mix sesame oil, mushrooms and salt in a saucepan set over medium heat.

3. Cook for 5 minutes, then add water as it is absorbed.

4. Drizzle the mushroom dressing over the kale, then toss to mix them.

5. Serve.

Nutrition:

- Calories: 271 kcal.

- Fat: 19.4g.

- Carbs: 20.3g.

- Protein: 10.2g.

- ## Blueberry and Fennel Salad With Miso Dressing

Preparation Time: 10 minutes

Cooking Time: 0 minutes

Servings: 1

Ingredients:

For the dressing:

- ½ cup avocado oil

- ¼ cup water

- 2 tablespoons organic white miso

- 2 tablespoons freshly squeezed lime juice

- 1 teaspoon ground black pepper

For the salad:

- 2 cups mixed salad greens

- ½ cup blueberries

- ¼ cup finely sliced fennel

- 1 tablespoon fresh mint leaves

- 1 to 2 teaspoons chia seeds for garnish

Directions:

The dressing:

1. In a blender, blend together the avocado oil, water, miso, lime juice, and pepper until well combined and smooth.

2. Adjust seasonings to your preference.

The salad:

1. Add the mixed salad greens to your serving bowl, and top with the blueberries, fennel, mint, and chia seeds.

2. Drizzle the salad dressing over the top, or add it to the salad and toss it in so the entire salad is covered with the dressing.

3. Garnish with chia seeds and enjoy.

Nutrition:

- Calories: 174 kcal.

- Fat: 12.2g.

- Carbs: 16.1g.

- Protein: 8.3g.

Chapter 7: Dessert

• <u>Coconut Chip Cookies</u>

Preparation Time: 10 minutes

Cooking Time: 15 minutes

Servings: 4

Ingredients:

- 1 cup spelt flour
- ½ cup coconut flakes, unsweetened
- 4 tablespoon honey
- ¼ cup Brazilian nut butter, melted
- ¼ cup coconut milk
- ¼ teaspoon of sea salt

Directions:

1. Preheat your oven to 350 degrees F.
2. Layer a cookie sheet with parchment paper.
3. Add and then combine all the dry ingredients in a glass bowl.
4. Whisk in coconut milk, and nut butter.
5. Beat well, then stir in the dry mixture. Mix well.
6. Spoon out a tablespoon of cookie dough on the cookie sheet.
7. Add more dough to make as many as 16 cookies.
8. Flatten each cookie using your fingers.
9. Bake for 25 minutes until golden brown.
10. Let them sit for 15 minutes.
11. Serve.

Nutrition:

- Calories: 192 kcal.
- Total Fat: 17.44g.
- Saturated Fat: 11.5g.
- Cholesterol: 125mg.
- Total Carbs: 2.2g.
- Sugar: 1.4g.
- Fiber: 2.1g.
- Sodium: 135mg.
- Protein: 4.7g.

• <u>Brazilian Nut Butter Bars</u>

Preparation Time: 10 minutes

Cooking Time: 10 minutes

Servings: 6

Ingredients:

- 3/4 cup spelt flour
- 2 oz. Brazilian nut butter
- 2 tablespoon honey
- 1/2 cup Brazilian nut butter

Directions:

1. Combine all the ingredients for bars.
2. Transfer this mixture to a 6-inch small pan. Press it firmly.
3. Refrigerate for 30 minutes.
4. Slice and serve.

Nutrition:

- Calories: 214 kcal.

- Total Fat: 19g.

- Saturated Fat: 5.8g.

- Cholesterol: 15mg.

- Total Carbs: 6.5g.

- Sugar: 1.9g.

- Fiber: 2.1g.

- Sodium: 123mg.

- Protein: 6.5g.

• Berry Sorbet

Preparation Time: 10 minutes

Cooking Time: 20 minutes

Servings: 6

Ingredients:

- 2 cups water

- 2 cups strawberries

- 1 ½ tsp. spelt flour

- ½ cups date sugar

Directions:

1. Add the water into a large pot and let the water begin to warm.

2. Add the flour and date sugar and stir until dissolved.

3. Allow this mixture to start boiling and cook for around ten minutes.

4. It should have started to thicken.

5. Take off the heat and set it to the side to cool.

6. Add in the strawberries and stir well to combine once the syrup has cooled off.

7. Pour into a freezer-safe container and put it into the freezer until frozen.

8. Take sorbet out of the freezer, cut into chunks, and put it into a blender or a food processor.

9. Hit the pulse button until the mixture is creamy.

10. Pour this into the same freezer-safe container and put it back into the freezer for four hours.

Nutrition:

- Calories: 99 kcal.

- Carbohydrates: 8g.

• Apple Quinoa

Preparation Time: 15 minutes

Cooking Time: 30 minutes

Servings: 04

Ingredients:

- 1 tbsp. coconut oil

- Ginger

- 1/2 key lime

- 1 apple

- 1/2 cup quinoa

Optional toppings:

- Seeds

- Nuts

- Berries

Directions:

1. Fix the quinoa according to the instructions on the package.

2. When you are getting close to the end of the cooking time, grate in the apple and cook for 30 seconds.

3. Zest the lime into the quinoa and squeeze the juice in.

4. Stir in the coconut oil.

5. Divide evenly into bowls and sprinkle with some ginger.

6. You can add some berries, nuts, and seeds right before eating.

Nutrition:

- Calories: 146 kcal.

- Fiber: 2.3g.

- Fat: 8.3g.

• <u>Hot Kamut With Peaches, Walnuts, and Coconut</u>

Preparation Time: 10 minutes

Cooking Time: 35 minutes

Servings: 04

Ingredients:

- 4 tbsp. toasted coconut

- 1/2 cup toasted and chopped walnuts

- 8 chopped dried peaches

- 3 cups coconut milk

- 1 cup kamut cereal

Directions:

1. Mix the coconut milk into a saucepan and allow it to warm up.

2. When it begins simmering, add in the Kamut.

3. Let this cook for about 15 minutes while stirring every now and then.

4. When done, divide evenly into bowls and top with the toasted coconut, walnuts, and peaches.

5. You could even go one more and add some fresh berries.

Nutrition:

- Calories: 156 kcal.

- Protein: 5.8g.

- Carbohydrates: 25g.

- Fiber: 6g.

• <u>Overnight "Oats"</u>

Preparation Time: 5 minutes

Cooking Time: 0 minutes

Servings: 04

Ingredients:

- 1/2 cup berry of choice

- 1/2 tbsp. walnut butter

- 1/2 burro banana

- 1/2 tsp. ginger

- 1/2 cup coconut milk

- 1/2 cup hemp seeds

Directions:

1. Put the hemp seeds, salt, and coconut milk into a glass jar. Mix well.

2. Place the lid on the jar, then put it in the refrigerator to sit overnight.

3. The next morning, add the ginger, berries, and banana.

4. Stir well and enjoy it.

Nutrition:

- Calories: 139 kcal.

- Fat: 4.1g.

- Protein: 9g.
- Sugar: 7g.

• Blueberry Cupcakes

Preparation Time: 15 minutes

Cooking Time: 40 minutes

Servings: 04

Ingredients:

- Grapeseed oil
- 1/2 tsp. sea salt
- 1/4 cup sea moss gel
- 1/3 cup agave
- 1/2 cup blueberries
- 3/4 cup tef flour
- 3/4 cup spelt flour
- 1 cup coconut milk

Directions:

1. Warm your oven to 365. Place paper liners into a muffin tin.

2. Place sea moss gel, sea salt, agave, flour, and milk in a large bowl.

3. Mix well to combine. Gently fold in blueberries.

4. Gently pour batter into paper liners.

5. Place in oven and bake 30 minutes.

6. They are done if they have turned a nice golden color, and they spring back when you touch them.

Nutrition:

- Calories: 85 kcal.
- Fat: 0.7g.

- Carbohydrates: 12g.
- Protein: 1.4g.
- Fiber: 5g.

• Brazil Nut Cheese

Preparation Time: 2 hours

Cooking Time: 0 minutes

Servings: 04

Ingredients:

- 2 tsp. grapeseed oil
- 1 ½ cups water
- 1 ½ cups hemp milk
- 1/2 tsp. cayenne
- 1 tsp. onion powder
- 1/2 lime juice
- 2 tsp. sea salt
- 1 lb. brazil nuts
- 1 tsp. onion powder

Directions:

1. You will need to start by soaking the Brazil nuts in some water.

2. You just put the nuts into a bowl and make sure the water covers them.

3. Soak no less than two hours or overnight.

4. Overnight would be best.

5. You need to put everything except water into a food processor or blender.

6. Add just 5 cups water and blend for two minutes.

7. Continue adding the 5 cups of water and blending until you have the consistency you want.

8. Scrape into an airtight container and enjoy.

Nutrition:

- Calories: 187 kcal.

- Protein: 4.1g.

- Fat: 19g.

- Carbs: 3.3g.

- Fiber: 2.1g.

- ## Fancy Coconut Date Bars for a Lovely Evening

Preparation Time: 10 minutes

Cooking Time: 30 minutes

Servings: 4

Ingredients:

- 1/3 cup of slivered walnuts

- ½ a cup coconut, flaked

- 10 dates, pitted

- ¼ cup of walnuts

- 1 teaspoon of coconut oil

Directions:

1. Take a food processor and, add the walnuts, blend them.

2. Add dates and pulse until mixed well.

3. Add coconut oil and walnuts until the mix is thick and sticks together.

4. Transfer the mixture to wax paper and form nice squares.

5. Fold up the sides of the waxed-on top.

6. Serve and Enjoy!

Nutrition:

- Calories: 154 kcal.

- Fats: 0g.

- Carbs: 39g.

- Protein: 0.1g.

- ## Sea Salt Brazilian Nut Butter Cookies

Preparation Time: 15 minutes

Cooking Time: 0 minutes

Servings: 9

Ingredients:

- 1 cup of walnuts

- ½ a cup of Brazilian nut butter (creamy and unsalted)

- 1 cup of pitted Medjool dates

- Sea salt as needed

Directions:

1. Take a food processor, add walnuts, nut butter, and dates, and blend the whole mixture until a dough-like texture comes (should take a few minutes).

2. Add some more Brazilian nut butter if you want a stickier dough.

3. Form balls using the dough and press down using a fork to create a coarse cross pattern.

4. Sprinkle salt generously.

5. Serve instantly or allow it to chill for crunchiness.

Nutrition:

- Calories: 350 kcal.

- Fat: 17g.

- Carbs: 27g.

- Protein: 18g.

Conclusion

Dr. Sebi was a man who learned traditional medicine from his grandmother. His real name was Alfredo Darrington Bowman. He had a health condition until he purportedly grew tired of Western healing methods. He returned to his home in Honduras, and there he developed his infamous 'alkaline diet.' He wished to be an "African in Honduras" and not an African Honduran. He claimed to have healed various terminal diseases such as cancer, asthma, diabetes, and AIDS with his "Cell Food" diet. Michael Jackson, Eddie Murphy, and Lisa Lopes were among his patients. Because of his numerous claims of curing terminal illnesses, law enforcement in New York City investigated him and found that he had no license to practice medicine. Although he was charged and arrested, he invited some of his clients to his hearing, who claimed he healed them, and with that, he won the case.

Sometime later, he was charged with money laundering and was arrested. While in jail, his family tried to get him out, but they couldn't because a court date was not set, and neither was bail. Later on, he became ill with pneumonia, and while in police custody, he died at the age of 82.

Even though Dr. Sebi placed a lot of accent on the consumption of a lot of vegetables and fruits, which is a good idea for a healthy diet, it has a little flaw; the regular consumption of only vegetables and fruits will not be sufficient enough to provide the required nutrients which the body needs. In this, the diet and nutrition guide that Bowman offers is overly restraining, as has been advised by professional nutritionists. These nutritionists state that there is nothing wrong with including whole foods since following Dr. Sebi's diet down to the letter denies the body some certain nutrients.

Even though there aren't enough proteins contained in the foods advocated in the nutrition guide for Dr. Sebi diet, there are particular nutrients like beta carotene, potassium, and vitamins C and E; they are also low in omega-3, iron, calcium, and vitamins D and B12, which the body needs but may pose issues, especially when one is trying to follow a diet that is based on plants thoroughly.

On the internet, you will find a lot of self-taught "gurus" who claim that they have discovered what is truly behind every disease and developed the ultimate medicine or treatment to cure them. On the other hand, science seems sluggish, has a subtle difference in opinion, and portrays the world as a complex environment with different diseases arising from varying causes. The treatment of these diseases is not perfect and usually harms the side. These so-called "gurus" like Dr. Sebi, for instance, take advantage of this fact and then try to deceive people that they have the ultimate cure and solution to all health problems, so they make up any concoction and sell them at high prices and make a lot of money off of people who believe them. Results from research have shown that the pH of urine can change a little. For a short period as a result of a change in diet, however, this is not true for blood pH because the diet does nothing to affect the pH of the blood, which means that following the diet of Dr. Sebi will not make the body more alkaline.

Furthermore, there is no greater blunder than the claim that African genes resonate (vibrate) at a higher frequency than the genes of others. Research that has been done in the field of gene variations for a long time has only led to one point, which is that differences in genes do not occur between geographic locations or civilizations but within them.

Many times over, people who have been thinking about attempting Dr. Sebi diet in a bid to alleviate their health condition or ailment have been advised to seek the counsel of a professional in health care with the list of the nutrition guide so that they can get a professional opinion on either following the diet or not. The major thing that nutritionists find disturbing are the claims that Dr. Sebi diet can heal might cause a lot of people who have been trying to deal with a medical condition to completely espouse the diet and its nutrition guide and abandon the prescribed medicines that they were taking before, which might have adverse effects on them. Therefore, it has also been recommended that people dealing with a health condition consult their doctors first and foremost before changing the medicine they are taking or switching over to a new diet.

BOOK 8: <u>DR. SEBI'S ALKALINE AND ANTI-INFLAMMATORY DIET</u>

HOW TO NATURALLY REDUCE INFLAMMATION AND BOOST IMMUNITY FOR LIFE-LONG HEALTH | ALKALINE PLANT-BASED RECIPES, 28-DAY DETOX PLAN & MORE

Introduction

Dr. Sebi is the inspiration for the alkaline diet. He was a natural healer from Honduras, recognized as an herbalist and an intracellular therapist. His diet is influenced by his home nation. It contains a broad range of natural alkaline foods which assist in reducing the negative effects of excessive acidity levels in the body. He created the eating plan after doing significant study and learning how acidic levels affect the body & why it's crucial to defend the body from acid levels & mucus that may lead to numerous illnesses.

Several people's lives have been enriched by his teachings, which have aided in promoting healthy living. For example, he developed an alkaline food plan that helped treat the most life-threatening disorders and helped reduce the danger of such diseases. It also assisted patients in better coping with their illnesses. As a result, the alkaline diet effectively reduces weight. In addition, it treats diabetes, epilepsy, arthritis, cancer, and sometimes even AIDS. Dr. Sebi spent more than 40 years investigating how alkaline foods may help people live healthier lives. He ultimately developed a nutrition plan that helps people lose weight and heal their bodies from the inside out.

We need to modify the lifestyle that Western globalization has disseminated. Hybrids, GMO meat, milk products, packaged foods, & plant foods are the primary targets. Alkaline plant foods are recommended. We need to revert to a diet that concentrates on the whole, non-hybrid plant-based foods to promote the healing and balance of all organs and functions. It's the foundation of both health and medicine. We should reuse natural, vital, and non-hybrid plant elements to speed up the cure or reversal of complicated disorders. According to Dr. Sebi, Herbal therapy is vital in reviving the belief that non-hybrid plant foods have chemical elements beneficial to the body and restore health. The African mineral balance treatment approach is based on the concept that any meal that raises the body's acidity and generates excess mucus formation is the basis of the disease.

In other words, meals high in acids and toxins infiltrate the body, triggering long-term inflammatory responses and chronic inflammation. Inflammation during sleep is a healthy, natural process that helps the body fight illness and restore physical damage. If acute inflammation is not treated, it affects healthy cells in numerous body sections, resulting in various disorders. For example, it impacts the mucosa of the protecting organs. It stimulates excessive mucus generation, compromising the health of the organs.

As a result, we must start eliminating certain things from our diet, particularly: dairy, processed meats, and artificial hybrid foods. Although you may lose weight by adopting Dr. Sebi's diet, it is not intended to be a weight-loss plan. Western cuisine isn't designed for your meal; it's full of salt, sweet, fat, and calorie-dense fried items. A plant-based diet is advised in its stead.

Eliminate the mucous if you wish to end the sickness. Order certain "electric" foods and agree to ingest these substances to remain alive. He paid special attention to pH values and said alkaline foods were more vibrant. The alkali plus viscous idea has multiple flaws. Lastly, the immune system creates mucus to combat illness, and our acid production is necessary for cardiovascular digestion and breathing.

Dr. Sebi's life was tumultuous, and many individuals considered his ideas were harmful in some manner. However, he was audacious enough to proclaim out loud that he could discover a solution for deadly illnesses such as cancer, AIDS, and diabetes, which had eluded medical study for years. His major goal was to persuade people to live a healthy lifestyle and recognize the relevance of alkaline foods in a balanced diet. People assumed Dr. Sebi was attempting to trick them into becoming vegans, and he suffered a lot of anger as a result. But, after people saw how efficient his techniques were, he became a celebrity and one of the most well-known herbalists in the world.

Chapter 1: Dr. Sebi

Who Was Dr. Sebi?

Alfredo Bowman, commonly known as Dr. Sebi, was a self-taught herbalist born in Honduras. He went to the U.S and then was inadequately treated for diabetes, asthma, frailty, and obesity, among other chronic diseases. Finally, according to his website, an herbalist in Mexico cured him, inspiring him to make his personal herbal concoctions, which he termed Dr. Sebi's Cell Food.

Dr. Sebi's life was tumultuous, and many individuals considered his ideas were detrimental in some manner. He was audacious enough to declare publicly that he could discover a solution for deadly illnesses such as cancer, AIDS, as well as diabetes, which had eluded medical study for years. He initially claimed that his herbs might treat chronic diseases, including AIDS, sickle cell anemia, and lupus. He was jailed in 1987 for practicing medicine without a license (however, the court acquitted him). Sebi consented to avoid making claims that his medicines might heal any ailments after another litigation by the state of New York a few years later.

His major goal was to persuade people to live a healthy lifestyle and recognize the relevance of alkaline foods in a balanced diet. People assumed Dr. Sebi was attempting to trick them into becoming vegans, and he suffered a lot of criticism as a result. But, after people saw how efficient his techniques were, he became a sensation and one of the best-known herbalists in the world.

Among the many allegations leveled against Dr. Sebi, one was carried all the way to court. This claim was made in response to a 1988 commercial claiming to heal patients of fatal diseases. The Court thought they had a good case and intended to imprison him. However, a whopping 77 individuals appeared in court, claiming to have been healed after adopting Dr. Sebi's instructions and integrating his diet into their daily routines. According to the witnesses, 77 individuals declared him not responsible. They also highlighted that his diet plan was a medical marvel and undervalued.

Despite the controversy, Sebi's clientele allegedly included Michael Jackson, John Travolta, and Steven Seagal. He caught pneumonia while imprisoned in Honduras and starved to death in the hospital. Life went on, yet people never forgot regarding Dr. Sebi and his incredible healing abilities.

Teachings of Dr. Sebi

When toxins plus mucus build up in the body, the body becomes more vulnerable to illness. Therefore, he claimed that those suffering from various ailments and those involved in disease prevention should constantly consume an alkaline diet, keeping in mind that the body becomes free of diseases when the increasing quantity of acidic chemicals and mucus is removed.

He also claimed that bodily cleaning and detoxification is an important and required technique for dealing with any ailment in the body.

Purification of the body aids in eliminating mucus collected in the liver, lungs, and many other bodily organs and removing excess acidic chemicals, making the body disease-free. Dr. Sebi also used herbs beneficial to the body's re-energizing and revitalization.

When human health improves, the body's organs function adequately, showing that the body is free of ailments.

Food classification by Dr. Sebi

Food was divided into six categories by Dr. Sebi:

- Drugs

- Food that has been genetically modified

- Hybrid foods

- Defunct foods

- Living foods

- Raw foods

He concluded that the first 4 food groups on this list should be avoided since they bring more harm than benefit to the body. For example, acids & mucus might build up in the body due to these foodstuffs. However, the remaining two kinds of foods he defined as healthy are the greatest since the nutritious value is not compromised in any manner. Foods that have been extensively cooked, hybridized, or modified, for example, have lost the needed quantity of nutrients. As a result, rather than providing health advantages, the body suffers. Raw foods, particularly vegetables, fruits, & herbs, are, on the other hand, beneficial for maintaining good health.

Dr. Sebi's Point of View

The world is increasingly afflicted with debilitating diseases that directly consequence the addictive, poisonous, industrially-processed foods that indicate the Standard Diet.

The African Bio-Mineral Balance Protocol was created by Dr. Sebi to tackle the chronic health difficulties caused by contemporary diets' inadequate nutrition.

Mucus & Acidification

Dr. Sebi realized that illness is a sign of the body's deposition of mucus & acid. He was certain that just one disease is caused by consuming acidic foods. The body must take minerals from bones to reinstate alkalinity once it becomes acidic. Mucus is generated to protect cellular membranes against acidic erosion. The cell's capacity to absorb nutrients and eliminate poisonous waste products is hampered by impaired membranes and sticky mucus. Blood flow is hindered, pressure rises, oxygenation drops, and waste builds up. This creates ideal circumstances for diseases to develop because the body's natural healing processes cannot function efficiently without appropriate nourishment.

Electrification

Most foods that we assume organic have been genetically modified in labs to modify their electrical characteristics. "Cell nutrition needs to be electrical," he said, "since the body of humans is electrical." "For chemical affinity to exist, the food must be electrical."

Consequently, we resist and warn against using genetically engineered organisms (GMOs). Plants genetically modified plants lack the chemical affinity that allows humans to absorb their nutrients. Real plants, created by Mother Nature, supply the body with all of the minerals and nutrients it needs to survive in an easily absorbed form.

Nourishment & Cleansing

The African Bio-Mineral Balance Program was created by Dr. Sebi to address difficulties impacting the nutrition of the African genome while also providing significant nourishment for the entire human community.

On two levels, the Balance Diet works:

- On an intracellular level, it removes toxins and mucous from the body & organs.

- Second, it replenishes the human body with the minerals required for normal electrical activity and alkalinity.

Dietary adjustments are also encouraged as part of the program to help you on your path to self-healing. Dr. Sebi recommends a plant-based diet rich in nutrient-dense vegetables, nuts, seeds, fruits, and herbs to replenish the body and preserve the alkaline balance essential for optimal health.

Eating Organic Foods: A Philosophical Approach

You should be consuming a broad range of plant-based foods. He does not push you to adopt a vegan diet, even if he feels it is sensible to solve all of your health issues. This alkaline diet's main emphasis is on eating natural and nutritious foods, which allows your body to reduce its acidic level and recover from within. Consuming the alkaline diet is based on the idea that the metabolic system would work properly again. Once the body has significant acidic content, it disrupts your metabolic system, which means that much of the food you consume is stored as fat instead of being converted into energy. While the acid levels are at their highest, it's challenging for the metabolism to function properly, creating issues with the digestive system. Suppose you really want to lead a healthier life. In that case, you must start consuming foods that help with digestion so that your physiological functions might work properly.

The first step involves improving your metabolism and converting the food you consume into energy instead of storing it as fat in the body. Your pH level begins to balance when you begin consuming nutritious meals. This process is slow, but it gradually shifts you toward an alkaline lifestyle, which is beneficial in the long term. Natural food philosophy states that you should not skip meals to lose weight. Instead, incorporate foods abundant in calcium, magnesium, and natural fat to alkalize the body. While you maintain a healthy regular diet, you reap many advantages that enhance your body and make you feel much better.

What are Dr. Sebi's eight diet rules?

Rule 1: Only consume the items mentioned in the nutritional guide.

Rule 2: Every day, consume 1 gallon (3.8 liters) of water.

Rule 3: Consume Dr. Sebi's pills one hour before taking your medication.

Rule 4: There are no animal products allowed.

Rule 5: No alcoholic beverages are permitted.

Rule 6: Limit wheat products as well as stick to the guide's list of "natural-growing grains."

Rule 7: If you don't want to kill your meal, don't use the microwave.

Rule 8: Stay away from canned and seedless fruits.

Chapter 2: The Alkaline Diet

The alkaline diet is designed to help adjust the pH of the fluids in the body, such as the urine and blood. Therefore, this diet is also known as the alkaline ash eating plan, alkaline acid diet, acidic ash diet, pH diet, and Dr. Sebi's alkaline diet. The diet is based on the African Bio-Mineral Balance philosophy and was created by self-taught herbalist Alfredo Darrington Bowman, known as Dr. Sebi.

He created this diet for anybody who wants to organically treat or prevent sickness while improving their general health without depending on Western medicine. As per Dr. Sebi, diseases are caused by mucus build-up in a certain body location. For instance, pneumonia is caused by the accumulation of mucus in the lungs. Still, diabetes is caused by excessive mucus in the pancreas. He claims that diseases cannot survive in an alkaline condition. They begin to manifest themselves when the body gets too acidic. Therefore, he claims to revive the body's natural alkaline condition and cleanse your sick body by rigorously adopting his diet and utilizing his patented supplements.

Dr. Sebi originally stated that this diet might treat AIDS, sickle cell anemia, leukemia, and lupus. However, following a lawsuit in 1993, he was forced to stop making such assertions.

A precise list of vegetables, fruits, cereals, hazelnuts, seeds, oils, and herbs is allowed in the diet. The Dr. Sebi program is vegan since animal products aren't really allowed. According to Sebi, for the body to repair itself, you must stick to the diet for the long - term.

Finally, although many individuals say that the method has helped them recover, no scientific studies support their claims.

The Alkalinity Quest

Sebi's primary idea seems to be that alkaline foods and herbs (pH > 7) are required to manage acid in the body and that sustaining this alkaline condition protects us against disease-causing mucus build-up. Alkalinity's consecration as our long-awaited rescuer reveals a fundamental ignorance of the human body. The pH of our blood cannot be changed greatly; in fact, blood includes carbonic acid & sodium bicarbonate molecules that are particularly designed to regulate the pH between 7.35 & 7.45. Then there's disease and death. On the other hand, Sebi continued to market a broad range of herbal extracts despite that piece of high school biology.

How Does the Alkaline Diet Work?

Here's some information on acidity and alkalinity in the diet of humans, as well as some essential aspects regarding how alkaline diets might assist:

Once it comes to the overall acid content of the human diet, researchers think "there have been significant shifts from hunter-gatherer societies to the present." In comparison to diets of the past 200 years, the food supply contains far less potassium, magnesium, & chloride, and significantly more salt, thanks to the agricultural revolution & subsequent vast industrialization of the food supply.

The kidneys generally keep our electrolyte levels in check (calcium, magnesium, potassium & sodium). These electrolytes are utilized to fight acidity when subjected to highly acidic substances.

According to a study, the potassium-to-sodium proportion in most people's diets has shifted dramatically. Then, potassium seemed to dominate sodium by a factor of 10:1, but currently, the ratio is 1:3. As a result, those who follow a "Standard American Diet" generally ingest three times as much salt as potassium! This considerably adds to our bodies' alkaline environment. Nowadays, most adults and children eat high-sodium diets deficient in antioxidants, fiber, vital vitamins, and magnesium and potassium. Furthermore, processed fats, simple carbohydrates, salt, and chloride are abundant in the average Western diet.

These dietary modifications have led to a rise in "metabolic acidosis." To put it another way, many people's pH levels are no longer appropriate. Furthermore, many people have inadequate food intake and issues like potassium and magnesium deficiencies.

Health Advantages

Because alkaline meals include key elements that aid in the prevention of premature aging and the loss of organs & cellular functioning, as stated below as well, alkaline diet advantages may include assisting in the prevention of tissue and bone deterioration, which may be harmed when excessive acidity depletes us of essential minerals.

1. Bone mass & muscle mass are protected

Mineral intake is critical for the formation and preservation of bone structures. According to research, the more alkaline fruits and veggies a person consumes, the less likely they will develop sarcopenia or a loss of bone strength & muscle mass as they age. In addition, an alkaline diet may help with bone health by regulating the proportion of minerals like calcium, magnesium, and phosphate, which are necessary for forming bones and preserving lean muscle mass.

The diet might even aid in the synthesis of growth hormones and the consumption of vitamin D, which preserves bones while also reducing the risk of many other chronic illnesses.

2. Reduces Hypertension & Stroke Risk

Reduced inflammation and increased growth hormone production are two of the anti-aging benefits of an alkaline diet. This has been demonstrated to boost cardiovascular health and protect against excessive cholesterol, high blood pressure, kidney problems, stroke, and sometimes even memory loss.

3. Reduces Inflammation and Chronic Pain

According to research, an alkaline diet has been linked to lower levels of chronic pain. Backaches, headaches, muscular spasms, menstruation symptoms, inflammation, and joint pain have all been linked to persistent acidosis.

According to research, people with chronic back pain who were administered an alkaline tablet daily for four weeks reported substantial reductions in pain as evaluated by the "Arhus low back pain assessment scale," according to research.

4. Helps to prevent Magnesium Deficiency by increasing vitamin absorption

Magnesium is necessary for the proper functioning of thousands of enzyme systems and biological functions. Unfortunately, many individuals are magnesium deficient, resulting in heart problems, muscular pains, migraines, sleep problems, and anxiety. Magnesium is also needed to stimulate vitamin D and avoid vitamin D insufficiency, which is critical for general immunological and endocrine health.

5. Assists in the strengthening of immune function and the prevention of cancer

If cells have little or no minerals, they need to dump waste effectively or adequately oxygenate the whole body's struggles. Mineral loss impairs vitamin absorption, while toxins and infections build up in the body, weakening the immune system. An alkaline change in pH owing to an adjustment in electric charges and the discharge of primary elements of proteins is thought to be linked to cancer prevention. Alkalinity has been demonstrated to be more advantageous for certain chemotherapeutic medicines that need a higher pH to act properly and reduce inflammation and the risk of conditions like cancer.

6. It may assist you in maintaining a healthy weight

Although the diet isn't primarily for weight reduction, sticking to an alkaline diet dietary pattern for weight loss will assist you in avoiding becoming obese. Due to the diet's tendency to lower leptin levels and inflammation, limiting acid-forming meals and consuming greater alkaline-forming foods might make it simpler to lose weight. This has an impact on your appetite as well as your fat-burning ability.

Because alkaline-forming foods are anti-inflammatory, following an alkaline diet allows your body to attain normal leptin levels and feel full with eating the right calorie count.

How to Follow It?

1. Purchase organic alkaline foods wherever feasible.

One crucial factor in adopting an alkaline diet, according to experts, is to learn about the sort of soil your food was produced in since fruits and vegetables cultivated in organic, mineral-dense soil are more alkalizing. However, according to research, the kind of soil in which plants are cultivated greatly impacts their vitamin & mineral content; therefore, not all "alkaline foods" are made equal.

For the best adequate amount of vital nutrients in plants, the pH of the soil should be between 6 and 7. Acidic soils with a pH below 6 may have lower calcium and magnesium levels. In contrast, soils with a pH of more than 7 may contain chemically inaccessible iron, manganese, copper, and zinc. In addition, the healthiest soil is well-rotated, organically supported, and vulnerable to wildlife/grazing cattle.

2. Consume alkaline water.

The pH of alkaline water ranges from 9 to 11. Therefore, it's perfectly safe to consume distilled water. Although reverse osmosis filtered water is somewhat acidic, it is still preferable to tap water or purified bottled water. Alkalinity may also be increased by adding pH drops, lime or lime, and baking soda to drinking water.

3. Measure your pH level (optional)

You may test your pH level by buying strips at the local health food shop or pharmacy if you're wondering about the pH level before adopting the instructions below. Saliva or urine may be used to determine your pH.

The finest benefits will come from your second urination of the morning. The colors on the test strip are compared to a chart included with the test strip kit. 1 hour before a meal and 2 hours after a meal is the optimum times to test your pH throughout the day. If you're testing your saliva, aim for a reading of 6.8 to 7.2.

Is It Safe to Follow an Alkaline Diet?
The alkaline diet is essentially a reinforcement of excellent, ancient healthy habits. The diet encourages people to consume more vegetables, fruits, and water while avoiding sweets, alcohol, meat, especially processed meals. All of these factors would help you improve your general health, lose weight, and even reduce your cancer risk — but not for the purposes that diet proponents claim.

This diet may also aid in the reduction of inflammation. Although inflammation is a normal reaction to injury and illness, too much inflammation, usually known as chronic inflammation, may damage DNA & lead to cancer. As a result, consuming anti-inflammatory foods may help lower your cancer risk.

Foods to Avoid
The pH of specific foods is used to regulate the diet. Some variants are less rigorous, allowing grains despite their moderately acidic pH for health advantages. However, if you're on an alkaline diet, you would like to stick to the list of foods below, limiting acidic meals, limiting or eliminating neutral foods, and concentrating on alkaline foods.

Foods to Stay Away From

- Meat
- Poultry
- Fish
- Animal-based Milk
- Cheese
- Yogurt
- Ice-cream
- Eggs (especially yolks)

- Grain products (rice (brown & white), rolled oats, pasta, cornflakes and whole-wheat bread)
- Alcohol
- Soda
- Lentils
- Peanuts
- Other cooked, packaged foods

Is This What Our Forefathers ate?

The paleo diet, which aims to emulate our gatherer ancestors' nutritional patterns, has a lot of similarities with the alkaline diet's focus on fruits and vegetables over manufactured meals. However, the evidence does not necessarily support the notion that our forefathers ate alkaline diets. According to an earlier study, almost half of the 229 ancient diets studied constituted acid-producing, whereas the other half constituted alkaline-forming.

Another research revealed that the disparity might be due to location. The researchers discovered that the further individuals lived from the equator, the greater acidic the diets were.

Principles of an Alkaline Diet

Most people find it challenging to eat healthily. However, with all of the food options available, it's critical to keep concentrated on what matters most — your health! "The Alkaline Way" is based on seven principles. Employ these principles to build and experience an Alkaline Diet that is delicious and healthful.

Consume a diverse range of fresh, high-quality whole foods.

The first principle in perusing the Alkaline Way is to consume mostly whole foods. This is the foundation of the Alkaline Diet. Fresh fruit and veggies, gently roasted nuts and seeds, slightly cooked vegetables, grain & bean sprouts, cultured foods, freshly squeezed juices, as well as vegetable juices must all be high on your list of "life-ly" foods. These foods are high inactive enzymes, which help indigestion.

Eat a broad range of whole foods to get the most health benefits. When digestion is poor, agitated, or weakened, consuming the same foods repeatedly restricts digestive and nutritional diversity and raises the risk of being allergic to those foods. Instead, diversify your diet selections to include items that are simple to digest, absorb, and remove. Experiment with different flavors—and you'll frequently get a health benefit in the process.

Consume 60-80% alkaline-forming foods.

The second principle is to eat mostly alkaline foods. If you are in excellent health, it is suggested that you consume at least 60percent alkaline-forming foods. Experts recommend an 80 percent alkalinizing diet to assist in soothing the immune system and improving digestion if the immune system is impaired or responding to anything or if the health requires to be preserved in any manner.

Consume foods that are good for your immune system.

Avoiding foods that cause your immune system to respond is the 3rd Alkaline Method principle for eating healthy. When overweight persons replace reactive foods with nonreactive foods and follow the Alkaline Way, they lose weight easily (even if they consume more calories), and their metabolism improves. On the other hand, most underweight persons achieve a healthy weight due to a health-promoting diet that boosts protein synthesis and repair.

Consume 60-70% plant-based, complex carbohydrates; 15-20% protein; and 15-20% healthy fat.

The fourth Alkaline Method principle promotes a balanced ratio of complex carbs, proteins, and fats. Ratios to Consider:

- Whole food (plant-based) complex carbs provide 60–70% calories.

- Protein accounts for 15–20 percent of total calories.

- Healthy fats account for 15–20 percent of calories (including most of the omega-3 fats)

Complex Carbohydrates from Whole Foods (Plant-Based)

Your Alkaline Way meal plan should be high in complex carbs from veggies, whole grains, plus legumes (beans, peas, & lentils). Also, spices, seasonings, and herbs, except the healthcare professional advise differently. 60-70 percent of your daily calories should come from these sources.

Protein:

Protein should account for around 15-20% of your total calorie consumption. For most individuals, 50 to 60 g of protein a day is a sufficient amount. Nuts & seeds, sprouts, nutritional yeast, blue-green algae, miso, and mushrooms are all good protein sources.

Beneficial fats:

Fat should account for 15-20% of the caloric intake. So make sure to eat enough omega-3 healthy fats, which help your body produce energy protein and rebuild tissue. Fresh nuts and seeds and cold-pressed natural oils are food-based resources of beneficial omega-3 essential fats.

Combining foods to make complete proteins:

Plant proteins, unlike animal proteins, lack some necessary amino acids. Therefore, you can get a complete protein by combining meals depending on the amino acid content. Brown rice and roasted beans, for example, are insufficient proteins when consumed alone because they lack a key amino acid; yet, while eaten simultaneously, they support each other and constitute a full protein intake.

The body treats "trans" fatty acids as if they had been naturally saturated fats such as butter and coconut oil, yet these fats are more dangerous. Tran's fats penetrate the placenta, are preserved in fetal tissue and may affect cell membrane functioning in the long run. However, "trans" fats may be found in fried meals like French fries, as well as many processed foods, including anything from name-brand oils to bakery products and confectionery.

Use unsaturated, non-hydrogenated "expeller-pressed" oils such as olive, grape seed, coconut, and exotic oils like avocado's.

Hydrogenated oils have increased cholesterol levels and interference with liver enzymes. In addition, these synthetic oils are also known to harm immunological function and encourage the growth of some kinds of malignancies.

Consume foods and beverages that are probiotic and fermented (cultured).

The Alkaline Way's fifth principle is to establish a habit of eating and drinking a wide variety of probiotics (cultured/fermented) foods and beverages. The word probiotic refers to a bacterium that aids in the growth of living organisms. A normal gastrointestinal tract is home to a diverse range of beneficial (probiotic) bacteria that help maintain the balance of the body and immune systems. Poor nutrition, stress, illnesses, and medications may reduce good bacteria, allowing infections to flourish. Probiotics are used to populate the stomach with good microorganisms.

Probiotics should be consumed in food or drink since this gives the maximum amounts and diversity of probiotics.

Drink plenty of water and consume plenty of fiber.

The 6th Alkaline Way principle is to drink enough water and eat plenty of fiber. Ordinary people drink far too little water and eat far too little fiber. Traditional civilizations ingest 40-100 grams of dietary fiber per day from real, active foods to avoid developing Western degenerative illnesses. Fiber's "roughage" makes the stool thick and mushy, which focuses on maintaining a reduced transit time—the frequency between eating and eliminating waste. Adequate fiber supports waste elimination daily simply and comfortably. It's less probable that poisonous waste would be recycled back into circulation if you keep the body clean and clear.

A good transit time is between 12 and 18 hours. This minimizes the chances of harmful germs and yeast taking over the body.

Water and its importance:

Drinking enough water is essential for good health, particularly if you eat a high-fiber diet. Water aids fiber in effectively passing wastes thru the body, and water is required for the proper functioning of every system in the body. Experts suggest drinking a minimum of one 8-ounce glass of filtered water eight times a day while implementing The Alkaline Way plan.

Consume more nutritious food combinations.

The Alkaline Way's last principle is effective food mixing, a crucial element of the Alkaline Way. The way we mix meals at mealtime may significantly influence digestion and, as a result, general health.

The skill of healthy meal combining is an essential part of balanced nutrition since it reduces digestive system wear and strain. If you're prone to stomach issues, pay special attention to how you combine foods (acid reflux, cramping, leaky gut syndrome, indigestion, irritable bowel syndrome, diverticulosis, as well as other digestive issues).

The Importance of a Balanced PH

The lungs and kidneys are mostly responsible for keeping the body's pH in check, and it's a fine line to tread. The pH of the blood varies from 7.2 to 7.45. The kidneys also aid in the pH balance of urine. For example, a urine pH of 4 indicates that it is very acidic. In contrast, a pH of 7 indicates neutral, and 9 indicates strongly alkaline.

But here's the catch: you can't modify your body's pH with a diet. Although you may notice a variation in the urine pH that can be determined with a basic dipstick test (commonly known as a urine test strip), urine pH does not represent your body's pH. This is because excessive acid may be ejected via the urine to rectify the body's pH levels.

If the body's pH fluctuates, it's a sign of a major health problem. For example, urine with a high pH may suggest a UTI or kidney stones. In contrast, urine with a low pH may indicate diarrhea, hunger, or diabetic ketoacidosis.

What is "pH Level," and What Does It Mean?

The potency of hydrogen is referred to as pH. It's a measurement of the acidity and alkalinity of the fluids and tissues in our bodies. It's assessed from 0 – 14 on a scale of 1 to 14. The lower the pH of a solution, the more acidic it is. The higher the value, the more alkaline the body is. A pH of approximately 7 is considered neutral; however, since the normal human body pH is around 7.4, we perceive a little alkaline pH to be the best.

The stomach is the most acidic part of the body, with varying pH values. Thus, even little changes in the pH of many organisms may create serious difficulties. For example, the ocean's pH has reduced from 8.2 to 8.1 due to environmental problems such as increased CO_2 deposition, and numerous ocean living organisms have suffered considerably as a result.

The pH level is really important for plant growth. Thus it has a huge effect on the mineral composition of the meals we consume. Nutrients in the ocean, soil, and human body act as buffers to keep pH levels in check; therefore, as acidity rises, minerals decline.

Acidity

What precisely is acidity?

The pH scale determines whether a substance is **acidic, basic, or neutral**.

- A pH level of 0 implies a strong acidity level.

- A pH level of 7 is considered neutral.

- A pH level of 14 seems to be the most basic/alkaline.

A tenfold imbalance in acidity and alkalinity of content is represented by the distance among two points upon the pH scale. The acidity of a pH level of 6 is 10 times that of a pH of 7, & so on. Acidity, as well as alkalinity, are measured using the pH scale. It determines if a solution contains both positively & negatively charged hydrogen ions. The more the hydrogen ions, the more acidic the solution.

Foods with a pH of 4.6 or below are considered acidic. This is because foods high in acid are far less to promote rapid microorganism development. Therefore they may take longer to break down.

The Human Body and Acidity

The pH of the body is around 7.40. This level is ideal for keeping the body's biochemical functions running smoothly. Blood oxygenation is among the most critical activities it regulates.

Despite the lack of compelling evidence that this helps maintain normal pH levels, many people choose to avoid meals that increase acidity in the stomach. Their major objective is to maintain their PRAL (potential renal acid load) under control. When you consume particular meals, your body creates a certain amount of acid, measured by the PRAL.

Excessive body acidity is regarded to become the first step in premature aging, vision and memory problems, wrinkling, age spots, hormone system failure, and a slew of other age-related issues. In addition, body acidity is linked to practically most diseases.

We get more acidic as we become older. Most elderly people's bodies are very acidic, with hazardous wastes accumulating in the bloodstream, tissues, and lymphatic system. Acidic wastes arise from a variety of places. Therefore, you could substantially slow down the aging process if you kept your skin, muscles, organs, as well as glands alkaline as they were when you were an infant.

The following are the first indications of acidity in bodily tissues:

- Feeling tired, weak, and short on energy
- Irritability, anxiety, panic attacks, and despair
- Having skin conditions such as eczema, psoriasis, acne, and hives
- Experiencing widespread aches and pains
- Diarrhea, constipation, or stomach pain

- Experiencing cramps before or during your period
- Feelings of heartburn
- Sleep deprivation
- Having an increased dental decay
- Feeling nauseous
- Experiencing libido loss

Long-term bodily acidity manifests itself in a variety of ways, including:

- Osteoporosis
- Immune system dysfunction
- Consistent digestive issues
- Arthritis, ligament and joint disorders

- Gout, kidney stones, and kidney disorders
- Problems with the heart and circulation
- Infections caused by fungi and bacteria
- Cancers

Limit or avoid acidic foods

Here's a brief rundown of the most acidic meals you should avoid. These items are acid-forming, and their consumption should be limited as part of a healthy diet:

- Convenience foods
- Alcohol
- Milk

- Caffeinated beverages
- Cereals that have been processed
- Pizza

- Sweeteners made from artificial sources
- Peanuts
- Cheese
- Pasta
- Rice
- Bread
- Products made from wheat
- Butter
- Cold cuts

- Vegetable oils that have been refined
- French fries
- Hot chocolate
- Red meat
- Beverages for sports
- Sugar (table)
- Corn syrup
- Pancakes
- Fried Foods

Take note that not every acidic food should be fully excluded from your diet. Some of the components on the acidic foodstuffs list are high in nutrients. Therefore, they may be incorporated into a balanced diet in moderation.

What is Acidosis?

Acidosis is a condition in which the body's acid levels are extraordinarily high. For optimum health, the body must achieve a balance of acidity. Too much acidity or alkalinity in the body may lead to major health concerns. When the body's acid levels are too high, it tries to adjust by removing the acid. Excessive acid in the body is normally excreted via the lungs and kidneys. Acidosis may produce major consequences if it puts excessive strain on these organs. Acidosis may be caused by various medical disorders, prescription medicines, and dietary variables. Although some forms of acidosis may be reversed, acute acidosis can be deadly if not treated.

Excessive acidity compromises the health of all physiological systems. To buffer (neutralize) the acid & safely eliminate it from the body, the body borrows minerals such as calcium, salt, potassium, and magnesium from essential organs, bones, and teeth. As a consequence of the excessive acidity, the body might suffer severe and long-term corrosion. This condition can go unnoticed for years. In addition, acidosis may cause catastrophic difficulties in key organs, including the liver, heart, and kidneys.

It causes obesity and diabetes.

An acidic pH may lead to weight issues, including diabetes and obesity. On the other hand, insulin Sensitivity is a syndrome that occurs when our bodies get excessively acidic. This causes an overabundance of insulin to be generated. Consequently, the body is bombarded with far too much insulin that each calorie is dutifully converted to fat.

An acid pH caused by an unbalanced diet is extremely likely to cause a state that triggers the planned genetic response to hunger and famine. Following that, the body will be forced to horde and store every calorie ingested as fat. Some believe that an acid pH triggers a strong genetic reaction to an imminent famine, directly interpreted by the all-important and extremely sensitive Insulin-Glucagon Axis. When this occurs, the body produces more insulin than normal, which causes the body to manufacture and retain extra fat.

A healthy, slightly alkaline pH, on either hand, will result in typical fat-burning metabolic activity, with no need for the body to manufacture additional insulin or lipids. As a result, fat may be burnt and removed naturally. A balanced pH diet is also less likely to result in yo-yo effects or weight gain after a diet. We should aim for a little alkaline pH to enable fats to be used naturally for energy rather than being hoarded and saved due to a faulty biochemical belief in a coming famine. Acidosis also damages the insulin-producing beta cells in the pancreas. The beta cells are extremely pH sensitive and cannot thrive in an acidic environment. Beta cells will lose sync with one another if this happens. Their cellular connection will be disrupted, and the body's immune system will begin to overreact. The cells' stress levels will rise, making it more difficult to function properly and live.

It hastens free radical damage as well as early aging.

Acidosis triggers lipid breakdown and harmful oxidative cascades, speeding up free radical damage to cell walls & intracellular membrane structures. Most healthy cells are killed as a result of this process.

Premature aging and enhanced oxidative pathways of cell wall degradation begin with acidosis. Wrinkling, dark circles, failed hormonal systems, interference with vision, memory, and other age-related issues are all signs of acidosis. Unwanted wastes that are not effectively expelled from the body poison the cells.

It causes lipid & fatty acid metabolism to be disrupted.

Acidosis impairs lipid & fatty acid metabolism, which is important for brain and nerve function. This disturbance results in neurological issues such as MS and MD and hormonal imbalances in the endocrine system.

In addition, an acidic environment induces LDL-cholesterol to be built down at a faster rate in the heart, lining and clogging the vascular network improperly. In other words, an acid pH causes electrostatic potential, which damages artery walls and triggers a PDGF-dependent immunological response, resulting in cholesterol oxidation and heavy metal plaque development.

It erodes the tissues of the arteries, veins, and heart.

Acidosis diminishes and eats away at the cell wall membranes of the heart, arteries, and veins, much as acid eats away at the marble. Our cardiac structures and interconnected tissues are weakened due to this erosion process.

The chemical environment of all biological tissues affects them. The cardiac muscle cells are no exception. Blood plasma pH affects the whole cardiovascular system, which functions as one vast functional "system of tubular muscles" to transport blood and nutrients to every living tissue in the body. The heart's pumping forces blood thru the arteries, veins, and capillary beds, assisting in regulating blood pressure and blood flow.

An acid pH disrupts free ionic balances in circulation, resulting in an increase in populations of positively charged particles, which interferes with heart and artery muscle excitability (contraction and relaxation).

Changes in blood pH are currently considered to cause the following:

- Arteriosclerosis development (tightening of the arteries)

- Aneurysm (widening as well as ballooning of artery walls)

- Arrhythmias (irregular heart beating including tachycardia)

- Myocardial infarction (cardiovascular attacks)

- Strokes (a heart accident).

- The anatomical deterioration of the cardio-vascularity ultimately causes blood pressure anomalies, exacerbating the issues mentioned above.

It affects the metabolism and reserve of energy.

Effective cellular and overall metabolism are hampered when your body's pH is too acidic. Acidosis disrupts cellular connections and functioning by causing chemical ionic disruptions. Acidosis lowers plasma protein plus calcium-binding, lowering the efficiency of such intracellular signal. It also causes a condition characterized by the admission of calcium cations via positive calcium channels. As a result, cardiovascular contractibility, or the heart's capacity to pump effectively and rhythmically, is reduced.

The "Sodium-Potassium pump" regulates intracellular protein activity and drives positive calcium plus hydrogen from the cells (Na-K pump). This pump creates a powerful inducement for sodium to be transported into cells. It also manages the amount of sodium & potassium in the body's reserves, and it consumes up to 25% of our daily calorie intake.

Positive calcium swaps plus sodium and is pushed out of cells. In contrast, the electrolytic cell for positive calcium promotes both positive hydrogen & positive calcium entrance into cells since cells contain less calcium & positive hydrogen than extracellular fluids. Therefore, the quantity of positive sodium in extracellular fluids is ten times higher.

Because less + sodium is accessible in acidic liquids, the digestion and induction of nutritious elements entering the cells are slow. This increases the amount of positive hydrogen plus calcium in the plasma, enabling LDL-Cholesterol to attach electrostatically. Due to the disruption of free positive calcium communities and channels, calcium may be excessively siphoned from bone masses. Osteoporosis is the result of this. In a word, an acidic pH depletes our energy stores and prevents us from using them.

It reduces the rate at which oxygen is delivered to the cell.

Acidosis lowers the amount of oxygen in the blood. Because all living tissues, particularly the heart and brain, need oxygen to thrive, a shortage will result in death. In addition, the quantity of oxygen given to the cells is reduced when the pH is acidic. As a result, they will perish at some point.

Acidosis is linked to a variety of diseases

It's vital to remember that the body's biochemistry is simply one of several tools that a physician may use to better comprehend the whole body. A pH result is neither a diagnostic tool nor a clinical diagnosis of any problem on its own. What happens if the body becomes excessively acidic? When you have an acidic balance, you'll be able to:

- Reduce the capacity of the body to retain minerals as well as other substances

- Reduce the amount of energy produced by the cells.

- Reduce the capacity of the body to fix the damaged cells

- Reduce the ability of the body to cleanse heavy metals

- Enable the tumor cells to proliferate.

- Increase your body's susceptibility to tiredness and diseases.

Anxiousness, diarrhea, dilated pupils, gregarious behavior, exhaustion in the morning, headaches, impulsivity, hypersexuality, sleeplessness, anxiety, racing heart, restless legs, breathlessness, sturdy appetite, hypertension, warm dry feet and hands are some of the symptoms that people with high acidity levels experience.

The body turns acidic almost all of the time due to a high-acid diet, mental stress, toxic overload, immunological responses, or any other activity that precludes the cells of oxygen & other nutrients. The body will attempt to counteract the acidic pH by consuming alkaline minerals like calcium. Unfortunately, calcium is lost from the bones, resulting in osteoporosis. Rheumatoid arthritis, diabetes, lupus, TB, osteoporosis, hypertension, and most tumors may be caused by acidosis, defined as a prolonged time in an acid pH condition.

An acidic pH, as well as oxygen deprivation, are two major causes of cancer. Cancer thrives and survives in an acidic, low-oxygen condition, as we all know. According to research, the acidity level of terminal cancer patients is 1,000 times higher than that of healthy persons. The pH level of the significant number of terminal patients is very acidic.

<h2 style="text-align:center">What is the reason behind this?</h2>

The reason is obvious. Lactic acid is formed when glucose is fermented without the presence of oxygen. The cell's pH drops to 7.0 as a result of this. The pH level drops to 6.5 in more advanced cancer situations. The level may even drop to 6.0, 5.7, or even lower occasionally. The simple reality is that human bodies cannot fight infections if our pH levels are out of whack.

<h2 style="text-align:center">The Long-Term Consequences of Living in an Acidic Medium</h2>

Structural System

While serum & soft tissue calcium levels drop, calcium held in bones is discharged, binding and neutralizing excessive acid in the tissues. Muscle cramps may result from the first calcium deficiency in the muscle. As more calcium is drawn from the bones to neutralize acid, the calcium deposits in the bones are depleted, resulting in osteoporosis, weaker and collapsed vertebrae, &, often, terrible posture and back discomfort. In addition, the calcium that is mobilized from the bones is accumulated in the joints as calcium-acid salts, causing degenerative arthritis.

Nervous System

When brain cells get overly acidic, they lose their capability to work properly. Consequently, the brain cannot create the necessary chemicals (neurotransmitters) to interact with neighboring brain cells. As a result, sleeplessness, anxiety, melancholy, neuroses, psychotic disorders, and memory loss are possible outcomes. In addition, because the brain is meant to interact with every cell in the human body (heart cells, intestine cells, muscular cells, epithelial cells, etc.) via the spinal cord as well as other nerves, if the neurological system is not operating effectively due to acidic imbalance, every bodily system might fail.

Circulatory System

Bacteria, fungi, and/or viruses may adhere themselves to the interior wall of arteries when the pH is too high. This subsequently recruits white blood cells, coagulation proteins, clotting cells, and other clotting factors to the region. This may result in plaque formation in the artery, narrowing it and reducing the blood flow, oxygen, and nutrients into the tissues served by that artery. A heart attack occurs when the coronary artery is obstructed.

Calcium, which was recruited from the bone to neutralize the acid, may accumulate in the arterial plaque if there is a surplus of acidity, transforming the plaque from floppy to stiff. As a result, the plaque stiffens the arteries, resulting in a rise in blood pressure.

Digestive System

The cells that make up the stomach & small intestine and the pancreas cells involved in creating and discharging digestive enzymes do not function properly when the pH is excessively acidic. Indigestion, heartburn, bloating, and stomach cramps are all symptoms. If the body does not absorb enough nutrients from the diet, malnutrition may occur throughout the body. In addition, foods that have not been digested might develop in the intestines, producing toxicity.

Intestinal System

Increased acidity induces colon cells to malfunction, resulting in diarrhea, irritable bowel syndrome, constipation, and diverticulitis. In addition, colitis, inflammatory bowel disorder (particularly Crohn's disease), and hemorrhoids may all be caused by a disrupted acid level in the colon, which allows unfavorable microorganisms to flourish and thrive.

Immune System

Antibodies & cytokines (chemical messengers that govern other immune cells) are not produced by immune cells that are overly acidic, and phagocytosis is impeded (the capability to ingest and spoilage microorganisms). Consequently, the person is vulnerable to viral, bacterium, fungal infections, and cancer.

Respiratory System

Oxygen adhesion to hemoglobin occurs across a very limited pH range in the lungs. Therefore, microbes in the airways may grow much more readily if the pH is excessively acidic, invading human cells and causing bronchitis, pneumonia, sinusitis, and other infections, as well as cough, bronchial spasms (asthma), and greater sensitivity to allergens (hay fever).

Urinary System

The urinary system aids in the removal of harmful waste from the body. However, due to their narrower urethra, which links the urine bladder to the outside of the body, women contain bacteria and/or fungus in their bladders. If the urine pH isn't in the correct proportions, these bacteria might multiply quickly. In addition, calcium, which is recruited from the bone to moderate the acid, may create calcium crystals and stones in the kidney's collecting system when the situation is too acidic.

Glandular System

Enzymatic activity is used by all endocrine glands to create hormones. However, the epithelial cells cannot create and release enough hormones to meet the body's demands if the pH is excessively acidic. As a result, changes in mood, blood sugar imbalances, exhaustion, reproductive problems, and other issues emerge.

Loss of weight

The metabolic enzymes within the cells do not perform correctly when the pH is excessively acidic, preventing the effective breakdown of fats and other nutrients.

10 Foods You Should Never Eat

Acid indigestion is spurred by the foods we eat. Acid-rich foods reduce the pH of your blood. Unfortunately, it also causes health issues such as stone development, decreased bone strength, and even boosts cancer risk. As a result, keep an eye on your food to keep yourself protected from all of these problems. Human blood pH levels should be between 7.35 and 7.45. As a result, any foodstuff below this amount causes acid reflux. So, here are the top ten foods to avoid if you want to reduce your acidity.

1. hydrogenated Vegetable oils

Hydrogenated oils are much more of a research project than food. Adding a hydrogen molecule into monounsaturated and polyunsaturated oils necessitates a slew of compounds, heavy metals, heat, and other procedures that turn the oil incomprehensible and harmful to your cells. Vegetable oils (hydrogenated) do not rot on the shelf. The premise that they do not split naturally implies that your body will have difficulty digesting them. Don't be fooled: these meals aren't good for your heart. They must be avoided at all costs.

Oils such as coconut oil, cacao butter, olive oil (extra virgin from Greece and Italy, to ensure it hasn't been tampered with), or even pastured organic butter are beneficial for your body since they are identifiable as food.

2. Vegetable oils that have been processed

Corn, canola, and 'vegetable oils are mono & polyunsaturated fats with compounds that do not have a hydrogen molecule connected to them. This allows them to easily react with several other environmental elements, such as free radicals, light, warmth, and air. Because these oils are so easily broken down, they are almost rotten by reaching the shelves. It is practically difficult to separate them from plants than put them into bottles without damaging them. These oils have been artificially deodorized and processed to make them seem and smell fresh, but they are still rancid.

Naturally saturated oils such as coconut butter are good substitutes, and so are complete food sources such nuts, seeds, avocado, and olives.

3. Standard dairy products

Traditional dairy cows are chemically fertilized for years to induce them to make milk - they are mammals, just like humans, and only produce milk once they have offspring to feed. Then, hormones, antibiotics, and other treatments are pumped into them to keep their milk production up and help them battle diseases and illnesses that they are susceptible to due to their disorders.

Because of the procedure to be rendered 'safe' for ingestion, traditional dairy is also exceedingly acidic for the body. Since your body must maintain an alkaline pH, the acidic composition of milk robs calcium and other alkaline elements from your body. When you eat acidic meals, your body uses alkaline reserves in the teeth and bones to counteract the acid, resulting in a net calcium loss. Overall, milk does not benefit the body in its present condition.

4. Flour (White)

Even though it has been fortified, white flour remains nutritionally deficient. This is because the germ and bran are removed from white flour during the manufacturing process, leaving just the endosperm. In addition, the bran contains nutrient-rich oils, whereas the germ contains most vitamins and minerals. When these two items are removed from the equation, you're left with only starch.

This starch is subsequently bleached, which decreases its nutritious value even further. Finally, you have a material in your body that transforms into paper Mache, which is very acidic and devoid of nourishment. Synthetic vitamins placed back into enhanced flour might not be as well utilized by your body as organic minerals and vitamins that would've been present in the plant if it had not been treated at all.

Whole grains may be used as a substitute! Whole wheat, spelt, rye, and oat is all good choices. You might also want to try sprouted grain goods and gluten-free options – just make sure your gluten-free options aren't also completely processed & comprised of refined grains.

5. Processed foods labeled as "low fat."

When you read the phrases 'low fat' or 'fat-free' on prepared or packaged goods (this doesn't include organically low-fat foods, including fruits and vegetables), you can expect that the items have gone through numerous steps of processing and include a myriad of chemicals, preservatives, and stabilizers. Your body will not recognize these meals as nourishment, and they will not help you shrink down your waistline. What they'll do is make your body struggle over time to break down the compounds and look for any remaining nourishment in the food. These goods are just unworthy of your body after the day.

Substitutes: Whole foods are best. Begin consuming more naturally reduced-fat foods, including whole fruits and vegetables, if you want to cut down on your fat consumption. Alternatively, consume naturally occurring fats such as nuts, seeds, avocado, and coconut, which your body will recognize and utilize to build a healthy body.

6. Aspartame

Aspartame has been identified as a neurotoxin. This implies that when you eat it, it essentially poisons your brain. It becomes more dangerous as it degrades in the presence of heat, and most aspartame-containing products have been heated via cooking or improper storage. It may be found in various foods, particularly those branded as "sugar-free." In addition, Aspartame may build up in the body over time and cause harm. The long & short of it is that you should never consume aspartame.

Natural sweeteners may be used as a substitute. Fruits, maple syrup, dates, and coconut sugar are good options for naturally sweetened dishes.

7. Meat

Meat that has been processed is not actually even meat. These is called 'meat' because it has meat as a component, but it also contain many artificial or toxic ingredients. The salt content in the deli and other processed meat items is quite high, which is bad for your heart. They're also loaded with toxins that are harmful to your health. Nitrates are one of the most bizarre substances found in deli slices, and they are well-known carcinogens. So the bottom line is: stay away from it!

8. Soda

It's largely made up of lab-created chemicals and flavored with excessive fructose corn syrup, which is known to be an empty calorie, meaning it delivers calories but no nourishment. The sugar concentration in soda, along with the absence of fiber that would typically limit the discharge of sugars in your system, will result in a large blood sugar surge. This puts a lot of strain on the liver & pancreas to get those sugars from the circulation into your cells.

Because soda is highly acidic, the body will have to draw from the alkaline mineral reserves in the bones and teeth to maintain the mild alkaline PH of the blood. And sugar-free drinks are no better: the artificial sugars in calorie-free sodas probably trigger your brain to crave sweets, causing you to consume more throughout the day than you might if you simply consumed a regular soda with regular sugar.

If you're looking for something effervescent, try kombucha, a traditional fermented tea drink. Tea, fresh juices, plus water may also assist your body stay hydrated.

9. Deep-fried foods

The oil that has been heated to frying temperatures is basically rancid. This is because the intense temperature denatures them and changes their chemical structure. When you mix this with the protein clumping and nutrient denaturing that occurs during the frying process, you end up with a food-like product that actually depletes your body of nutrients rather than delivering them. Therefore, fried foods must never, ever be eaten. In addition, Trans Fatty Acids are found in fried meals, and we already know that these are the fats that are the most harmful to your health. These fats are oxidized fats that induce cell damage and are associated with heart disease.

10. Genetically altered corn

<u>You should be aware of three things:</u>

1) Corn is grain rather than a vegetable

2) Because humans lack the digestive enzymes required to thoroughly break down corn, it usually passes via your digestive system undamaged

3) Pesticides have been transformed on a molecular level in GMO corn, which indicates the chemicals are not just on the ground but also part of the corn's genetic makeup.

All of this is really harmful to your health. When you consider that GMO corn is included in almost all processed goods, you may be consuming a diet mostly made up of GMO corn products. The majority of fast food buns, for example, are made out of 70-80% corn! There isn't even wheat.

Substitute: When choosing a side dish, use unprocessed bread/grain items and organic vegetables.

Other important foods to avoid includes:

- Excessive legumes
- Excessive nuts
- Alcohol

Approved List of Alkaline Foods by Dr. Sebi

Dr. Sebi was a fitness & wellbeing expert who developed a vegan diet centered on alkaline rather than hybrid foods. Dr. Sebi, a Honduran man from unfortunate conditions, made significant progress in the realm of natural health and wellbeing by developing his specialized diet, which contains seeded fruits (excluding seedless fruits), wild rice, syrup of agave, extra virgin olive oil, coconut oil, and other ingredients. Dr. Sebi believed in six basic food groups: living, raw, deceased, hybrid, genetically engineered, and drugs.

His diet virtually eliminated all food categories except live and raw, urging dieters to follow a vegetarian diet as precisely as possible. Foods like organically produced fruits and veggies and whole grains fall under this category. Dr. Sebi felt that raw and living meals were "electric" and helped the body fight acidic waste. Dr. Sebi created a list of foods he felt ideal for his diet, which he dubbed the Dr. Sebi Electric Food Guide. Dr. Sebi's product line continues to expand and adapt even after death.

If you eat out frequently, adhering to the Dr. Sebi Diet & Dr. Sebi Food List might be tough. As a consequence, you should get used to cooking a large number of vegan diet foods at home (using wild rice, extra virgin olive oil, syrup of agave, etc.).

Vegetables

Dr. Sebi believed that people should consume non-GMO foods, as he did with his electrified meals. Fruits and veggies which have been seedless or changed to include more minerals and vitamins than they do organically fall into this category. Dr. Sebi's vegetable list is rather extensive and diversified, giving you dozens of options for creating a variety of tasty meals.

This list contains the following items:

- Amaranth greens, popularly known as Callaloo
- Avocado
- Peppers (bell)
- Mexican Squash – (Chayote)
- Cucumbers
- Greens (Dandelion)
- Garbanzo beans
- Bananas, green
- Flower/ leaf of cactus - (Izote)
- Kale
- Lettuce (excluding Iceberg)
- Mushrooms of all kinds (excluding Shiitake)
- Mexican Cactus – (Nopales)
- Okra
- Olives (not drenched in vinegar)
- Onions
- Greens in a poke salad
- Purslane (Verdolaga)
- Sea veggies (Wakame/ arame/ nori and etc)
- Squash, except for pumpkin

- Tomatoes (just cherry & plum/Roma)
- Tomatillo
- Greens from turnips

- Watercress
- Zucchini

Fruits

Whereas the vegetable inventory is very extensive, the fruit selection is more limited. Several fruits are prohibited on the Dr. Sebi diet. On the other hand, the list of the fruit continues to provide a varied range of alternatives for diet adherents. For example, all berry kinds are permitted on the Dr. Sebi dietary list, except for cranberries, which seem to be a man-made fruit. In addition, the following items are also on the list:

(No packaged or seedless fruits are allowed)

- Apples
- Bananas
- Berries of all kinds (excluding cranberries)
- Cantaloupe
- Dates
- Figs
- Seeded grapes
- Limes
- Mango
- Seeded melons

- Orange
- Papayas
- Peaches
- Pear
- Plums
- Pear Prickly (Cactus Fruit)
- Prune
- Seeded Raisins
- Soursops
- Tamarind

Grains

- Amaranth
- Fonio
- Kamut
- Quinoa

- Rye
- Spelt
- Teff
- Rice (Wild)

Nuts and Seeds

- Seeds of hemp
- Sesame seeds, uncooked
- Tahini butter/raw sesame seeds
- Walnuts
- Brazil nuts

Oils

- Coconut oil (unprocessed)
- Olive oil (unprocessed)
- Avocado oil
- Oil made from grape-seeds
- Oil made from hempseed
- Oil extracted from sesame seed

Spices and Seasonings

- Bay leaf
- Cloves
- Basil
- Dill
- Oregano
- Parsley
- Savory
- Sweet basil
- Tarragon
- Thyme
- Sea Salt (Pure)
- Finely ground Coarse Seaweed
- Agave Syrup
- Achiote
- Coriander (Cilantro)
- Habanero
- Powdered onion

What Is Mucus and Its Relation to Different Diseases

Mucus is a preventive substance secreted from the mouth, nose, throat, lungs, stomach, and intestines, among other areas. Mucus is made up of many different components, but the most important is a molecule called mucin. Based on their structure, mucins in mucus may act as a physical barrier, lubricating content, or viscous substance. Mucus covers surfaces across our body when its structure and production are normal, allowing us to live alongside various microbes. However, when mucin structure, as well as synthesis, are abnormal, diseases might result.

Mucus is responsible for more than just congestion. It is very good for our health since it traps pathogens and protects the body from infections.

Dr. Sebi remarked, "Mucus is the source of all diseases," "Get rid of the mucus, and you'll get rid of the sickness." Dr. Sebi claimed mucus & acidity induced illness.

According to experts, variations in the type and amount of mucus may contribute to suffering in several chronic conditions. However, the sticky substance that lines our lungs, digestive tracts, and other sections of our bodies are, for the most being, a symptom of the problem rather than a cause.

However, if an improper quantity of mucus is present, it can make things difficult. The quantity of mucus required is comparable to the 'Three Bears' concept, in which too much and too little is a problem, and it must be exactly perfect. For the most being, excessive mucus is a side effect of being unwell, such as when you have a cough and a runny nose. It is not the primary cause of disease. Mucus irregularities or overproduction, on the other hand, may lead to illness in specific cases.

Abnormal mucus is a pathological aspect of some disorders, like asthma and cystic fibrosis, leading to disease. For example, too much mucus builds up in cystic fibrosis, a genetic illness that impairs mucus production all across the body, and chronic bronchitis, a lung infection in which bacteria thrive. Every day, the average human produces more than a liter of mucus. This comprises snot, saliva, cervical mucus, digestive, urinary, pulmonary, nasal, and protective eye layers.

Excessive Mucus Production: Causes & Risk Factors

Excessive mucus, also known as excess sputum, is a symptom of several chronic respiratory disorders, acute infections, and environmental irritants. Some varieties of COPD (chronic obstructive pulmonary disease), for example, are characterized by excessive mucus production and a reduced capacity to filter mucus from the lungs.

Mucus is frequently confused with saliva. However, the two are not quite the same. Saliva is a liquid generated in the mouth that aids in digestion and swallowing meals. Mucus traps dead cells & detritus from the respiratory tracts, allowing it (along with any organisms, like bacteria) to be ponied up and out of the lungs.

While this is good for your body, excessive mucus production, especially unclaimed and continuous, may lead to respiratory problems and a high chance of infection.

The Most Common Causes

Excessive sputum may be present all of the time with several chronic respiratory disorders. At times, you may have severe flare-ups with considerably more sputum than normal. Even if your lungs are in good condition, you may have excessive sputum throughout a respiratory disease. Goblet cells, as well as sub-mucosal glands, create mucus. Failure of these cells, infection, swelling, irritation or residue in the respiratory tract may cause overproduction or hyper-secretion.

Smoking and some medical diseases may cause damage to the cilia, which are microscopic hair-like structures that assist the transport of mucus out of the lungs. Coughing ability may also be hampered by atrophy (shrinkage) of the muscles involved in coughing. Excessive respiratory mucus is usually associated with the following conditions:

Infection of the lungs

Anyone may have a short-term respiratory disease that causes mucus to build up in the lungs. A minor bacterial or viral respiratory system infection and serious bacterial pneumonia may cause this. Infectious organisms cause the lungs to produce an immune response to clear themselves of the infection. Once you have an illness, your sputum output rises to eliminate invading bacteria. In most cases, the mucus should return to normal following a few days of your recovery.

Asthma

Asthma is characterized by respiratory distress brought on by environmental factors, including airborne particles, pollen, and pet dander. In addition, you might well have hyper mucus secretion throughout an asthma attack.

Bronchitis

Excessive mucus synthesis in the lungs is linked to chronic bronchitis, a kind of COPD. Therefore, coughing with sputum production daily for a minimum of three months is one of the diagnostic criteria.

When the situation worsens, the mucus might thicken considerably more than normal.

Emphysema

Emphysema is a COPD characterized by extreme mucus secretion, coughing, and susceptibility to lung infections.

Bronchiectasis

Bronchiectasis is a disorder in which recurring infections cause the airways to enlarge permanently. As a result, Bronchiectasis causes thick, foul-smelling sputum to be produced.

Edema of the lungs

A hazardous rise in lung fluid may occur due to pulmonary edema. Sputum is frequently frothy and may be pink in color, attributed to the existence of blood.

Genetics

Increased mucus is linked to several genetic illnesses. Some illnesses directly impact the lungs, whereas others wreak havoc on the muscles that control breathing, increasing respiratory mucus.

Cystic fibrosis

It is a hereditary condition that affects the respiratory and gastrointestinal systems, among other bodily systems. One of the most distinguishing features of this illness is increased mucus production.

Primary ciliary dyskinesis

It is a hereditary illness characterized by faulty cilia, resulting in excessive mucus in the lungs and susceptibility to infections and breathing problems.

Excess mucus may also be caused by neuromuscular diseases, including muscular dystrophy and spinal muscular atrophy, which impede muscle function and diminish lung movement during inhaling and exhaling, as well as your strength and capacity to cough. Mucus accumulates in the lower lung as a result of this.

Chapter 3: Detoxification and Cleansing

What is Detoxification?

Detoxification is a naturally occurring phenomenon in our bodies that eliminate and convert toxins and undesirable elements. It is our body's major function, and it continually functions and integrates with the remaining body's functions. As a result, it is a mechanism that maintains our bodies healthy and enhances and optimizes their performance. This is accomplished by reducing the toxins we introduce into the body and simultaneously providing its removal and detoxification processes with the nutrients they need to function properly.

The liver is where detoxification begins. Your liver basically achieves this in two steps, although it's a difficult procedure. First, toxic chemicals are converted to highly reactive metabolites, eventually excreted. Second, detoxification is supported by the kidneys, lungs, or even the gut. Toxins may have an immediate and long-term effect on these organs. The long-lasting, low-grade toxins found in commercially farmed fruits and vegetables are more harmful, such as residue. Because reactions aren't instantaneous, you can overlook the link between persistent low-grade toxins and weight loss struggles.

Although the detoxification process is the most neglected by today's healthcare system, it is an important functioning element. The majority of the molecules produced in our bodies daily are used to eliminate waste products. The body needs hundreds of enzymes, vitamins, and many other compounds to help it eliminate waste and toxins. We need to make these molecules to help us focus on the good according to what we eat and leave the harmful. However, the liver and the digestive tract do the majority of the job; the kidneys, lymph system, lungs, and skin are all engaged in the complicated detoxification system.

The major goal of detoxification systems is to assist the organs and digest and eliminate the toxins in the human body. So it's necessary for optimal health.

What exactly does a full-body detox entail?

A whole-body detox is a method that some individuals think may help them get rid of toxins. It might include following a certain diet, fasting, supplementing, or utilizing a sauna.

Detoxes may promote healthier habits like eating a balanced diet, exercising regularly, and being hydrated, which can help the body's natural detoxification mechanisms. A complete body detox, often known as cleansing, is a program individuals undertake to rid their bodies of toxins. Toxins are chemicals that harm one's health, like poisons and pollutants. The liver, kidneys, gastrointestinal system, and skin are all capable of removing these chemicals on their own.

There is no one-size-fits-all explanation of what a full-body detox entails, although it may entail:

- Stick to a strict diet

- Fast
- Increase your intake of water or juices.
- Make use of supplements
- Utilize laxatives, suppositories, or colonic irrigation
- Use a sauna
- Decrease the exposure to environmental contaminants

There are, however, certain hazards, as well as some detox products that might be dangerous.

How does the detoxification process work?

Detoxification is the process of purifying the blood. This is accomplished by eliminating pollutants from the bloodstream in the liver, which also processes toxins for excretion. Toxins are also eliminated via the kidneys, intestine, lungs, lymphatic vessels, and skin during a physical detox. Unfortunately, impurities aren't effectively filtered when these pathways are weakened, and the body suffers as a result.

A body detox program may assist the natural cleaning process of the body by:

- Fasting to allow the organs to rest

- Helping the liver to eliminate toxins

- Facilitating elimination via the intestine, kidneys, as well as skin

- Boosting blood circulation; and

- Recharging the body with nutritious foods

How do you know if you really need a body detox?

Everybody must detox a minimum of once a year. However, detoxing is not recommended for nursing women, children, or people with chronic degenerative disorders, cancer, or TB. If you're unsure whether or not detox is appropriate for you, talk to your doctor.

"It's vital to detox today," explains Linda Page, N.D., Ph.D., publisher of Detoxification: Strategies to Cleanse, Purify, and Renew, since there are more toxins in the surroundings than ever before.

Detoxing is recommended by Page for symptoms like:

- Fatigue that isn't explained
- Sluggish expulsion
- Irritated skin
- Allergies
- Infection at a low level
- Bags beneath the eyes or puffy eyes
- Bloating
- Menstrual issues
- Mental anguish

What is the best way to begin a body detox?

To begin a physical detox, you'll need to reduce your toxic load first. Remove alcohol, caffeine, cigarettes, refined carbohydrates, and saturated fats from your diet since they all function as poisons in the body and obstruct your recovery. Also, replace natural alternatives for chemical-based home cleaners, including personal health care items (household cleaners, conditioners, deodorants, and toothpaste).

Stress is another barrier to good health since it causes your body to produce stress chemicals into your system. While these hormones might give you an "adrenaline high" to help you win a race or make a deadline, they also generate toxins and shut down the liver's detoxifying enzymes in large doses. Yoga, Qigong, and meditation are all easy and effective strategies to reduce stress by adjusting your physical & mental responses to the stress that life will inevitably bring.

Which detox plan suits you best?

Depending on the specific requirements, there are a variety of detoxification regimens and detox recipes available. However, a 3 to 7-day juice fast (drink only vegetable and fruit juices and water) is recommended by Page as an efficient technique to eliminate toxins.

The following are the top five detox diets:

1. Detox with Fruit and Veggies
2. Cleanse with a Smoothie
3. Cleanse with Juice
4. Detox from Sugar
5. Detoxification using Hypoallergenic Ingredients

Difference between Detox and Cleansing

While the phrases cleanse and detoxification are often used simultaneously, they are not the same thing! While both eliminate toxins from the body, detoxification or cleanse is not the same! Clean is at the core of the term "cleanse," and you must think of it as a means to clean your body. A cleansing usually focuses on the digestive system and employs supplements or tablets to expel toxins directly. Detox procedures, on either hand, aim to aid your body's natural toxin-removal mechanisms. Because the kidneys and liver are the body's primary detoxifying organs, excellent detox programs involve supporting the liver & kidneys by providing them with the nutrients and supplements they ought to perform at their best.

So, what exactly are toxins?

Heavy metals, such as mercury, are at the forefront. Still, contaminants, plastics, and pesticides are also on the list. Toxins are hazardous particles that may remain in your body for long periods, aggravating cells, causing inflammation, & interacting with your body's natural activities.

The following are symptoms of toxicity or an extremely toxic load (and consequently the necessity for a detox or cleanse):

1. Fatigue

2. Headaches

3. Joint discomfort

4. Depression

5. Anxiety

6. As well as constipation

The Cleansing Process

Cleansing is linked to maintaining intestinal health. The process of digestion is the system that delivers nutrients to the body. It becomes sluggish in fulfilling its responsibilities if it becomes unwell. An accumulation of waste in the intestines may become poisonous, causing pain and sickness. Bloating is among the symptoms of a sick stomach. Gas builds up whenever the body doesn't even get rid of toxins as quickly as it should. After then, the food starts to decompose. Food ought to be organic and as close to organic as possible.

There are both useful and dangerous bacteria in the digestive system. When the ratio of these microorganisms is disrupted, problems emerge. Purging is by far the most fundamental kind of cleaning. A laxative is used to eliminate wastes, parasites, and other unpleasant substances. However, the difficulty with this technique is that it would be non-selective and eliminate the good and the bad. It might also be problematic since you can lose too much water in the process, leaving you dehydrated. One of the body's techniques is getting rid of toxic toxins is by drinking enough water.

According to Marie Spano, a nutritionist & vice president of the International Association of Sports Nutrition, exercise and good sleep are crucial to making your cleaning program work for you.

It's a good idea to start the cleaning process by mending the gut by watching what passes into it. Unhealthy food is so termed because it lacks the body's minerals to function properly. Instead, it clogs the digestive system, causing it to malfunction. Gluten, soy, fructose, dairy, and caffeine-containing foods should be avoided and substituted with organic, additive-free alternatives.

The cleansing process does not end with removing waste from the digestive system. Instead, it must be repaired by supplying nutritious food that helps the intestines function optimally. This includes fiber-rich, nutritious foods that aid in restoring adequate levels of organisms, such as beneficial bacteria in the gut. Natural beverages, including unflavored probiotic yogurt, may also help.

You must have been through a pre-cleanse period to begin the cleaning regimen. In addition, you must abstain from drinking alcohol and eating various harmful foods. Therefore, the first few days in the program were difficult. However, when the body adapted and began to work better, a significant increase in overall energy levels can be seen.

The Detox Technique

Detoxification is another method of removing hazardous substances from the body. Toxins are normally eliminated from the body via the skin, liver, and kidneys. Detox is intended to help these organs work more efficiently. So, which toxins are the procedure aimed at? For one thing, the oxygen you breathe contains toxins that make their way into the body and cause irritation. In addition, pesticides, preservatives, and flavors are all found in many foods.

Gwyneth Paltrow is among the celebs that have found success with detox. It takes place over 21 days. The Clean Program is the name given to it by the doctor who created it. To get rid of pollutants, he recommends a diet of smoothies, clean meals, plus supplements. The majority of the patients say they lost weight due to the approach.

Your skin is also exposed to a toxic cocktail contained in the creams, lotions, and other products you use. As a result, the organs in charge of detoxification might sometimes get overworked. You should talk to a dietitian about them since some might cause problems. Garlic, for instance, thins the blood, putting people whose blood clots slowly in danger. Food supplements may also help the kidneys & liver function better.

Cleanse the Body Naturally with Food

The essential technique to detox is to eat a balanced diet. To begin, eliminate foods that obstruct detoxification or leave you highly toxic. Fructose, which is present in soda (as high-fructose syrup of corn or HFCS) and fruit juices & commercialized juice cleanses, is one. According to research, this simple sugar might have a role in chronic disorders, including obesity. Fructose increases persistent inflammation and oxidative stress, leading to obesity.

Reducing Tran's fats and degraded fats is also part of natural cleansing. Even though the front label reads "low in fat," these fats may be found in processed goods that have "partially hydrogenated" in the components. Damaged fats, such as poached eggs on the banquet table, have been damaged and should be avoided.

Food allergies may impede weight loss and aggravate toxicity by rendering your gut more porous and enabling toxins to access the bloodstream. Common food sensitivities include gluten, milk products, soy, and corn. Try avoiding these meals for 3 - 4 weeks if you're thinking of detoxing.

"The reasonable strategy is to use a focus on food to assist the incredibly complicated mechanisms of detoxification and biotransformation," says John Cline, MD. "It's preferable to consume an apple as part of a range of meals than to attempt to imitate its advantages with specific nutritional supplements if an apple includes at least 700 distinct phytochemicals."

The Safest Foods for Detoxification

Oils and Fats

Olive oil and organic coconut oil are natural fats and oils that give energy for the detoxification and biotransformation mechanisms.

Seeds & Nuts

For a nutritious snack, try Brazilian nuts, sunflower seeds, walnuts, as well as flax seeds. Nuts & seeds are high in fiber, which helps with normal excretion and elimination.

Proteins

Protein is required to efficiently function the two primary detoxification routes found inside the liver cells, known as Phase 1 & Phase 2.

Legumes

Insoluble and soluble fiber, and a spectrum of amino acid precursors, may be found in beans, lentils, and other legumes.

Fruits

Fruits include a range of phytonutrients with antioxidant qualities, like beta-carotene, lutein, & anthocyanin's. They're also rich in water and an excellent source of soluble & insoluble fiber.

Vegetables

Non-starchy veggies are high in phytochemicals and fiber, among other nutrients.

A body-cleanse diet consists mostly of nutrient-dense, low-sugar, high-fiber plant-based foods and high-protein and healthy nutrition fat sources. Most food products, especially inflammatory fats, would be eliminated in favor of whole, unadulterated, natural foods.

Consume organic plant foods wherever feasible. According to the Environmental Working Group, normal food includes 178 pesticides. If organic isn't an option due to cost or availability, consult the EWG's list of the most — & least — pesticide-laden fruits and vegetables, labeled the Dirty Dozen as well as Clean 15, respectively.

Food contains nutrients that aid in detoxification, but therapeutic amounts of particular nutrients may also effectively cleanse the liver and other detoxifying organs naturally. Therefore, a complete variety of nutrients to promote liver function and detoxification should be tailored to the individual's requirements.

Chiropractors assist patients in selecting the proper nutrients ineffective levels to detoxify daily. A chiropractor or even other physicians may also create a personalized detoxification approach for you that incorporates a healthy diet.

10 Natural Techniques to Aid Your Body's Detoxification Process

Make regular detox a priority to promote liver health and the body's natural detoxification processes so you may achieve (and remain) lean, healthy, as well as enthusiastic while lowering your disease susceptibility. Here are some methods for getting rid of toxins.

1.   Consume the appropriate meals

Numerous studies have shown that whole food like green vegetables, berries, and seasonings like turmeric might assist detoxification in numerous ways. When combined with protein and good fat, these whole foods form an ideal detox and weight-loss diet. When feasible, choose natural plant foods and high-quality animal meals.

2. Trust your gut.

GI Renew is a supplement that replenishes intestinal flora.

A dysfunctional detoxification system is caused or exacerbated by gastrointestinal disorders. Therefore, optimizing the digestive system necessitates reducing the impediments that cause dysbiosis (gut abnormalities) and other issues and consuming the right gut-supporting foods and minerals.

See your chiropractor and other health professionals if you anticipate intestinal permeability (leaking gut) or other digestive issues.

3. Lower the level of inflammation

Toxicity causes inflammation, which leads to a higher toxic load and, as a result, fat loss is hindered. Omega-3-rich plant foods like flaxseed & chia seeds, non-starchy veggies, and spices like turmeric are all part of an anti-inflammatory diet.

Integrate anti-inflammatory ingredients such as resveratrol, as well as curcumin into the diet with the help of your chiropractor and other healthcare providers.

4. Maintain a healthy immune system

At the very least, make sure you eat properly, get enough sleep, control your stress, practice appropriate hygiene, such as hand washing, and receive adequate nutrients to promote healthy immunity.

5. Increase the effectiveness of your natural detoxification process.

While the cells are continually detoxing, consider undergoing a full-body detox in the spring (or autumn). These two- to three-week regimens contain everything you need to help your liver and other organs detox properly, such as protein, minerals, and a detox-minded food plan.

6. Keep your exposure to a minimum

The first line of defense is always prevention on offense and defense. Toxins may be found in home cleaners, construction materials, plastic, junk foods, and other sources. The Environmental Working Group (EWG) is a wonderful place to start since it has various information, including how to detect toxins in your life.

7. Drink lots of water that is free of contaminants

Hydration maintains your cellular machinery working smoothly, allowing it to cleanse and perform various other activities. To prevent additional contaminants, use water that has been adequately filtered.

8. Wipe the toxins out

Exercise has a range of benefits, including assisting the body better, eliminating toxins & burning fat. Find a regular fitness routine that matches your preferences and schedule, whether it's hot yoga as well as high-intensity interval training.

9. Have plenty of rest

A few years ago, researchers discovered the glymphatic system, a brain detoxification mechanism that happens when sleep. Unfortunately, as per Andy R. Eugene and Jolanta Masiak, insufficient sleep causes toxin build-up by impairing the glymphatic system. Therefore, the body cannot adequately detoxify if you do not get enough decent sleep in the necessary proportions regularly.

10. Make an appointment with a chiropractor

The neurological system, which governs all metabolic routes, such as detoxification pathways, is affected by chiropractic adjustments. Adjusting your perspective will allow your body to cleanse and operate at its best. Toxic overload is a common cause of obesity. The correct detoxification plan may supply your body with the nutrients it needs to repair and lose weight. While these tactics are a fine place to begin, a chiropractor and another healthcare expert can help you create a detoxification strategy suited to your specific needs.

Detoxification Through Fasting

Fasting throughout Ramadan is directed in Islam, but it is both curative and preventative for several diseases that individuals suffer from due to poor eating and living patterns. Fasting was suggested by traditional healers hundreds of years ago due to the outstanding health advantages of willingly giving up meals and drinks for extended periods. However, fasting is perhaps the most important natural healing remedy unavailable in Western culture. The recent rise of affluent disorders like atherosclerosis, hypertension, cardiovascular disease, infections, diabetes, and cancer may be linked to the abandonment of this age-old practice in the West.

These ailments are becoming increasingly widespread in Muslim communities, resulting from not fasting appropriately and deviating from the original aim of fasting.

For centuries, fasting has been adopted in Jews, Christians, Islam, and Eastern cultures as a therapeutic, spiritual, religious, and cleansing. In addition, fasting therapy has been employed and believed in by Socrates, Plato, Aristotle, and Hippocrates to restore health where there was disease.

Fasting's therapeutic properties are since it is a sort of detoxification from gluttony and susceptibility of our bodies to harmful substances in our diet and surroundings. But, of course, we can't live in bubbles to shield our bodies from these pollutants. Still, we can use fasting properly to benefit from its cleansing benefits.

Detoxification is a popular and trendy term, but what exactly does it imply? Detoxification is the procedure of lowering toxins' intake and expelling them from the body or changing them & eliminating excessive mucus and congestion to restore the body's natural functioning and healing abilities.

Nicotine and other dangerous medications, air pollution, lipids, cholesterol, even free radicals are all examples of toxins. Fasting promotes excretion processes and increases the discharge of pollutants from the colon, kidneys, bladder, lungs & respiratory system, sinuses, and skin. In addition, we enable the digestive tract to rest by not constantly eating throughout the day.

By reducing the amount of effort required for the digestive organs, such as the intestine, stomachs, liver, gallbladder, pancreas, as well as the kidneys, to heal and restore themselves, eliminate underlying toxins, and mop up the flowing blood & lymph, the body can heal and restore itself. The body expends a lot of energy in the process of breaking down meals. The energy that would typically be spent on digestion is now offloaded and may be utilized to improve health and vitality, as well as enhance mental abilities

Fasting may help with a variety of health issues. For example, indigestion, impaired bowel function, and extra belly fat put pressure on the back muscles, leading to various back problems. Fasting and a reduced diet in the evenings may help with this sort of back pain. In addition, allergies & sinus congestion may be alleviated by fasting, which helps the body clear itself of extra mucus.

- Weight reduction may be achieved throughout the month of Ramadan as long as people do not overindulge in meals and desserts after the fast is completed.

- Fasting is an effective way to break coffee, cigarettes, and even narcotics addictions.

- Fasting for 5 to 7 days will greatly diminish the intense desire for hazardous drugs.

- Fasting is a powerful motivation to break unhealthy habits and a catalyst for transformation and personal development.

Fasting is a great approach to cleanse, particularly if you can eat fruits & light veggies throughout your fasting routine. The list of items to avoid throughout a detox program is almost identical to shun during a fast. The key is to consume light, fresh, and unprocessed food. This may differ based on people's beliefs and practices. However, that's precisely what a detox suggests as well.

Consider the fact that the human body detoxes naturally daily. For example, the digestive system removes undigested food while the lungs expel carbon dioxide-rich air. The skin, too, uses pores and sweat glands to remove waste and perspiration. Besides these natural detox mechanisms, the body may need extra assistance eliminating toxins accumulated over time.

How Frequently Should You Do It?

Excessive mucus, food scraps, sludge, old feces, and artificial mineral deposits may all be removed with a 3- to 7-day detox. Even a quick fast removes toxins from the body. While fasting may be a fantastic method to cleanse and reset your system, it's critical to make sure the water you're drinking has a high nutritional content.

Fasting with water:

Fasting with water has been and remains to be among the most powerful healing methods in history. Several debates on water fasting by prominent ancient figures such as Plato, Aristotle, Socrates, Leonardo Da Vinci, and Pythagoras. Furthermore, there is a variety of fresh material on water fasting accessible on the Internet, which may assist in self-education about the various methods of fasting and the advantages of fasting.

Scientific studies have shown that your brain develops when you fast, and you'll be cleverer. Furthermore, according to recent research, three-day water fast resets your immune function by stimulating stem cells, allowing you to function at your best. Every day, we perform a range of activities, such as breathing contaminated air, and drink tainted beverages, and so on, clogging the body filters, including the lungs, mouth, liver, as well as kidneys. Human bodies heat up with time, and indeed the immune system suffers as a result. Fevers cause the body to sweat off toxins and generate a natural fasting response. In such situations, three-to-four-day water fast is beneficial. This will aid in the cleansing of your system. So, should you simply let the body go through the biological cycle of being really ill and in agony to properly cleanse the system? There's no need to become ill if you clean the cleaners constantly by conducting water fast.

Intermittent fasting is a more convenient alternative to complete water fast. Essentially, you don't eat anything at all for one day in a week, allowing the kidneys and liver to properly detoxify and eliminate any pollutants. It is, however, critical to properly hydrate oneself throughout those 24 hours, either via drinking enough water or through other means. You may also take a salt flush, an evacuation, breathing techniques, and natural skin washing to help flush out the toxins.

Fasting is frequently discouraged for diabetics and hypoglycemics. Still, it might help human bodies discharge stem cells and restore themselves with the correct assistance. For example, you may begin an intermittent fast at noon, skip supper, sleep, skip breakfast, and resume eating at lunch break. This is among the simplest methods, and providing you remain well hydrated; you should have no difficulty. If you can't commit to the whole 24 hours, omitting a small meal may be helpful.

Fasting on juice:

A juice cleanses a form of detox diet that entails drinking only vegetable and fruit juice for a certain time (typically 1 to 3 days). Some plans incorporate one or even more smoothies each day to deliver energy and hunger relief by providing protein, fat, and other nutrients. On certain plans, vegan meals, as well as snacks, are provided.

A juice cleanses, according to supporters, aids the body's natural detoxification processes, purifies the diet of sweets, caffeine, processed meats, and other foods and chemicals that diminish energy, & jumpstarts a healthier eating pattern.

Because the nutrients, phytochemicals, and antioxidants are readily absorbent liquid, unfiltered organic juice is a major cleansing component. For those who require more energy, are a novice to juice cleanses, or prefer a less severe experience, vegan, gluten-free snacks and meals may be included. In addition, a juicer/juice press may be used to do a juice detox at home.

Chapter 4: 28-Day Detox Plan

Tiredness, exhaustion, weight gain, sleep problems, thyroid problems, reduced libido, digestive problems, a loss of mojo, despair, anxiety, eczema, and addictions are symptoms your body needs to detox.

Getting rid of toxins

Keeping the colon and lymphatic systems more effective is a significant aspect of the detox. It allows them to start clearing out the ama (digestive toxins from unprocessed food & muck in the system) through the main detoxification. To do so, you'll need to free up the paths via the kidneys; blocked pipes can't be flushed out. You'll also be passing items through the colon more quickly while supporting your gut flora's garden.

How Are The 28 Days Divided?

The first phase, which lasts from day 1 to day 14: is all about removing toxins from your diet and lifestyle so that your body can prepare for what's ahead. After that, full-time fasting is required. After that, no food nor liquid (except water) is allowed.

The second phase goes from day 15 to day 28: the moment to truly build on the success you've achieved in the previous stage, which is the past 14 days. In this phase, you should aim to drink 3-4 different alkaline smoothies each day, selecting the recipes from the ones below.

Days	Breakfast	Lunch	Dinner
•	Water + Herbal Teas	Water + Herbal Teas	Water + Herbal Teas
•	Water + Herbal Teas	Water + Herbal Teas	Water + Herbal Teas
•	Water + Herbal Teas	Water + Herbal Teas	Water + Herbal Teas
•	Water + Herbal Teas	Water + Herbal Teas	Water + Herbal Teas
•	Water + Herbal Teas	Water + Herbal Teas	Water + Herbal Teas
•	Water + Herbal Teas	Water + Herbal Teas	Water + Herbal Teas
•	Water + Herbal Teas	Water + Herbal Teas	Water + Herbal Teas
•	Water + Herbal Teas	Water + Herbal Teas	Water + Herbal Teas
•	Water + Herbal Teas	Water + Herbal Teas	Water + Herbal Teas
•	Water + Herbal Teas	Water + Herbal Teas	Water + Herbal Teas
•	Water + Herbal Teas	Water + Herbal Teas	Water + Herbal Teas
•	Water + Herbal Teas	Water + Herbal Teas	Water + Herbal Teas

•	Water + Herbal Teas	Water + Herbal Teas	Water + Herbal Teas
•	Water + Herbal Teas	Water + Herbal Teas	Water + Herbal Teas
•	Alkaline Shake Post-Workout	Smoothie with Kale	Blueberry-Banana Smoothie
•	Smoothie with Kiwi & Cucumber	Turmeric Ginger Citrus	Melon Green Juice
•	Melon Green Juice	Blueberry Alkaline Smoothie	Vegetable Punch
•	Apple-Ginger Smoothie	Melon Green Juice	Kiwi Alkaline Smoothie
•	Cactus Smoothie	Blueberry-Banana Smoothie	Flax Seeds Alkaline Smoothie
•	Kiwi Alkaline Smoothie	Smoothie with Grapefruit	Detox Juice
•	Turmeric Ginger Citrus	Vegetable Punch	Avocado Blueberry Smoothie
•	Detox Juice	Collard Greens Smoothie	Cactus Smoothie
•	Melon Green Juice	Kiwi Alkaline Smoothie	Melon Green Juice
•	Vegetable Punch	Green Alkaline Smoothie	Apple-Ginger Smoothie
•	Green Juice	Flax Seeds Alkaline Smoothie	Turmeric Ginger Citrus

•	Blueberry-Banana Smoothie	Turmeric Ginger Citrus	Cactus Smoothie
•	Melon Green Juice	Vegetable Punch	Blueberry Alkaline Smoothie
•	Green Juice	Melon Green Juice	Detox Juice

Chapter 5: Smoothie Recipes

- ## Hemp Seed Milk Alkaline Smoothie

Ingredients

- Hemp seed milk, 1 cup

- 1 cup diced watermelon

- 5 iced strawberries

- 1/2 of a tiny banana

- Chia seeds, 1 teaspoon

- 1 cup crushed ice

Directions

- Combine the banana, chia seeds, half of the ice, and half of the milk in a blender. Blend until everything is properly incorporated.

- Blend in the remaining milk & ice with the watermelon and iced strawberries.

- Dump in the smoothie and stir until fully mixed.

- ## Kiwi Alkaline Smoothie

Ingredients

- Coconut milk (1/4 cup)

- 1/4 cup of cucumber

- Half of a banana

- One kiwi

- Ice cubes, a fistful

Directions

- Bring all of the ingredients together.

- Combine the coconut milk, 1/4 cucumber, banana, and kiwi in a blender and blend until smooth.

- Chill before serving.

- ## Green Avocado Smoothie

Ingredients

- 1 pitted and scraped avocado

- 1 cup coconut milk

- 1 lime's juice

- A couple of kale leaves

- A few mint leaves

- A few pieces of cucumber

Directions

- Combine all of the ingredients in a blender, and enjoy!

- ## Smoothie with Grapefruit

Ingredients

- 1 grapefruit juice

- Coconut milk (1 cup)

Directions

- Combine all of the ingredients in a blender, then serve and enjoy!

- ## Collard Greens and Grapefruit Smoothie

Ingredients

- Grapefruits, 2

- 3 leaves of collard greens (large)

- Coconut water, 1 cup

- 1/2 cup pomegranate pits

Directions

- Deseed, then peel the grapefruit.

- Collard greens should have their stems removed.

- Blend all of the components together until they make a creamy, foamy texture.

- ## Smoothie with Strawberries
Ingredients

- Strawberries (1/2 cup)

- 1 lime's juice

- One banana

- Coconut water, 1 cup

- Hemp seeds, 1 tablespoon

- 1 scoop powdered alkalizer & detoxifier

Directions

- In a blender, combine all ingredients and mix until creamy & frothy.

- ## Smoothie with Kale
Ingredients

- Kale (1 cup)

- One banana

- Strawberries (1/2 cup)

- 1/4 cup raspberries

- Orange juice, 1 cup

Directions

- Fresh as well as frozen berries and bananas may be used.

- Combine all of the ingredients in a blender and blend until smooth.

- If you want to be more invigorating, add ice if it's a hot day. Enjoy!

- ## Green Alkaline Smoothie
Ingredients

- Kale, 2 fistfuls

- Apple juice, 1 cup

- 1 tablespoon freshly squeezed lime juice

- 1/2 cucumber

Directions

- Take 1/2 medium cucumber, 1 cup of apple juice, and 1 tablespoon fresh lime juice.

- In a blender, combine all of these ingredients until smooth. Serve and have fun.

- ## Flax Seeds Alkaline Smoothie
Ingredients

- Flaxseeds, 1 tablespoon

- Kale, 1 cup

- Strawberries (1/2 cup)

- One banana

- Ginger, 1 teaspoon

- Coconut water, 1 cup

Directions

- Combine all of the ingredients in a blender and mix until smooth. Serve and enjoy your drink.

- ## Blueberry Alkaline Smoothie

Ingredients

- Blueberries (1/2 cup)

- 1 tablespoon walnut butter

- Chia seeds, 1 tablespoon

- 1 tablespoon flaxseeds, ground

- Coconut milk (1 cup)

- Coconut oil, 1 tablespoon

- 1 tablespoon powdered hemp seed

Directions

- Simply combine all of the ingredients in a blender and mix until smooth.

- Hemp milk may be substituted with coconut milk if desired.

- ## Alkaline Peach Smoothie

Ingredients

- Peaches (1/4 cup)

- 1/2 cucumber

- 1/4 cup of parsley

- One banana

- 1/2 cup water

- 1/2 of a lime's juice

Directions

- Peaches should be sliced and blended.

- In a blender, combine the other ingredients, mix until smooth, and serve.

- ## Berry Smoothie

Ingredients

- Blueberries (1/2 cup)

- 1 lime's juice

- Chia seeds, 1 tablespoon

- Strawberries (1/2 cup)

- 1/2 of a banana

- Coconut water, 1 cup

Directions

- In a blender, combine all of the ingredients.

- Fresh or frozen berries may be used.

- You may drink it straight from the blender or mix it with ice for a more delicious drink.

- ## Veggie Blast Smoothie

Ingredients

- 1 trimmed and chopped cucumber

- 4 flaked tomatoes

- 1/2 onion

- 1/2 cup chilled rosemary infusion

- To taste, black pepper and Himalayan salt

- 1 tablespoon extra-virgin olive oil

- 1 cup of kale

- 1 lime's juice

Directions

- Place the kale and lime juice in a large bowl and put them aside.

- Combine the cucumber, peeled tomatoes, clove, onion, rosemary infusion, and olive oil. Then combine them with kale as well as lime juice in a blender.

- Lastly, season with salt and pepper. Serve immediately this insanely healthy and tasty smoothie.

- ## Kale and Fruit Blast Smoothie
Ingredients

- 2 scraped and cored apples

- 1 flaked mango, cut into pieces

- One banana

- Lime juice

- 1 tiny ginger slice – to taste

- Water, 2 cups

- 4 kale leaves (no stems)

- A bundle of parsley (1/2)

Directions

- In a blender, combine all ingredients until they form a foamy texture. Serve and have fun.

- ## Super Smoothie with Strawberry
Ingredients

- 1/2 cup strawberry

- Lime (one)

- One banana

- Coconut water, 1 cup

- Hemp seeds, 1 tablespoon

- 1 scoop powder of alkalizer and detoxifier

Directions

- In a blender, combine all ingredients and mix until smooth. It's worth noting that the banana might be fresh or frozen. Instead of putting the entire lime in the blender, squeeze out the juice.

- ## Smoothie with Kiwi and Cucumber
Ingredients

- One kiwi fruit

- 1/4 cucumber

- 1/2 banana

- 3 to 4 walnuts

- 1/4 c. coconut milk

Directions

- Put all of the ingredients in a blender and mix until smooth. Put a few ice cubes into the blender if you really want to make the smoothie even more refreshing.

- ## Alkaline Breakfast Smoothie
Ingredients

- Grapefruits, 2

- 3 collard leaves, medium

- 1/2 cup arils of pomegranate

- Coconut water, 1 cup

Directions

- The grapefruits must first be peeled and the seeds removed. Next, ensure that the collard leaves are free of leaves. After you've finished these two processes, combine the ingredients in a blender.

- ## Smoothie with Alkaline Energy Boosters

Ingredients

- Kale, 1 cup

- One banana

- 1/2 cup strawberry

- 1 cup of orange juice

- 1/4 cup of raspberries

Directions

- You may use fresh or frozen raspberries strawberries, as well as bananas. In a blender, combine the ingredients and add several ice cubes to keep it more refreshing.

- ## Smoothie with Alkaline Greens

Ingredients

- 2 kale handfuls

- 1 cup of apple juice

- 1 tablespoon freshly squeezed lime juice

- 1/2 cucumber

Directions

- Combine all of the ingredients in a blender and mix until smooth.

- ## Alkaline Smoothie with Extraordaberries

Ingredients

- Blueberries (1/2 cup)

- Lime (one)

- 1 tablespoon of chia seeds

- 1/2 cup of strawberry

- 1/2 banana

- cup of coconut water

Directions

- Squeeze the lime into the processor and combine it with the other components.

- ## Alkaline Shake Post-Workout

Ingredients

- One avocado

- 1 tablespoon Brazilian nut butter

- 1 cup of coconut milk

- One banana

- 1 tablespoon of chia seeds

Directions

- Combine all of the ingredients in a blender and mix until smooth.

- ## Alkaline Smoothie with Peaches

Ingredients

- Peaches, 1/4 cup

- 1/2 cucumbers

- 1/4 cup of parsley

- One banana

- 1/2 cup of water

- 1/2 limes

Directions

- Squeeze approximately half of a medium-sized lime into a cup. Before placing the peaches in the processor, make sure they're sliced. Then, blend everything together with a couple of ice cubes.

- ## Alkaline Smoothie with Blueberries

Ingredients

- Blueberries (1/2 cup)

- 1 tablespoon walnut butter

- Kale, 1 handful

- 1 tablespoon of chia seeds

- 1 tablespoon flax seeds, ground

- 1 cup of coconut milk

- 1 tablespoon of coconut oil

- 1 tablespoon powdered hemp seed

Directions

- Simply combine the ingredients in a blender, and your smoothie is ready. Depending on your preferences, you may substitute hemp milk for coconut milk.

- ## Alkaline Smoothie with Anti-Inflammatory Properties

Ingredients

- 1 tablespoon flaxseed

- A cup of kale

- 1/2 cup strawberry

- One banana

- 1 teaspoon ginger powder

- 1 cup of coconut water

Directions

- Blend together all of the components until smooth. You may use any sort of berry in place of the strawberries.

- ## Healthiest Alkaline Juice

Ingredients

- One lime

- 1 pear

- 3 celery stalks

- A handful of fresh parsley

Directions

- All vegetables should be well cleaned.

- Reduce the size of the pear by chopping it into smaller pieces.

- If you're using a medium juicer, cut the stalks of celery into 1-inch chunks.

- If the lime isn't organic, peel it.

- All of the ingredients should be juiced.

- Stir it well.

- This alkaline juice should be consumed right away. Enjoy.

- ## Turmeric Ginger Citrus Miracle

Ingredients

- Three oranges

- One lime

- 1-inch slice of ginger

- 1/2 inch chunk of fresh turmeric

414

Directions

- Remove the peels from the oranges.

- If the lime isn't organic, peel it.

- Peel the turmeric as well as ginger.

- All of the ingredients should be juiced.

- ## Exhilarating Watermelon Juice

Ingredients

- 1 lime

- 1 tiny sweet watermelon

Directions

- The watermelon should be cut in half.

- If you're using a slow juicer, scoop out the pieces and discard the rind.

- You may juice melon pieces, along with the rind, using a rotating juicer.

- If the lime isn't organic, peel it.

- Everything should be juiced in your juicer.

- Enjoy.

- ## Green Juice for Glowing Skin

Ingredients

1. 2 apples, peeled and cut into pieces

2. Cucumber (one)

3. 1 lime and a handful of mint leaves

Directions

- Rinse the apples and cucumber.

- If the lime & cucumber aren't organic, peel them.

- Using a knife, slice the apple into pieces.

- In a juicer, blend all of the ingredients together.

- Enjoy.

- ## Detox Juice (Alkaline)

Ingredients

- 1 cucumber, medium

- 1 cup coriander

- 1 apple, peeled and cut into pieces

- Lime (one)

- 1/2 lime

- 1/2 teaspoon spirulina powder (organic) (optional)

Directions

- All vegetables should be well washed.

- Using a knife, slice the apple into pieces.

- If the lime, cucumber, and lime aren't organic, peel them.

- All of the ingredients should be juiced.

- Stir in 1/2 teaspoons organic spirulina powder thoroughly.

- Enjoy the alkaline juice while it's still fresh.

- ## Fruit Juice with Alkalizing Properties

Ingredients

- 1 orange

- 2 cups of mango, diced

- 1/2 lime leaves and several mint leaves (optional)

415

Directions

- Remove the peel off the orange

- Remove the skin from the mango and chop it into slices.

- If the lime isn't organic, peel it.

- Everything in the juicer should be juiced

▪ Basic Alkaline Juice

Ingredients

- 1 cup coarsely chopped kale

- 1 cucumber, tiny

- 2 cups of mango

- 1 inch of ginger

- 3 celery stalks

- One lime

Directions

- All vegetables should be well washed.

- Chop the kale into small pieces.

- If the ginger, lime, and cucumber aren't organic, peel them.

- Reduce the size of the celery stalks by chopping them into smaller pieces.

- Cut the mango into pieces after removing the skin.

- In a juicer, blend all of the ingredients together.

- Enjoy your alkaline-rich juice.

▪ Alkaline Diet Juice

Ingredients

- Cucumber (one)

- 1-inch ginger slice

- one lime

- A handful of fresh parsley

Directions

- Wash all fruits and vegetables thoroughly.

- Pare the cucumber, ginger, as well as lime.

- Everything should be blended in your juicer.

▪ Alkalizing Cleanse Juice

Ingredients

- One lime

- 1 cup coarsely chopped kale

- 1 piece of cucumber

- 2 apples, peeled and cut into pieces

- 1 teaspoon wheatgrass powder (organic) (optional)

Directions

- All vegetables should be well washed.

- Chop the kale into small pieces.

- If the apples, cucumber, and lime are not organic, peel them.

- Chop the apple to fit into the juicer's feed hole.

- Everything within your juice should be blended.

- Stir in 1 teaspoon organic wheatgrass powder well.

▪ Melon Green Juice

Ingredients

- 1/2 melon (honeydew)

- Cucumber (one)

- Lime (one)

Directions

- Remove the melon's flesh using a fork. The seeds may be juiced.

- If the cucumber isn't organic, peel it, as well as the lime.

- Everything should be juiced in your juicer.

- This delightful juice should be consumed immediately.

- ■ **Energy Shots with Turmeric and Ginger**

Ingredients

- 1/2 inch slice of fresh turmeric

- 1-inch slice of fresh ginger

- One lime

Directions

- If the turmeric root & ginger root aren't organic, peel them.

- End up leaving the peels on if you're blending organic veggies. Simply wash everything completely.

- Everything should be juiced.

- This invigorating turmeric ginger shot is a great way to start your day.

- ■ **Green Smoothie with a Boost**

Ingredients

- 2 large leaves of kale

- 1/2 cup diced frozen mango

- 1 whole banana

- 1 tablespoon lime juice

- 1 cup of water

Directions

- Place the greens in the processor after thoroughly washing them. Place the mango and a banana in the blender after peeling them. After combining the ingredients, drizzle in the water and combine until smooth.

- ■ **Alkaline Smoothie (Refreshing)**

Ingredients

- 1 fistful of fresh kale

- Strawberries, Chilled – 4

- 1 cup diced watermelon

- 1 whole banana

- 1 cup of hemp seed milk

- 1 cup of ice cubes

Directions

- Rinse the items before putting them in the processor to juice. If you don't really want a brown smoothie, puree banana, and kale with 1/2 a cup of milk plus ice cubes, combine the remaining halves with strawberries and watermelon.

- Blend until smooth, then combine the two smoothies in one glass & serve.

- ■ **Apple-Ginger Juice**

Ingredients

- 1 large apple

- 20 gram of ginger root, scraped

- 1/4 lime juice

Directions

- Wash all of your ingredients well and put them aside to cool.

- Combine the apple, and ginger root.

- Toss the lime juice into your cup.

- Toss with ice cubes and a lime slice as a garnish (optional).

▪ Vegetable Punch

Ingredients

- 1/2 cup romaine hearts, minced

- 2 tablespoons chives, diced

- 1 medium tomato

- A half of a medium deseeded jalapeno pepper

- 1/2 medium red bell pepper

- 1 celery stalk, large

Directions

- In a juicer, mix the lettuce, chopped chives, tomato, jalapeño, bell pepper, a stalk of celery.

- Serve chilled, adding ice cubes if desired.

- If you don't have a juicer, finely chop all of the ingredients & begin blending with the softer ones first. Blend in the larger and more difficult veggies, lastly. After everything has been mixed, filter the juice through a cheesecloth.

▪ Tropical-Kale Delight

Ingredients

- 1 small mango

- 1 banana, medium

- Kale leaves, 1 cup

Directions

- The mango should be cut into strips, and the kale should be coarsely chopped.

- These two should be blended first and then strained. Then, return the liquid to the processor, along with the banana.

- If you don't mind the chunks from the mango and kale, there's no need to filter the liquid.

▪ Orange Sunrise Mix

Ingredients

- 1 large tomato

- 1 medium orange

- 1 large apple

Directions

- Remove the peel from the orange and wash the rest of the ingredients.

- Cut all fruits and vegetables into bite-sized pieces and place them in the juicer.

- Serve the juice straight up or refrigerate with ice cubes.

▪ Green Juice

Ingredients

- One and a half cucumbers,

- Green apple, 3/4

- Kale leaves, a bunch

- 1/2 lime

- 15-gram ginger root,

- A handful of parsley leaves

Directions

- Clean all your items well, peel the ginger, and put everything through a blender afterward.

- Pour in half a lime's juice & enjoy.

▪ Super Alkaline Cherry Smoothie

Ingredients

- 1 1/2 cup of coconut milk

- 1 cup of seeded fresh cherries

- 1 cup of kale leaves (stalks removed)

- 1 peeled kiwi

- 2 tablespoons walnuts

Directions

- In a high-powered blender, combine all of the ingredients.

- Blend until completely smooth.

▪ Blueberry Banana Smoothie

Ingredients

- 1 banana, ripe

- Half cup of blueberries

- 1 tsp. powdered alkaline greens

- Optional: 1/2 tbsp. ground flaxseed

- Optional: 1/2 tbsp. hemp seeds

- Half cup of ice

- 1/2 cup of milk of your choice (plant-based)

- 1 cup of water

Directions

- In a blender, combine the banana, 1/2 cup of blueberries, 1 teaspoon alkaline greens powder, 1/2 tbsp. Flaxseed, 1/2 tbsp. Hemp seeds (if utilizing), ice cubes, milk, and water.

- Cover and mix for 1-2 minutes, or until the ingredients are completely processed and smooth.

Chapter 6: Switching From a Standard Diet

The Standard American Diet (SAD) is a contemporary eating pattern with long-term, negative health repercussions for American children and adults. The Standard Diet is high in ultra-processed products, refined sugar, fat, and salt. In addition, this diet is severely low in fruits, veggies, whole grains, legumes, and lean protein.

Making healthy meal choices might seem hard with fast-food chains on virtually every corner as well as fast foods crowding the grocery store shelves. Unfortunately, poor food choices may cause various chronic illnesses, placing pressure on the healthcare system. An overabundance of disinformation in the popular media and a significant lack of awareness among the general people exacerbates the problem. On the other hand, simple dietary modifications may enhance one's health and minimize the chance of acquiring a variety of chronic illnesses.

Switching from standard to alkaline

Shifting to an alkaline diet is the first step on the road to recovery from SAD. Shift to whole foods with high nutritional density instead of highly processed foods like white bread, white rice, and sugary items.

What do you mean by "whole foods"?

Unprocessed foods that are as similar to their original condition as possible, without the need for a tag or a barcode. There are no extra fats, carbohydrates, or artificial additives in these items.

Whole foods offer a higher ratio of vitamins, minerals, and phytonutrients over calories than prepared foods. Plant nutrients are referred to as phytonutrients. They've been examined extensively for their potential to decrease inflammation and improve overall health. Whole foods like fruit, vegetables, and legumes are the greatest way to receive a variety of phytonutrients.

In conclusion, the path to recovery from SAD starts with diet and lifestyle changes that may also help to reduce inflammation.

The following are some of the protective factors to shift from a standard diet to an Alkaline or plant-based diet:

- Consume greater anti-inflammatory phytonutrients such as carotenoids and bioflavonoids-rich fruits and veggies.

- Consume sufficient omega-3 fatty acids, such as those found in flaxseed, green vegetables, as well as sea vegetables.

- Increasing the amount of fiber consumed.

- 30 - 60 min of mild to intense aerobic exercise each day

- Eliminate your consumption of ultra-processed meals

- Fruits and vegetables should be prioritized

- Increase your intake of plant-based proteins

- Half of your grains should be whole

- Sugar additives must be avoided

- Make more meals at home

- Keep healthy foods more accessible

What To Expect While Switching?

Difficulties while changing to a new diet

When you start a new diet, you can feel a little nauseous at first. This is since your body may need some time to adjust to the new alterations. The incredible thing is that these negative effects are just temporary hurdles on your path to potential health, with most of them disappearing in 1-2 weeks.

Dietary changes may have the following side effects:Headaches

- Getting hungry

- Bloating or excessive gas

- Constipation

- Mood swings (irritability)

- Congestion or diarrhea

- Fatigue

- Dizziness

- Hunger pangs

- Concentration problems

- Disruptions in sleep

- Deficiencies in nutrition

These adverse effects are typically minor and only last a short time. However, if your symptoms continue, become severe, or include frequent vomiting, dizziness, or exhaustion, you should get medical help as soon as possible.

Why is it that switching our diet makes us feel uneasy?

The increased quantity of fiber and protein in the diet causes most of the adverse effects connected with altering the diet; however, occasionally, it's simply your brain needing caffeine or sweets.

Other factors that may cause irritation include:

- You're not getting enough calories.

- The diet is very restricted, with no fats, carbohydrates, or sweets allowed.

- You've cut out too many food categories from your diet.

- You are not getting enough nutrients from your diet.

- Your brain is yearning for the feel-good chemicals that your favorite meals provide.

- You're anticipating far too many beneficial improvements in your body, really too soon.

Common Mistakes to Avoid

1st Mistake: Trying to be perfect from the start

There is generally always one element that can be counted on. When individuals first begin following an alkaline diet, they strive for perfection. When they first start out, rationality vanishes as they strive to accomplish everything at once. This is undoubtedly true for most individuals when they begin making changes to their wellbeing or lifestyle, such as a diet program or gym routine. When you aim to be flawless from the start, you prepare yourselves for failure. When you're attempting to give up something, you have to deal with cravings, behavioral shifts, stress, psychological struggles, and trying to come up with alkaline foods to cook simultaneously.

Summary: Turning this weakness into a strength

- Don't attempt to accomplish everything at once, and don't aim to be great right away.

- Prioritize getting the Best in first, rather than limiting the BAD. This will render it more enjoyable and simple while still delivering tremendous results.

- When it comes to removing and switching away from harmful foods, take it one day & one week at a time: this week dairy, coming week caffeine. And don't go on to the next one since you've mastered the first.

- Focus on the Basics first: water, greens, oils, minerals, and moderate exercise are the 20% elements that will provide you 80% of the total benefit. When these five little modifications are added together, they add a significant advantage.

2nd Mistake: Lack of planning

Even the most veteran alkalizer will be undone by a lack of preparation. But, it's easy to be prepared. It's all about building a repertoire of simple, tasty alkaline meals that will become your go-to. Foods that you can rely on at any time.

Understanding what meals you'll eat in the coming days, planning ahead, and then, heaven forbid, buying the items you'll need to cook those meals are all part of being prepared. Everything is about a little forethought, planning, and preparation so that you may live alkaline comfortably and wonderfully.

Summary: Transforming this weakness into a strength

- Don't rely on the chance! If you live, shop, and eat daily, you will find yourself hungry, albeit with accessibility to acidic foods.

- A little planning makes a huge difference: plan your meals at least three days ahead of time and prepare for them!

- Always have a limited list of ingredients on hand — 8-10 items that you can prepare 5-6 easy alkaline snacks and meals at the stroke of a feather.

- Always have a few of 'get out of jail free' snacks on hand — nuts and seeds, sprout bread, avocados, and tomatoes are all good choices.

3rd Mistake: Digestion

The importance of the digestive system is underappreciated. Unfortunately, your digestive system becomes blocked and damaged after consuming an acidic, less-than-healthy diet for a long time. As a result, it becomes infected with yeast, germs, mycotoxins, and candida. Both of these scenarios are detrimental to your health and ambitions.

Worst of all, they'll imply that you're only reaping a small portion of the rewards of your efforts. So while being alkaline can help this cleaning process get started, there are several easy things you can really do to accelerate things - particularly if you're just getting started.

Summary: Converting this weakness into a strength

- Don't forget about your digestive system! Give it some love (particularly in the beginning), and the results will come in a flash!

- Green veggies, and other high-fiber foods should be prioritized first.

- Simple carbohydrates, refined meals, processed foods, and other items that increase yeast growth in your digestive tract should be avoided.

- Get yourself some psyllium husks.

- Slow down, relax, and appreciate your food.

- Hydration, hydration, hydration.

4th Mistake: Quantities

This is a humorous yet truthful statement. The majority of individuals who begin an alkaline diet consume very little! For some reason, portions are thrown out the window, and they consume these tiny small meals. The greatest way to alkalize, cleanse, and heal the body and the digestive system is to saturate the body with nutrients, which you can only accomplish by eating a lot!

Summary: Turning it into an advantage

- Never miss a meal.

- Eat a lot

- If you're ever concerned, ensure you're getting adequate oils, complex carbohydrates, and proteins.

- Make 2x the lunch and dinner and store some for later use as snacks or a second serving if you become hungry after an hour or two.

- Appetite is acidic; therefore, don't allow it to happen to you.

- When you're initially starting out, have alkaline foods on hand at all times.

These four typical mistakes have all been working together to provide you with a compounding advantage. As a result, these four actions will provide you with a better reward than the finished product.

What To Expect Following the Dr. Sebi Lifestyle

The long-term consequences of Dr. Sebi's alkaline diet might differ depending on whatever variation is followed. Protein, and also minerals and vitamins such as vitamin D, vitamin B12, calcium, as well as iron may be inadequate in a rigorous diet that excludes grains, dairy, & animal foods.

Human bodies are generally acidic due to Western diets, which are high in fatty foods, excessive protein, not enough fiber, and too much sugar. Inflammation and a greater risk of numerous illnesses and disorders occur when the body gets overly acidic. On the other hand, an alkalizing diet helps balance your pH level, lowering acidity. Your body can thrive at its best when you live in more alkaline conditions. For example, alkalinity may help reduce inflammation in the brain, stomach, skin, and muscles, all of which are often affected in autistic children.

An alkalizing diet reduces inflammation and prevents the formation of yeast and harmful bacteria, which are frequent in autistic children. Detoxification is also improved as a result of this. When individuals follow the right alkalizing diet and detoxification procedure, many of them thrive. This is an example of a lifestyle modification that may make a huge difference in one's life. It's also crucial to figure out whether you have any dietary allergies or intolerance that might be causing your symptoms.

A healthy body comprises organs and functions that precisely control pH balance & sustain an alkaline condition. Rather than relying on fad diets and quick fixes, nutritionists recommend implementing long-term lifestyle modifications to achieve long-term success. This involves eating a nutrient-dense diet that contains foods from various food categories. In addition, limit your intake of highly processed foods, high in empty calories and low in nutritional content.

Tips for A Good Kickstart And a Longer Life

Eating a nutritious diet is something that most of us don't think about until we're in our mid-to-late-thirties. When we're young, we can usually "get away" with eating whatever we want whenever we want. As a result, some of us disregard the potential to develop good eating habits while still young. So don't be disheartened if you've had a poor day packed with too many yummy foods. Instead, make a note of what went wrong so you may learn from it.

1. Don't rely on your willpower to get things done. That's a lot of work. Instead, try to stay away from people, places, & programs to encourage you to consume unhealthy foods.

2. Increase your water intake. While we are hungry, we are frequently thirsty. So instead of grabbing for a candy bar, try sipping some water. Also, wherever feasible, drink water instead of sugary drinks.

3. Limit your selections. Limit the diet to select things to avoid consuming out of curiosity.

4. Include green veggies. Include a green or leafy vegetable in your meal.

5. Limit your intake of fatty dressings, sauces, and other condiments. Adding ranch dressing, crackers, cheese, and bacon to a salad become a fatty/high-calorie meal. Instead, eat a lot of veggies.

6. Increase your intake of home-cooked meals. This is not only a healthy suggestion, but it is also cost-effective.

7. Order your food first if you're eating out. This will assist you in avoiding becoming influenced by the poor dietary choices of others.

8. Get plenty of rest. According to some studies, a Lack of sleep might boost your urge to eat. Because this is a difficult chore for some (due to family and/or professional responsibilities), take time to rest & unwind when you can. This might entail not watching television or using the Internet.

9. Discuss eating habits. & concerns with your doctor regularly during your consultations. Then, whenever it comes to health, there are no stupid questions.

10. Get started right away. Don't put off making New Year's Goals until January 1st. Immediate action has a lot of clouts.

BOOK 9: <u>DR. SEBI'S HERB ENCYCLOPEDIA</u>

THE COMPLETE COLLECTION OF DR. SEBI'S ALKALINE HERBS AND THEIR POWERFUL BENEFITS. DISCOVER THE SECRET PROPERTIES, WHERE TO FIND AND HOW TO USE THEM FOR WHOLE-BODY HEALTH

Chapter 1: Dr. Sebi's Diet Pillars

The Dr. Sebi diet concentrates on plant-based foods, which is one of the advantages. The diet encourages people to consume a lot of fruits and vegetables, which are abundant in fiber, vitamins, minerals, and plant components.

Diet Rules

You should follow these fundamental guidelines, according to Dr. Sebi's dietary guide:

Rule 1: Only eat the items mentioned in the nutritional guide.

Rule 2: Every day, drink 1 gallon (3.8 liters) of water.

Rule 3: Take Dr. Sebi's vitamins one hour before taking your prescription.

Rule 4: No items derived from animals are allowed.

Rule 5: No alcoholic beverages are permitted.

Rule 6: Avoid products made from wheat and stick to the guide's list of "natural-growing grains."

Rule 7: Don't use the microwave because it destroys food nutrients.

Rule 8: Do not use seedless or canned fruits.

Foods to Eat

Vegetable and fruit-rich diets have been linked to lower inflammation and oxidative stress and protect against various illnesses. In Dr. Sebi's nutrition guide, you'll find a list of items that are allowed on a diet, including:

- Apples, cantaloupe, dates, dates, figs, elderberries, berries, papayas, peaches, soft jelly coconuts, plums, pears, seeded key limes, seeded melons, mangoes, prickly pears, and tamarind.

- Avocado, bell peppers, chickpeas, cactus flower, cucumber, dandelion greens, lettuce, kale, olives, sea veggies, squash, tomatoes, mushrooms, okra, and zucchini.

- Some of the grains available are Fonio, amaranth, rye, Khorasan wheat (Kamut), wild rice, spelled, quinoa, and teff.

- Brazil nuts, raw sesame seeds, hemp seeds, raw tahini butter, walnuts are nuts and seeds that can be eaten.

- Avocado oil, grapeseed oil, uncooked coconut oil, sesame oil, hemp seed oil, and olive oil.

- Elderberry, chamomile, tila, fennel, burdock, ginger, achiote, raspberry herbal teas, cayenne, habanero, onion powder, tarragon, sage, pure sea salt, pure agave syrup, thyme, powdered, granulated seaweed, date sugar, oregano, cloves, basil, bay leaf, dill, cayenne, sweet basil, habanero, and tarragon.

- In addition, you can eat grains in the form of cereal, pasta, bread, or flour. However, food having yeast or baking powder is prohibited.

- You are permitted to consume water in addition to tea.

Dr. Sebi Ideology Fundamentals

The acid-alkaline diet, or alkaline ash diet, is another name for the alkaline diet. The food you consume can change your body's pH value, a metric of acidity or alkalinity. When food gets converted to energy, it is known as metabolism. Chemical processes in your body are gradual and regulated. Whenever things are burnt, they leave behind an ash deposit.

Similarly, the meals you eat leave a deposit known as metabolic waste, which is referred to as "ash." This metabolic waste might be alkaline, acidic, or neutral. Supporters of this diet argue that metabolic waste directly impacts your body's acidity. The alkaline diet is based on the concept that eating alkaline foods instead of acid-forming meals can enhance your health. Supporters of this diet even say that it can aid in treating major illnesses such as cancer.

Acidity

The pH of your body changes a lot. There is no defined degree of acidity or alkalinity; certain sections are acidic, while others are alkaline. Your stomach is full of hydrochloric acid, which gives it an extremely acidic pH of 2–3.5. This acidity is required for food digestion. Human blood is mildly alkaline with a pH of 7.36–7.44.

If left untreated, it can be deadly when your blood pH goes outside of the usual range. However, this only occurs in particular illness situations, such as diabetic ketoacidosis, malnutrition, or excessive alcohol use. The pH of your blood is closely controlled by your body. Diet has no effect on blood pH in healthy persons, but it can modify urine pH.

Mucus

Dr. Sebi felt that the illness was caused by mucus and acidity. He believed that consuming some foods and avoiding others may help the body cleanse, resulting in an alkaline condition that would minimize illness risk and symptoms. An alkaline diet will assist you in naturally detoxing your body, removing excess mucus, reducing inflammation, cleansing your liver and reversing diabetes.

Diseases

Osteoporosis is a bone disease that causes a reduction in bone mineral content over time. It's more frequent among postmenopausal women, and it raises your risk of fractures significantly.

Many supporters of the alkaline diet think that your body uses alkaline minerals, like calcium in your bones, to neutralize the acids from the acid-forming foods you eat to maintain a steady blood pH.

Acid-forming diets, such as the traditional Western diet, are thought to induce a decrease in bone mineral density. This idea, however, ignores the function of your kidneys, which are critical in the removal of acids.

Controlling blood pH is also a job for your respiratory system. When bicarbonate ions in your kidneys react to acids in your blood, water and carbon dioxide are produced, and you breathe out and urinate out.

Sugars and starches, also known as carbohydrates, can assist you in losing weight by curbing your hunger, lowering your insulin levels, and lowering your insulin levels.

Chapter 2: Sourcing Herbs

Wildcrafting

Wild crafting is a skill that entails gathering medicinal plants in the wild. Humans have already been wildcrafting ever since the beginning of time. Still, when medications are so readily available, the work and time necessary to harvest your own may be questioned in this day and age. I can promise you several advantages to gathering and producing medication from wild herbs. Using medicinal plants that thrive in our local areas is more environmentally friendly. Still, it also ensures that the herbs we collect are fresher and more effective. Local plants are also more likely to provide profound therapeutic benefits to our bodies, brains, and souls since they are formed of the same energies that give birth to our own spiritual and physical beings.

Legal issues and responsibilities

Wildcrafting appears to be in perfect harmony with nature at first look. What can be more resourceful, natural, and practical than foraging for your herbal plants there in the wild?

It's a little more complicated than that. You must ensure that you do not take more than what the habitat can maintain; in other terms, your harvest must be sustainable. You must also ensure you're following all applicable laws and respecting the property interests of governmental and private landowners.

- **Be extremely cautious**

This is a hybrid of the precautionary approach and the camping rule: first, do no damage, and then leave things in better condition than you got them. Wildcrafting is a significant responsibility; if done incorrectly, you risk damaging or destroying plants, as well as harming the local environment. You might potentially endanger yourself and others (by handling or swallowing dangerous plants, for example) and possibly break the law.

- **Know the plants**

First and foremost, ensure that you know any rare or endangered species of plants in your region and that you do not pick them. United Plant Savers, the well-known group, has an up-to-date watch list of endangered plant species across the United States plus Canada; even novice wildcrafters should be familiar with it.

- **Know the land**

To begin, you must ensure that the land is in good condition. Toxic chemicals and pesticides are frequently found around busy roadways and electricity lines. It's better to avoid the area if it was formerly an industrial location. If you're doing wildcrafting near a creek, make sure you know where it comes from.

- **Be aware of the rules.**

Trespassing on private land would be a no for anyone who isn't a wildcrafter or even a genius. Wild crafting is frequently outlawed or severely restricted on public lands.

- **Take a little**

It's crucial to come down on the way of caution while gathering plants within the wild since the health of a local ecosystem is almost always a top consideration. Take just as much as one can reasonably utilize but not more than 10% if you've concluded that harvesting is both sustainable and ethical.

Useful Tools

A few tools are required for wildcrafting. Everything you don't yet have may be purchased at a local hardware/garden store for a reasonable price. You'll probably create a set of preferred tools for the plants you harvest regularly over time.

- **Mesh Bags**

They're little and light, and they let the plants breathe on their way back. Mesh bags are frequently available at natural health stores and easily acquired online.

- **Baskets**

When harvesting with two hands, a basket comes in handy since it can merely be set on the ground or the plants dropped into the aperture.

- **Pruning Sheers**

Harvesting tiny branches necessitate the use of pruning shears. However, you could make a clean incision that a plant may readily heal from with this instrument.

- **Sickle or Scissors**

Scissors are required for collecting plant aerial parts. You may locate a rising quality scissors collection at a garden center that might be better than regular kitchen shears. Cleanly trimming aerial areas permits roots to remain in the ground & the plant's life to continue, allowing the plant to repair more quickly than ripping or torn portions.

- **Digging Stick**

A digging stick is typically more useful than a shovel that accidentally cuts roots.

- **Appropriate clothing**

Be mindful of the topography and likely weather conditions in the location where you'll be harvesting, and dress appropriately.

- **Medicine-Making Supplies**

Some individuals like to brew tinctures using herbs as clean as possible. If you're interested in doing so, you might wish to carry your medicine-making materials with you to the field.

- **Guide to the Field**

I usually bring my preferred field guide when I go out, specifically into the wilderness.

- **Record Sheet**

We'll have a check sheet and then a record-keeping worksheet later throughout this series. You might wish to bring them, as well as a pen and a clipboard.

- **Gloves**

Gloves aren't always required, but they're always a good idea to have on hand "just in case."

Harvesting

The gathering of the ripe rice crop from the field is known as harvesting. Reaping, stacking, handling, threshing, cleaning, and transportation are all part of paddy harvesting. These could be done one at a time, or a mutual harvester could be used to do all of them at once.

We optimize grain output while minimizing grain damage and quality deterioration; proper harvesting procedures must be used.

Harvesting process

- Cutting the straw and ripe panicles above ground are known as reaping.

- Threshing is separating paddy grain from the rest of the cut crop.

- Immature, unfilled, non-grain elements are removed during cleaning.

- Hauling is the process of transporting the cut crop into the threshing area.

- Field drying entails letting the cut crop just on the field dry out under the sun (optional).

- Stacking/piling entails storing the harvested produce in stacks or mounds for the time being (optional).

- Bagging is the process of placing threshed grain into bags for transportation and storage.

Field drying/stacking/piling are not suggested since they might result in quick quality degradation and significant harvest losses.

Aside from this, harvesting can entail a range of other actions like gathering, reaping (cutting standing grain), bundling, and different modes of conveying the grain and crop.

Growing and Propagation

Herbs are frequently the first plants that inexperienced gardeners try since they are so simple to grow. Herbs bring beauty to your environment, discourage unwelcome garden pests, and greatly enhance your meals and drinks, in addition to becoming simple to care for. Perhaps you're considering extending your herb garden now that you've established a few plants. It's not as complex as you would assume.

What Does Propagation Mean?

Propagation is the procedure of growing new plants from bulbs, cuttings, seeds, and other plant components. Herbs may be propagated in three ways: cuttings, seeds, and division. All three approaches may be used to start most plants. Stem cuttings are the easiest approach to acquiring extra plants for herbs.

When Should You Grow Herbs?

Taking a cutting from the plant during its primary growth season, which is normally between spring and autumn, is the optimal time to do it. Take cuttings from herbs that aren't blossoming right now.

You'll need to pluck a few flowers off the stalk if there are any.

How to Cut and Where to Cut

There'll be a "softwood" segment and a "hardwood" portion on each given stem. Softwood has a lighter hue and a more flexible stem. That's the new development. Old-growth is more difficult to dig out than new growth.

Taking your cuttings first thing in the morning would put a lesser strain on the herbs. To avoid disease transmission, use rubbing alcohol to disinfect your cutting equipment before and after every cut. Cut a node. Cut a 4-6 inch piece of wood. Pinch off the lowest 2 inches of the cutting's leaves. The new roots will sprout from this area.

Eliminate the Cuttings

You may either root the cuttings into a cup of water or otherwise plant them inside a growth medium after they've been prepared. You'll need to cover your cuttings using plastic for both techniques to keep them wet.

Inside a Water Glass:

Fill a glass with enough water to cover the stems and put the cuttings in it. There should be no leaves in the water. Place your jar of cuttings in a light spot and cover it using the plastic zip bag. In 3-4 weeks, the cuttings should have enough roots to be useful. You may now put them in a pot.

In the Growth Medium:

Your cuttings can also be planted straight in pots with growth material. Use a soilless growth medium (the same sort you'd use for seed beginning). Dip the stems with rooting hormone before one-pot them up to pace up their rooting process. Water the cuttings, then cover them in one plastic zip bag once they've been potted. In 3 to 4 weeks, the cuttings would root.

Following-up

The cuttings must be kept moist but not soggy. Take the plastic cover & flip it inside out every couple of days to remove the dampness. When the soil seems dry, or even the water level inside the glass jar reaches below the stems, water them. Keep the young cuttings away from direct sunshine and heat. The plastic functions like a mini-greenhouse now for the herbs, which you don't want to get too warm since they'll cook. You may transplant the herbs to your garden and perhaps a larger container once they have rooted.

Collecting Herbs

Pick healthy flowers, leaves, or seeds for drying. Clip the stems carefully using scissors. Any sick, moldy, or insect-damaged pieces should be discarded.

Collecting techniques

- **Leafy Annual Herbs**

Pinch off leaves from the tops of the stems immediately above a set of leaves to collect leafy annual herbs, including basil and marjoram. The plant will continue to develop and produce two branches just above leaves. This is also known as "pinching off," It stimulates the plant to grow more bushy and sensitive leaves. To keep your plant productive, harvest green tips often and trim off flower buds. Before the first frost, harvest an entire plant.

- **Leafy Perennial Herbs**

Thyme, tarragon, and sage are perennial herbs that a stem or sprig can collect. Cut the stems 3 to 4 inches out from the plant's base to harvest the herb. Cut the stem at the plant's base to harvest herbs having long stems as oregano and parsley. Cut the stems above a set of leaves to harvest rosemary, which would branch out & continue to grow. Harvest perennial herbs till the first frost, typically four weeks before the first frost. Let the plant concentrate on winding down over the season before falling dormant as winter approaches.

- **Blossoms**

Some herbs have solitary flowers, while others have clusters or spikes of flowers along the stem. Single flowers like chamomile, feverfew and calendula are gathered by selecting individual flowers after they have fully opened. Cut the stem a few inches out from the base of your plant or above its top set of leaves to harvest spiky flowers when several of the petals are open.

- **Seeds**

Anise, coriander, dill and caraway, for example, are typically dried on the plant after being collected for their seeds. Let the herb blossom and seed on its own. Seeds grow from green to brown or black while they dry after blooming. When the seeds are dry, they are ready to harvest. When a seed head is tapped, the seeds usually flow out. Hold a container beneath the seed head, then snip the stem so that the seed cluster and any seeds released fall through into the container.

Storing Herbs

Herbs should be dried after harvesting to retain their essential oils and maximize flavor intensity and therapeutic benefits. There are a few different ways to really dry herbs for storage:

- **Herbs to Hang & Air Dry:** The simplest way to dry herbs containing stems is to air-dry them. Tie the stems into little bundles, then hang them upside down from direct sunlight in a dry, warm, dust-free, and airy location.

- **Using the Drying Screen to Air Dry Herbs:** Alternatively, you may air-dry the herbs by spreading them over on the window or drying screen. Allow air to travel above and below across the drying screen by suspending it over two chairs.

- **Use the Food Dehydrator:** When dry herbs faster, use the food dehydrator. A dehydrator operates by passing air through screens inside a moderate flow.

How to Store your Dry Herbs

Remove the leaves out from stems, then store loosely inside clean glass jars/containers having airtight lids after the herbs are dried and brittle. Crush and crumble the herbs immediately before using them to preserve their taste and strength. Label your jars with the herb's name and the date.

Keep your jars away from humidity, heat, and temperature changes in a cold, dark spot. Dry herbs should not be kept in the kitchen cupboard, trust it or not. Most herbs are kept in huge jars in a cold, dark cupboard rarely used. Instead, fill little herb jars with roughly a month's supply of herbs for your kitchen cupboard. When kept correctly, dried herbs will last a minimum of six to twelve months.

Please remember that dried herbs have a higher strength concentration than fresh herbs. Therefore, when a recipe asks for fresh herbs, use roughly one-third of dried herbs instead.

Chapter 3: Alkaline Herb List

IRISH SEA MOSS

Description

Irish moss-Chondrus Crispus is a kind of algae/ seaweed, not being Moss, despite its name. The red, branching seaweed may be found along the Atlantic Ocean's coasts in Great Britain, Europe, and North America. Irish moss is used in various sectors, but the food industry is one of the most popular.

Carrageenan, a jelly-like material found in Irish moss, gives wide applications. Carrageenan may be used in anything from ice cream to just infant formula since it can be utilized as a vegan replacement for gelatin and also a general emulsifier.

Benefits

- Iodine is a vital nutrient for the thyroid and is high in it. Iodine aids thyroid hormone production, regulating metabolism, nerves, and bone development.

- Irish moss, in particular, has been one of the finest plant sources for omega-3s. These fats are necessary for heart health. Getting adequate omega-3 has been linked to a decreased risk of developing high cholesterol, heart disease, blood pressure and blood clots.

- Fucoxanthin, a chemical found in Irish moss, may be beneficial. This carotenoid is responsible for the deep red-brown color of Irish moss.

- Fucoxanthin has been proven to help control blood sugar levels within studies. It appears to aid the body's response to insulin, implying that your body can better manage its very own blood sugar levels with less effort.

- Consumption of Irish moss by diabetics may assist in avoiding blood sugar rises and crashes.

- Irish moss contains antioxidants such as fucoxanthin and other carotenoids, which help combat free radicals. Free radicals that aren't regulated can harm cells, leading them to increase in harmful ways – damaged cells eventually turn cancerous. You might well be able to lower your chance of acquiring certain cancers by consuming Irish moss.

Dosage and Preparation

- Once the sea moss has been soaked, take it from the liquid, then place it on a cleaned, dry plate. The water, which now includes lots of nutrients from sea moss, should not be discarded since it will be needed to yield the gel. (If your water has a lot of debris or is murky, dump it and create your fresh sea moss gel with fresh spring/alkaline water.)

- Combine the sea moss and the water inside your high-powered blender. Start with one cup of water, plus add more as needed to achieve the desired consistency for your gel.

- Blend for 1-3 minutes, or till smooth. Refrigerate the Sea Moss inside an airtight container like a Mason jar. After 2 hours in the fridge, our sea moss gel would thicken.

- 4 - 8 grams of soaking sea moss can be added directly to a smoothie.

- Alternatively, 1-2 tablespoons of your sea moss gel can be added.

- A daily dose of 1-2 tablespoons (4 -8 grams) containing sea moss gel is advised.

Possible side effects/ drugs interaction

Carrageenan can adhere to medicines within the stomach and intestines. When you take carrageenan with oral medicines, your body absorbs less of the medication, which reduces its efficacy.

Poligeenan can cause intestinal inflammation, making it difficult to absorb nutrients. This might cause bloating and discomfort over time. It's also been related to colitis and Crohn's disease symptoms.

CASCARA SAGRADA

Description

Cascara sagrada seems to be a plant that grows in the form of a shrub. Medicine is made from dried bark. The shrub Cascara sagrada is native to western North America, and its bark is used for medicinal purposes. Anthraquinones, which are found in Cascara sagrada, are strong laxatives.

The U.S. Food & Drug Administration (FDA) approved cascara sagrada and over-the-counter (OTC) drugs for constipation. However, doubts concerning cascara sagrada's efficacy and safety have been raised throughout time. Therefore, the FDA allowed manufacturers to submit efficacy and safety data to address these concerns. However, the companies determined that the expense of conducting safety and efficacy studies would certainly outweigh the profit from cascara sagrada sales. As a result, they failed to cooperate with the request.

Consequently, the FDA warned manufacturers that such OTC laxative products comprising cascara sagrada must be removed or reformulated from the U.S. market on November 5, 2002. Cascara sagrada is now available as just a "dietary supplement" and not as a drug. The FDA does not require "dietary supplements" to satisfy the same requirements as OTC or prescription medications.

Benefits

- Cascara sagrada is widely used as a laxative through the mouth to relieve constipation. It acts by inducing intestinal muscular contractions. These muscular contractions aid in the passage of feces through the bowels. Anthraquinones are compounds found in the bark that give it a certain color and laxative properties.

- Cascara sagrada extract is sometimes employed as a flavoring ingredient in beverages and foods since it is bitter.

- Some sunscreens contain cascara sagrada, which is utilized in their manufacturing process.

Dosage and Preparaion

- If you're going to utilize the shrub's bark, make sure it's been aged for at minimum a year.

- Boil one teaspoon of well-dried bark into three cups of water for 30 minutes to prepare your tea.

- Take one-two cup of tea at ambient temperature each day before bedtime.

Possible side effects/ drugs interaction

When taken orally, Cascara sagrada is Potentially SAFE for most people when used for less than a week. Stomach pain and cramps are common side effects.

Cascara sagrada seems to be POSSIBLY UNSAFE when consumed for more than a week. Dehydration, low potassium levels, sodium, chloride, and other "electrolytes" within the blood, heart difficulties, muscular weakness, and other significant adverse effects are possible.

If you have stomach discomfort, nausea, or vomiting, you shouldn't use it as you should with any laxative. If you have chronic intestinal problems like ulcerative colitis, Crohn's disease, irritable bowel syndrome and sprue, avoid using cascara.

Cascara sagrada should not be used by pregnant or nursing women.

RHUBARB ROOT

Description

Rhubarb, also known as sweet round-leaved pieplant or dock, is sometimes mistaken for a fruit. Yet, it is among the several perennial vegetables. Rheum rhaponticum is the scientific name for ordinary garden rhubarb. However, other members of such a plant group are also utilized for therapeutic purposes. Rheum palmatum is the scientific name for Chinese rhubarb, known as da Huang within traditional Chinese medicine. The flavor and characteristics of Chinese rhubarb are far superior to those of the typical American type. Rhubarb belongs to the Polygonaceae family, which includes buckwheat. It originated in Mongolia, within northern Asia, and was brought to India and Turkey many years ago. It was previously known as Turkey or India rhubarb.

Benefits

- Stomach bleeding may be helped by taking this herb.

- Rhubarb powder or extract is taken orally appears to assist with gastrointestinal bleeding.

- Sores caused by the cold. Applying rhubarb and sage over herpes cold sores appears to help them recover faster. It may be just as beneficial as acyclovir cream.

- Kidney failure is a serious condition. According to most studies, rhubarb extract enhances kidney function in renal failure patients, both with and without captopril.

- Gum disease is one condition that affects the teeth and gums. Early study shows that rhubarb extract rinses can aid in treating gum disease.

- Having high blood bp during pregnancy is a common occurrence. Early study suggests that commencing 28 weeks into the pregnancy till delivery, consuming rhubarb extract can lower the likelihood of high blood bp throughout pregnancy.

- Early study shows that eating a mixture of ten herbs, including rhubarb, daily for three months can help patients with glomerulonephritis improve their kidney function.

- Using a Chinese herbal medicine called Danning Pian, which contains giant knotweed, rhubarb, old dried orange peel and green orange peel, may help patients suffering from non-fatty hepatic disease improve their liver function.

Dosage and Preparation

- A tea or decoction can be made by combining 1.5–1 teaspoon (2.5–5 cc) of crushed rhubarb root with 1 cup of water. The mixture is boiled and simmered for 10 minutes over low heat.

- Rhubarb tea could be consumed two times per day. The tincture will be taken three times per day at a dose of about 1–2 ml.

Possible side effects/ drugs interaction

Uterine contractions, intestinal discomfort, severe stomach cramps and watery diarrhea. Muscle weakness, potassium loss, bone loss and irregular heart rhythm are frequent adverse effects of rhubarb root usage over time. This issue is frequently solved by decreasing the dosage.

Rhubarb root must not be used with diuretics, cardiac medicines, other cathartics or laxatives, or steroids due to the risk of potassium loss. When rhubarb root and licorice root are combined, potassium loss from the system is reduced.

PRODIGIOSA

Description of the herb

The dark green leaves of this bushy perennial have a grayish-purple color underside. Its leaves are big, serrated, and drooping, with unique cream, white, yellow, and green flowers that resemble tassels that bloom all year. Its other names include Brickellia arguta, Athanasia Amarga, Brickellia cavanillesii. It grows between one foot and three feet tall throughout Southwestern North America, covering Mexico and New Mexico.

The lovely herb is simple to grow and thrives inside a container garden.

Benefits

- It aids in dealing with the Diabetes issue.

- It is found to be effective against diarrhea.

- It aids in relieving stomach pain.

- It aids in fighting against Gallbladder disease and other conditions.

- It reduces your blood sugar level.

Dosage and Preparation

- The ratio for making a tincture or some herbal bitter is 1:5. (plant matter to the liquid solvent like apple cider vinegar/alcohol).

- Prodigiosa tea is made by combining one teaspoon of your herb with eight ounces of boiling water. Wait 10 minutes for the tea to steep.

- Take the tea two times per day.

Possible side effects/ drugs interaction

- Brickellia usage during pregnancy and breastfeeding: Little is known regarding the usage of Brickellia through pregnancy and breastfeeding. Avoid using to be in a safe place.

- Diabetes: Animal studies show that some compounds in Brickellia may be able to decrease blood sugar levels. Brickellia risks interfering with blood sugar regulation and lowering blood sugar far too much. If you have diabetes and take Brickellia, keep a close eye on your blood sugar levels.

- Brickellia may help to decrease blood sugar levels after surgery. It has been suggested that it may affect blood sugar management after and during surgery. Brickellia should be avoided for at least two weeks before a scheduled surgery.

BURDOCK ROOT

Description of the herb

Burdock root is another vegetable that originated in Northern Europe and Asia but has now spread to the United States. The deep roots of your burdock herb are quite lengthy and range in color from beige to brown to practically black on the outer. Burdock has purple flowers during the spring and fall and has big heart-shaped leaves.

Burdock root has been utilized in holistic medicine for centuries to treat various ailments.

Traditional medicine believes that it has been the dark roots of the plant, not the plant itself, which provide health advantages. Burdock includes oils, tannins, plus plant sterols, among other things. Doctors are unsure whether which of the plant's constituents are beneficial to one's health. The reason is that most studies focus on the burdock root overall as a whole rather than a single component.

Benefits

- Burdock root has been proven to prevent critically high blood glucose levels in a petri dish and a live tissue specimen during a 2014 study. Researchers discovered no advantages linked to raw burdock root during a 2015 trial of mice. However, in mice, fermented burdock root decreased blood sugar levels substantially.

- Traditional healers have used burdock root for generations to treat common sore throats, colds and other illnesses. Burdock may be able to combat infections, according to scientific studies. It possesses antibacterial properties, according to certain research. It seems to be very effective in destroying biofilms, which are huge, sticky bacterium colonies. A biofilm is something like the oral plaque which causes cavities. Biofilms may be found throughout the body. Burdock root was effective in treating biofilm-related UTI in a 2015 research. Burdock may also destroy other germs, according to one research published during 2017.

- Even though there is no scientific evidence in the West to support the necessity for detox, it has long been a part of traditional Chinese medicine. Burdock may cleanse the blood, according to traditional medicine practitioners. Alternative health professionals frequently talk about detoxifying the body and purifying the blood.

- Burdock roots potentially have diuretic properties. Diuretics aid in removing the excess water from the body, providing relief to those who are retaining water.

- Antioxidants aid in the battle against free radical damage. Free radicals are substances in the body that cause cell damage and are linked to various diseases such as aging, cancer, and inflammatory illnesses. Antioxidants are thought to delay the aging process because they accumulate as people age. Burdock root has been proven to be an antioxidant in several studies. Burdock may alleviate diabetic symptoms, according to the 2014 research in rats, due to its antioxidant qualities.

- Chronic inflammation can be caused by free radical damage, auto-immune disorders, and other medical problems. Many medical disorders, including osteoarthritis, are connected to inflammation. Burdock root dramatically reduced measures of inflammation among patients with knee osteoarthritis, according to the 2k14 study Trusted Source.

- Both free radicals plus inflammation have been related to cancer growth. Burdock's antioxidant and anti-inflammatory properties may thus aid in cancer prevention. According to a preliminary study, burdock may also help delay cancer progression. In addition, burdock was proven to decrease the development of breast cancer tumors during 2016 research.

Dosage and Preparation

- To prepare burdock root tea, start purchasing 8- 10 fresh burdock roots. Cut them in 1-2 inch slices to begin. Shred the root pieces into thin strips that might resemble bark peelings. Place it outside to dry for several hours in the sun.

- Put them inside a frying pan after they are dry and heat up without using any oil. Heat them for about 5-10 minutes, they should readily roast, and the color should be a deep golden brown. They may be brewed for making burdock root tea once they've cooled. Keep the leftovers inside a mason jar in a cold, dark, and dry location for later use.

- Inside a teapot, put your burdock root strips into two cups of water and boil.

- Allow a 5- to 10-minute steeping period.

- After that, shift the tea into a cup, and put one teaspoon of honey as a sweetener.

- One teaspoon of burdock root into seven ounces of water should be taken daily.

Possible side effects/ drugs interaction

Burdock can induce allergic responses as well as other adverse side effects. Therefore, the following people should avoid burdock root:

- The women who already are pregnant, expecting to get pregnant, or those who are nursing.

- The children under the age of 18 years.

- The individuals who have a history of plant allergies, unless a doctor advises otherwise.

- Individuals using diuretics, diabetic medications, or blood thinners.

- Before taking burdock root, anyone with persistent or life-threatening medical issues should see their doctor.

DANDELION

Description of the herb

Dandelion, often called 'yellow gowan' /'lion's tooth,' is a flowering plant. This plant originated in Eurasia and is still found there today. It's found in over 60 nations worldwide, mostly within the northern hemisphere's moderate temperatures. The above flowering plants have been used for centuries to relieve inflammation-related pains, treat pancreas swelling (inflammation), treat & prevent skin disorders, cancer, bladder/ urethra disorders, tonsils (tonsillitis), digestive and digestive liver problems, and improve the overall digestive system & liver health. Due to the chemical compositions plus nutrients, researchers have proven it's a very powerful cleansing/detoxification herb.

Benefits

- It aids in the detoxification and cleansing of the liver and kidneys.

- It aids in the treatment and prevention of diabetes by controlling blood sugar levels. It aids in the fight against and relief of inflammation-related aches.

- Its antioxidant qualities aid in deactivating and limiting the damaging impacts of free radicals within the body.

- It helps to lower cholesterol levels.

- It reduces blood pressure by removing extra fluid from the body.

- It aids in the natural loss of extra weight by boosting glucose metabolism.

- It aids in the improvement of the digestive system.

- It aids in the immune system's improvement.

- It aids in maintaining healthy skin and the treatment and prevention of skin problems.

Dosage and Preparation

- Take some fresh dandelion leaves and wash them under running water to remove any dirt.

- Put 1/2 - 1 glass of cleaned dandelion into your pan once it has been washed.

- Boil 4-5 cups water, then pour it into the saucepan with the dandelion, covering it for about 12-15 hours and otherwise overnight.

- After straining out your dandelion leaves the next day, you'll get dandelion tea/infusion.

- Take 1/2 tablespoon Dandelion for each 3/4 glass of water three times every day. If you bought the dandelion online, you might consume 4-10 grams of dried dandelion leaf three times a day.

Possible side effects/ drugs interaction

Dandelion is completely safe as of the period of writing the book, however taking too much of it might cause certain unpleasant side effects, such as:

- Gastrointestinal discomfort or irritation

- Allergic responses

The following specific precautions are needed to be taken before using or ingesting dandelions:

- Pregnant and nursing mothers should avoid dandelion since no study has been done to determine whether it is dangerous for them or not.

- If you have Eczema, avoid dandelion since it causes an allergic reaction in more than 85 percent of persons with Eczema.

ELDERBERRY

Description of the herb

The Sambucus tree, a flowering plant within the Adoxaceae family, is known by various other names, including elderberry. Sambucus nigra, often called European elderberry and black elder is the most prevalent kind. The plant is native to Europe, although it is also commonly grown in other regions of the globe. Elderflowers are clusters of little cream or white-colored flowers that grow up to 30 feet tall on S. nigra. Tiny black or sometimes blue-black clusters of berries might be found. The berries are rather sour and must be cooked before being consumed. Raw or cooked, the flowers have one subtle muscat scent and could be eaten either raw or cooked.

Benefits

- Aids in the battle against cancer. Both American and European elders were revealed to have cancer-fighting qualities in test-tube experiments.

- Inhibits the growth of dangerous bacteria. Elderberry has been shown to stop bacteria such as Helicobacter pylori & may help with bronchitis symptoms and sinusitis.

- It may help your immune system. For example, elderberry polyphenols were discovered to boost immunological protection in rats by raising the amount of Wbcs.

- U.V. protection may be possible. The sun protection factor of your skin product, including elderberry extract, was determined to be 9.88.

Dosage and Preparation

- Mix 2 tbsp of your dried elderberries and 2 cups of water inside a kettle. The berries will begin to release their color almost immediately.

- Over high heat, bring the kettle to a boil. Lower the heat and let the tea simmer about 15 minutes after boiling.

- When the tea has completed simmering, remove it from the heat and set it aside for 5 minutes to cool.

- Pour the tea into a glass using one fine-mesh strainer and drink!

- 1-4 cups per day are recommended.

Possible side effects/ drugs interaction

Although there are contrasting views on whether elderberry is beneficial, most doctors feel it is safe to use in modest doses. However, the plant's unripe or raw berries or flowers can cause vomiting, nausea, and diarrhea. Larger doses might result in much more severe toxicity.

- Other considerations include not taking one if you're pregnant or nursing.

- The elder tree's other components are poisonous, such as the twigs, branches, roots, leaves, and seeds. A glycoside is a form of cyanide that they have.

- Elderberry may cause allergic responses in those with weakened immune systems.

- You can be allergic to that if you acquire a rash or even have difficulties breathing after eating it.

GUACO

Description of the herb

Guaco, bejuco, vejuco, and huaco, are words used to describe a variety of vine-like South American, Central American, and West Indian climbing plants that are said to have medicinal properties. The genus Mikania has many species that are known as guaco. Guaco can be utilized to refer to a Rocky Mountain bee plant, Cleome serrulata, even though it is not any real vine.

The guaco was called after a kind of kite, according to Colombians and Native Americans, in a copy of its cry that they think it employs to lure the snakes it eats.

Benefits

- This unusual vine has several advantages, including curing snake bites. In addition, Palo guaco can aid in the treatment of the following ailments:

- Bronchitis, Flu, Common Cold, Scabs, Asthma Allergies, Ulcers, Athlete's Foot, Liver Issues, Constipation, Tumours, Malaria, Infection, Diarrhea, Stomach Pain Chest Pain.

- It also aids in reducing fevers, works as a blood purifier, and aids in the healing of wounds. Anti-inflammatory, anti-fungal, antibacterial, plus pain-relieving activities are also present. Palo guaco is a classic tropical vine with many potential health advantages. It's worth adding to our natural remedies arsenal.

Dosage and Preparation

- The bark of the Palo Guaco is historically used to make tea.

- Put 1-2 teaspoons Palo Guaco Bark into 8 ounces boiling water to make your tea. Steep about 5-10 minutes, covered. After that, strain and enjoy.

- Take 4.0z of guaco per day.

Possible side effects/ drugs interaction

Pregnant and lactating women, children under 18, and those with known medical issues should get medical advice before using this product.

MULLEIN

Description of the herb

Mullein is another plant that is used in the production of medicine. Some individuals take Mullein by mouth to treat coughs, asthma, pneumonia, colds, and sore throats. However, there is a scarcity of scientific evidence to back up these and other claims.

Mullein is utilized as a flavoring component in alcoholic beverages during production.

Benefits

- There is insufficient information to rate effectiveness (otitis media). However, an early study suggests that using a specific product into the ear for three days lowers ear discomfort in children and teens having ear infections. Such product includes, Mullein, St. John's wort and calendula.

- Creams can also be made from dried and natural forms (leaf or flower).

- Mullein is recommended by certain naturopathic physicians and herbalists for respiratory & inflammatory problems. Still, there isn't enough scientific information to back it up.

- It also aids in dealing with wounds, colds, flu, diarrhea, asthma, gout, migraines, tuberculosis, cough, Croup, hemorrhoids, inflammation of airways, sore throat.

Dosage and Preparation

- Mullein tea can be made using dried loose leaves or manufactured mullein tea bags. For example, 1–2 teaspoons dried mullein flowers or leaves in one cup of water.

- Allow it to steep for about 10-15 minutes just before consuming. The tea can be consumed three-four times each day.

Possible side effects/ drugs interaction

- Mullein is potentially safe when administered to the ear for a short period. For up to three days, a special preparation including Mullein, St. John's wort and calendula was utilized in the ear.

- Pregnancy/breastfeeding: There's not enough credible information on the safety of mullein consumption while pregnant and lactating women. Avoid using to be in a safe place.

Chamomile

Description of the herb

Chamomile is a herb used to treat various ailments since ancient Egypt. Chamomile is an Old World native with highly fragrant leaves and flowers with white petals plus golden centers. It belongs to the daisy family. Chamomile herb comes from the Asteraceae plant family's daisy-like flowers. It's been used as a natural cure for various ailments for millennia. Chamomile tea is popular as a caffeine-free substitute to green or black or green tea, and it's an earthy, mildly sweet flavor.

Furthermore, chamomile tea contains antioxidants, which may help reduce the risk of various ailments, namely heart disease.

Benefits

- Chamomile contains certain special qualities that may help you sleep better.

- The importance of proper digestion to your overall health cannot be overstated. According to limited data, chamomile may help promote improved digestion by lowering the risk of some gastrointestinal diseases.

- Chamomile tea contains antioxidants that have been linked to a decreased risk of some cancers.

- Chamomile tea has been shown to help reduce blood sugar levels.

- The anti-inflammatory characteristics may protect the cells of the pancreas from damage caused by chronically high blood sugar levels.

- Flavones, a kind of antioxidant found in chamomile tea, are plentiful.

- Flavones have been researched for their ability to decrease blood pressure plus cholesterol levels, both of which are crucial indicators of the risk of heart disease.

Dosage and Preparation

- Boil 200 ml of water.

- Put 3 tablespoons of dried chamomile flowers inside your teabag/ infuser.

- Put tea bag inside a cup and pour over hot water.

- Let it steep for around 5 minutes.

- Take out the infuser and enjoy the tea with any sweetener of your choice.

- Take the tea twice daily.

Possible side effects/ drugs interaction

- There have been cases of chamomile allergies that are most likely to arise insensitive to daisy plants like chrysanthemums and ragweed.

- Furthermore, chamomile-containing cosmetics may irritate the eyes whenever they come in direct contact with them. This can cause conjunctivitis, an inflammation of the eye's lining.

- It's also worth observing that the efficacy of taking chamomile tea in young children, nursing women or pregnant, or persons with liver or renal illness has yet to be determined.

RED CLOVER

Description of the herb

The dark-pink herbaceous red clover is native to Asia, Europe, and North Africa. Furthermore, it is currently widely used as the fodder crop in South America to enhance soil quality. Red clover's flowering section is used as a beautiful garnish or extract. At the same time, it may also be extracted from essential oils. Red clover seems to be a short-lived perennial or cool-season biennial with a variety of ascending stems or leafy erect that grow 4 - 8 inches long from the woody crown of the root. The stems and leaves are pubescent. The stems and branches of plants are hollow and hairy.

Benefits

- Osteoporosis is a disorder where the bones have lost their strength and poor bone mineral density. When a woman enters menopause, her reproductive hormones, particularly estrogen, diminish, resulting in accelerated bone turnover and BMD reduction. Isoflavones, a kind of phytoestrogen that can partially imitate estrogen within the body, can be found in red clover. In several studies, isoflavone consumption has been linked to a lower risk of osteoporosis.

- The high isoflavone content of red clover is said to help alleviate menopausal symptoms, including night sweats and hot flashes. Other menopausal symptoms, including sadness, anxiety, and vaginal dryness, were mildly improved by red clover.

- Traditional medicine has employed red clover extract to boost hair health and skin.

- According to early studies, red clover may help postmenopausal women's heart health.

- Many people believe that red clover can aid with cancer, weight reduction, whooping cough, arthritis, asthma, and other ailments.

Dosage and Preparation

- Put 4 grams of the dried flower tips (or even red clover bags of tea) to one (250 mL) cup with boiling water, then steep around 5–10 minutes to produce red clover tea.

- It's advised to restrict your daily intake between (240–720 mL) 1–3 cups due to reports of negative effects from (1.2 liters) 5 cups each day.

Possible side effects/ drugs interaction

- Due to the estrogenic activity, people having hormone-sensitive conditions like ovarian cancer, endometriosis, or breast cancer should consult their medicare provider before considering taking red clover.

- Furthermore, there is little information on the safety of red clover in young pregnant mothers or breastfeeding. As a result, it must be avoided.

- Finally, red clover might impede blood coagulation, so it's best to avoid it if you have a bleeding issue.

BLUE VERVAIN

Description of the herb

Vervain is a perennial plant native to Asia and Europe called Verbena officinalis and verbena, an herb of the same cross.

The plant has serrated lobed leaves and pale-purple silky flowers, and it belongs to a Verbenaceae family. Because of the numerous medicinal chemicals, it is utilized as a herbal treatment worldwide. Vervain refers to the kinds of verbena used for medicinal purposes in the hundreds.

Benefits

- Vervain's glycosides, essential oils, and triterpenoids have been shown in test tubes and animal studies to help prevent tumor development and promote cancer cell death.

- Certain brain-related and neurological conditions may benefit from vervain extract.

- According to the study, the substance encourages the formation of new blood arteries within the brain, which provide it with oxygen and enhance its mitochondrial function.

- Vervain, however, has long been employed in traditional medicine as a nerve tonic or relaxant, and animal studies now support this claim.

- Antibiotic resistance is becoming a major worldwide issue. However, according to research, vervain appears to defend itself from antibiotic-resistant fungus and bacteria.

Dosage and Preparation

- Have some sifted and sliced blue vervain, irradiated.

- Make your tea by adding 1 teaspoon of blue vervain inside one cup of boiled water.

- Steep around for 10 minutes.

- Best results can be obtained by drinking 1-2 cups on a routine basis.

Possible side effects/ drugs interaction

- Vervain extract during pregnancy may result in poor weight gain and fetal malformations such as decreased bone ossification (hardening). As a result, all vervain-containing substances should be avoided by pregnant women.

- Furthermore, it is uncertain if the plant's components pass into breast milk. Therefore, to guarantee the safety of mothers and their kids, nursing moms should err on the way to caution and resist ingesting the plant.

- Furthermore, a prior study suggests that consuming vervain tea alongside meals can prevent 59 percent of iron absorption. Therefore, people suffering from anemia/iron deficiency must avoid the plant.

BLADDERWRACK

Description of the herb

Bladderwrack (Fucus vesiculosus) seems like a brown seaweed with a long history of use in traditional medicine. Rockweed, dyers fucus, red fucus, black tang, rock wrack, and bladder fucus are other names.

Bladderwrack grows about (90 cm) 35 inches tall over the Pacific and Atlantic Ocean coasts, the Baltic and North Seas, and other waterways within U.S. and Canada.

Many individuals feel that bladderwrack's outstanding nutritional profile can give health advantages, despite others maintaining that the claims go ahead regardless of the evidence.

Benefits

- Despite numerous health claims, there is little proof that bladderwrack can help with weight reduction, arthritis, joint discomfort, urinary tract infections, and fertility.

- Bladderwrack is abundant in iodine, a trace nutrient that helps maintain thyroid function by creating thyroid hormones such as thyroxine (T4) and triiodothyronine (T3). These hormones aid in metabolic regulation, proper growth, and neurological development.

- Antioxidants like fucoxanthin, phlorotannins, fucoidans, alginic acid, and vitamins C and A are abundant in bladderwrack.

- Cellulite, burns and skin aging have all been treated using bladderwrack like a topical therapy.

Dosage and Preparation

- Put one tea bag in (236 mL) 8 ounces of boiling water for 4–5 minutes to get bladderwrack tea. Alternatively, (5 mL) 1 teaspoon dried bladderwrack can be added to boiling water then simmered for almost 10–15 minutes.

- To prevent taking too much iodine and other active elements in bladderwrack, restrict your intake to not more than (500ml) 2 cups a day until additional safety studies are available.

Possible side effects/ drugs interaction

- It is most likely safe to apply bladderwrack into the skin. However, avoid using it on cuts and open wounds. Also, stop using it if you have any negative responses, including a skin rash.

- Like some other edible seaweeds, Bladderwrack is fine to consume modestly. It does, however, contain significant quantities of salt, iodine, and heavy metals, all of which can be harmful to one's health, especially when taken as a supplement.

- Bladderwrack may be harmful to pregnant or breastfeeding women and individuals with thyroid issues. Avoid consuming bladderwrack supplements till further information is available, and ask your healthcare practitioner before consuming or drinking them.

PAU PEREIRA

Description of the herb

Pao Pereira belongs to the species of tree. Medicine is made from the bark. An apocynaceous Brazilian tree, located within states of the Minas Gerais, Rio de Janeiro, Bahia, and Espirito Santo, is extensively employed as an embellishment of squares & public spaces for its beauty, broad and beautiful canopy, and flowers that bloom in the winter months of June and May. Hence, Pau-Pereira is a popular nickname for this species. Moreover, the bohemians of that period thought consuming the drink near the tree's wood would increase their sexual appetite since it contained vital ingredients.

Benefits

- It aids in relieving Cancer, Fever, Constipation, Malaria, Liver disease, Stomach problems, Sexual arousal.

- Pao Pereira may be able to stop cancer from spreading. It may also aid in the eradication of the parasite which causes malaria.

Dosage and Preparation

- Add ¼ cup of water to 2 tbsp of Pau Pereira.

- Allow it to simmer for almost 10 minutes after it begins to boil.

- Turn off the heat and then set aside for 10 minutes, covered.

- It has been strained and is ready to use.

- Take 2–3 cups per day.

Possible side effects/ drugs interaction

Little is known regarding the usage of Pao Pereira throughout pregnancy and lactation. Therefore, to be in the safe zone, avoid using it.

PAU D'ARCO

Description of the herb

Pau d'arco is a nutritional supplement derived from the inner bark of Tabebuia trees native to South and Central America. Its name alludes to the supplement and the trees it is made. The name "pau d'arco" means "bow tree" in Portuguese, which is an apt description given the tree's usage by South American indigenous peoples for creating hunting bows. Medicine is made from barks and wood. It may reach a height of 125 feet and contains pink-purple flowers that bloom before fresh leaves emerge.

Pau d'arco, also referred to as taheebo/ lapacho, has traditionally been used to cure various illnesses. In addition, it's touted as a weight-loss supplement that claims to alleviate inflammation.

Benefits

- Pau d'arco extract contains antibacterial and anti-fungal effects, according to research.

- Inflammation, your body's biological response to damage, is thought to be inhibited by Pau d'arco extract.

- While modest amounts of inflammation are good for you, chronic inflammation is linked to disorders including cancer, heart disease and obesity.

- Pau d'arco may help you lose weight.

Dosage and Preparation

- Put Two-three tsp (10–15 gms) of bark boiled in water for at least 15 minutes and drink it up to three times a day as tea.

Possible side effects/ drugs interaction

- When consumed by mouth, Pau d'arco seems POSSIBLY UNSAFE. Pau d'arco may induce severe nausea, vomiting, diarrhea, disorientation, and internal bleeding when taken in large dosages. In usual dosages, the efficacy of pau d'arco is unknown.

- Pau d'arco is considered UNSAFE when taken orally in normal levels during pregnancy and Probable UNSAFE when taken in greater dosages. The safety of putting it all to the skin is not well understood. If you're pregnant, stay safe and avoid using it.

SARSAPARILLA

Description of the herb

Sarsaparilla seems to be a tropical plant belonging to the Smilax genus. The climbing, woody vine could be found deep within the rainforest canopy. South America, Jamaica, the Caribbean, Mexico, Honduras, and the West Indies are all home to this species.

Sarsaparilla was later imported to European medicine and then listed as a syphilis treatment herb within United States Pharmacopoeia.

Sarsaparilla was also the name of a famous soft drink during the early 1800s. Its drink was popular in taverns and was utilized as a home cure.

Benefits

- Saponins are chemicals that may alleviate joint pain and irritation while also killing microorganisms. Other compounds may aid in the reduction of inflammation and the protection of the liver from harm.

- The use of sarsaparilla root to cure psoriasis has been recorded for decades. Sarsaparilla significantly alleviated skin lesions in psoriasis patients.

- Sarsaparilla has anti-inflammatory properties. This property makes it an effective therapy for inflammatory disorders such as rheumatoid arthritis, other sources of joint pain, and gout-related edema.

- Sarsaparilla has been demonstrated to have antibacterial and antimicrobial properties against bacteria and other microbes that have infiltrated the body. Although it might not be as effective as current antibiotics or antifungals, it's been used to treat serious ailments such as leprosy & syphilis for millennia.

- Sarsaparilla was found to have anticancer activities in cell lines from various tumors and animals in a recent survey.

- Sarsaparilla has also been demonstrated to preserve the liver.

- Sarsaparilla is employed as a "synergist" in herbal blends. In other words, sarsaparilla saponins boost the absorption and bioavailability of other herbs.

Dosage and Preparation

- Boil 2 cups (16. oz) of water till it gets to a boil.

- Bring the flame to its lowest, then put sarsaparilla root into it.

- Brew it for almost 10- 12 minutes.

- Strain the tea into your cup (reaching around 8-9 ounces now).

- You can also put one whole lime.

Possible side effects/ drugs interaction

- Sarsaparilla has no recognized negative side effects. Taking an excessive amount of saponins, on the other hand, may induce gastrointestinal discomfort.

- Certain drugs may interact with sarsaparilla. It can improve your body's capacity to absorb other medications. Contact your doctor immediately if you have any negative effects while consuming sarsaparilla.

- Studies have not suggested sarsaparilla would be safe for pregnant /nursing moms. So if you want to be safe, stay away from medicinal herbs, including sarsaparilla, unless a doctor tells you to.

HIERBA DEL SAPO

Description of the herb

Hierba del Sapo (Eryngium heterophyllum Engelm) does seem to be a humid-growing Mexican plant. The herb has been examined in clinical practice and laboratory studies with volunteers for over 22 years, confirming its therapeutic usefulness in various medical disorders. Lowering cholesterol plus triglycerides has become one of the greatest successful uses. Hierba del Sapo could also help with type 2 diabetes, gallstones and renal disease, atherosclerosis, osteoarthritis, and other degenerative diseases. New Mexico, Southeastern Arizona and Mexico are all home to this lovely thistle. During the summer then in October, its blue flowers could be found blossoming in meadows, open forests, along watercourses, and even in the highlands. But take a look down! It is a thick, bristle-toothed perennial that is only 1 1/2 - two feet tall.

Benefits

- This product's ingredients are typically used for: High triglycerides, High cholesterol, Diabetes type 2, Kidney disease, Gallstones, Osteoarthritis.

Dosage and Preparation

- The finely sliced plant is steeped over 5-10 minutes topped using 2 teaspoons every 8 ounces of water to make your tea.

- Take it twice per day.

Possible side effects/ drugs interaction

- It is unknown whether or not the plant is safe to use during pregnancy and breastfeeding.

- It's best to avoid it if you're pregnant because it might trigger uterine contractions.

- It's best not to use it for over 8 weeks at a time because it might harm your kidneys.

- In persons who are allergic to this plant, its products may induce skin reactions.

EUCALYPTUS

Description of the herb

Eucalyptus is really an evergreen tree whose therapeutic benefits are well known. Although it flourishes in many parts, the popular tree is native to Australia. It possesses rich gum-infused bark, lengthy stems, and round leaves that, if eaten whole, are difficult to digest. On the other hand, eucalyptus leaves may be brewed into the safe tea to drink. The leaves could also be turned into essential oil for topical or inhalation applications.

Benefits

- Antioxidants, notably flavonoids, found in eucalyptus leaves defend your body from oxidative stress as well as free radical damage. On the other hand, children are at significant risk of further eucalyptus toxicity. They, therefore, should seek medical advice before consuming this tea.

- Eucalyptus is a frequent component in cold & cough treatments and is commonly seen as a natural cure for a cold.

- According to some studies, eucalyptol helps to improve cold symptoms, including coughing, nasal congestion, and headaches, by reducing inflammation and mucus accumulation.

- Eucalyptus oil can help dry skin by raising ceramide levels. Ceramides are one type of fatty acid found in the skin that helps it keep its barrier intact and retain moisture. Ceramide levels are frequently lower in those who have dandruff, dry skin, or skin illnesses, including dermatitis and psoriasis.

- Many anti-inflammatory chemicals in eucalyptus, like cineole and limonene, may work as pain relievers.

- Eucalyptus has a reputation for reducing stress symptoms.

- Eucalyptus leaf extract, often known as eucalyptol, has been shown to help with tooth health.

- Due to the presence of eucalyptol, eucalyptus oil is an essential insect repellant.

Dosage and Preparation

- Wash your four eucalyptus leaves and put them inside a pan with enough water to cover them. Bring to the boil.

- Remove from the flame, then put aside for 15 minutes to steep. When necessary, reheat and pour into a cup.

- You can take the tea twice daily.

Possible side effects/ drugs interaction

- Although eucalyptus leaves are typically considered harmless, consuming eucalyptus oil carries some major health hazards since it can cause poisoning.

- It's also worth noting that youngsters are more susceptible to toxicity. Seizures, breathing difficulties, a loss of consciousness or even death have all been documented.

- Furthermore, there is insufficient research to evaluate if eucalyptus oil seems to be safe for pregnant or nursing mothers. As a result, these populations should avoid it.

CORDONCILLO NEGRO

Description of the herb

Cordoncillo Negro popularly known as Matico (Piper aduncum), is a potent plant praised by Dr. Sebi (the late) for its numerous health advantages. Cordoncillo Negro is a powerful herb that provides a slew of health and therapeutic advantages. It's a Jamaican native, and we get it from the quiet virgin woods where it grows organically. It is most commonly used to treat stomach and upper respiratory problems.

Benefits

- Relieves stomach pains, digestive problems, nausea (especially pregnancy-related sickness), vomiting, and flatulence.

- Cancers of the stomach

- Treats a variety of upper respiratory problems.

- It soothes the throat.

- The cough is relieved.

- Mucus is expelled from your respiratory tract.

- Decongestion

- Relief from pain (includes menstrual cramps)

- Accelerates Healing Wounds

- Toothaches are relieved.

- Inflammation is addressed.

Dosage and Preparation

- Make your tea by adding 1 gram of cordoncillo negro inside one cup of boiled water.

- Steep around for 10 minutes.

Best results are achieved when it is taken 2-3 times each day, 1 cup.1 gram of herb per cup

Possible side effects/ drugs interaction

- There are no known health risks associated with the correct administration of prescribed therapeutic amounts.

SOURSOP

Description of the herb

Soursop seems to be known for its exquisite flavor and numerous health advantages. Also, it's nutrient-dense, with plenty of fiber plus vitamin C for a small number of calories.

A fruit of genus Annona muricata, commonly called Graviola, is a tree endemic to tropical parts of the Americas. This spiky green fruit's creamy texture and rich flavor are typically compared to strawberry or pineapple.

Soursop is normally eaten raw, with the flesh scooped out after cutting the fruit in half. Fruits come in various sizes and can be fairly huge, so it's preferable to divide them into many servings. This fruit has a low-calorie content in its usual serving.

Niacin, folate, riboflavin, and iron are all found in small amounts in soursop.

Many fruit components, including the fruit, leaves, and stems, are used medicinally. However, it can also be applied directly to the skin and cooking.

Research has shown a range of health advantages for soursop in recent years.

It may even assist with anything from reducing inflammation to delaying cancer growth, according to several test-tube and animal studies.

Benefits

- Soursop's strong antioxidant content is responsible for many of its stated health advantages. Antioxidants are molecules that aid in neutralizing dangerous substances known as free radicals that can cause cell damage. According to some studies, antioxidants may help reduce the risk of various ailments, including cancer, heart disease, and diabetes.

- Soursop may also have antimicrobial qualities, according to certain research.

- Multiple bacteria strains, including those that cause gingivitis, tooth decay, and yeast infections, were shown to be successfully killed by soursop.

- In animal experiments, Soursop and its constituents have been shown to help combat inflammation. Although inflammation is a natural immune response to damage, growing evidence suggests that persistent inflammation may play a role in illness.

- In animal tests, soursop has been demonstrated to help manage blood sugar levels.

- Graviola can cause nerve damage and movement issues, especially if taken long. It can also cause severe neuropathy, which can cause symptoms similar to Parkinson's disease, like tremors and stiff muscles. In addition, Graviola may exacerbate the symptoms of Parkinson's disease in people who have it.

470

Dosage and Preparation

- Remove the core from 1 big ripe soursop.

- Put the soursop pulp inside a large mixing basin (the fleshy part containing the seeds).

- Fill your blender with soursop pulp (not more than 3/4 filled).

- Fill the blender halfway with 4 to 6 cups of water to fully cover the pulp.

- Blend on high till the pulp is completely liquefied.

- Strain your soursop juice in a bowl to separate the pulp and seeds out from the juice.

- Stir the juice with a big spoon and pour it through a strainer, adding extra water if needed.

- Choose whether you want soursop juice alongside lime, then flavor with the ingredients listed above.

- Limit yourself to 1/2 cup a couple of days a week.

Possible side effects/ drugs interaction

- Graviola can be harmful to the kidneys and liver if used often. Therefore, Graviola should not be used by anyone with liver or renal disorders.

- If you have elevated blood pressure or are using blood pressure medication,

- suffer from diabetes

- , are going to have a baby

- If or are nursing a baby, you should see your doctor before using Graviola.

VALERIAN ROOT

Description of the herb

Valerian dietary supplements have been commonly offered as sleeping aids in the U.S. However, people in Europe are more likely to use them for anxiety and restlessness.

Although there are over 250 varieties of valerian, Valeriana officinalis is the most often utilized for medical purposes.

Though medicinal valerian has been used since ancient Greece and Rome, there is little scientific proof that it treats anxiety and insomnia.

Nonetheless, the Food and Drug Administration considers valerian safe and milder than synthetic medications like barbiturates and benzodiazepines. As a result, valerian may be worth a shot if you're suffering from anxiety or sleeplessness.

Benefits

- For ages, herbal medicine practitioners had given valerian root treating insomnia and sleep problems. Modern scientific research has not confirmed the slight sedative effect of valerian root. However, several studies have shown evidence of the impact, although further studies are required.

- During II World War, people in the United Kingdom employed valerian roots to ease stress induced by air attacks. Before then, it was utilized to treat anxiety issues by doctors during the 1500s. Early study suggests that valerian root has an anxiolytic impact, another word for anti-anxiety properties, but further research is needed.

- According to one research, taking valerian root reduced the intensity and likelihood of hot flashes among women going through menopause. Sweating, a quick pulse, and sudden warmth are all symptoms of hot flashes, which some people find bothersome. Hot flashes are caused by hormonal changes.

- Premenstrual syndrome (PMS) symptoms are experienced by 90 percent of menstruate women. PMS may be so severe in some people that it interferes with their ability to maintain a regular life during their period. PMS symptoms include Bloating, Cramps, Headache, Irritability, Swollen & tender breasts, Anxiety, Back pain, Depression, Excessive tiredness. According to one research, ingesting valerian root can help with both physical and mental symptoms of PMS.

- In the United States, Valerian root is classified as a dietary/herbal supplement and is controlled like a food product. However, the FDA doesn't really allow its use as a supplement in medical treatments since it is not classed as a medication.

Dosage and Preparation

Soak 2–3 grams of herbal dried valerian root into 1 cup of boiling water over 10–15 minutes to make a tea. Valerian root appears to function best after two weeks of consistent use.

Possible side effects/ drugs interaction

Some mild adverse effects may occur after using valerian root, including Dizziness, Headaches, Upset stomach, Pruritus / uncomfortable, itchy feeling, Feeling tired during the morning, Swelling of lips/ tongue, Mood swings, Confusion, Forgetfulness, Yellow skin/ eyes, Fast heartbeat, Dark urine, Skin rash/ hives.

ASHWAGANDHA

Description of the herb

The evergreen plant Ashwagandha grows across Asia and Africa. It's a popular stress reliever. But unfortunately, there isn't much proof that it can be used as an "adaptogen."

Chemicals in Ashwagandha may aid in relaxing the brain, decrease edema, lower blood pressure, also change the immune system.

Ashwagandha is utilized for various stress-related illnesses since it is traditionally an adaptogen. Adaptogens are substances that are thought to assist the body cope with high-stress levels. Insomnia, anxiety, aging, and various other illnesses are among the ailments for which it is prescribed; however, there is no scientific proof to back up most of these claims. In addition, there is no strong evidence to support the use of Ashwagandha on COVID-19.

Physalis alkekengi is not the same as Ashwagandha. However, both are referred to as winter cherries. Also, Ashwagandha should not be confused with Panax, American ginseng, eleuthero or ginseng.

Benefits

- In Ayurveda, an alternative medication founded on Indian natural healing concepts, Ashwagandha is among the essential herbs. It's been used to reduce tension, promote energy, and improve attention for over 3,000 years. Sanskrit, meaning "horse's breath," Ashwagandha alludes to the herb's distinct aroma as well as its ability to boost vigor. The ashwagandha plant seems to be a tiny shrub native to North Africa and India with yellow flowers. Several ailments are treated with powder or extracts made from the plant's roots or leaves. Its high content of withanolides, which have been demonstrated to combat inflammation and tumors, is responsible for many of its health advantages.

- According to limited data, Ashwagandha lowers blood sugar levels by affecting insulin secretion and sensitivity.

- Withaferin, a bioactive molecule found in Ashwagandha, has been proven in animal & test-tube experiments to accelerate tumor cell death and might even be beneficial against various cancers.

- Cortisol is called a stress hormone as it is released by your adrenal glands in reaction to stress and when your blood sugar goes too low. Unfortunately, cortisol levels can become persistently excessive in some people, leading to elevated blood sugar plus increased abdominal fat accumulation. Ashwagandha has been found in studies to help lower cortisol levels.

- In both human and animal research, Ashwagandha has been demonstrated to lower anxiety and stress.

- Several studies show that Ashwagandha may help reduce depression, while further research is needed.

- In males, Ashwagandha increases testosterone levels and improves sperm quality & fertility.

- In men, Ashwagandha has been demonstrated to boost muscular mass, lower body fat, and improve strength.

- Ashwagandha has been proven to boost the activity of natural killer cells while also lowering inflammatory indicators.

- Ashwagandha could assist in lowering the risk of cardiovascular disease by lowering triglyceride and cholesterol levels.

- Supplementing with Ashwagandha may help improve memory, brain function, response speed, and task performance.

Dosage and Preparation

- Inside a saucepan, bring one mug of water to a boil. Put a teaspoon of your ashwagandha powder or a few ashwagandha roots if you have them. Allow 10-15 minutes for the water to boil. Strain into a cup and season with a squeeze of lime juice plus a pinch of honey to taste.

- Over 60 days, a daily dose of 250 to 500 mg ashwagandha is suggested.

Possible side effects/ drugs interaction

- When taken orally, Ashwagandha may be safe for up to three months. However, Ashwagandha's long-term safety is unknown. Ashwagandha at high dosages might induce stomach distress, diarrhea, and vomiting. Liver issues are a rare occurrence.

- There isn't enough credible evidence to say whether Ashwagandha is harmless or the potential adverse effects when used topically.

- When you're pregnant, Ashwagandha is probably not a good idea. Some data suggest that Ashwagandha might induce miscarriages.

- There isn't enough credible information to say whether Ashwagandha is advisable to take during breastfeeding. Avoid using to be in a safe place.

- Ashwagandha may enhance the indications of auto-immune illnesses by causing your immune system to be more active. Therefore, it's advisable to avoid Ashwagandha if you get one of these disorders.

- Ashwagandha may cause your central nervous system to slow down during surgery. In addition, anesthesia and other drugs used before and after surgery, according to healthcare practitioners, may exacerbate this impact. Therefore, stop taking Ashwagandha two weeks before the first scheduled surgery.

LILY OF THE VALLEY

Description of the herb

It is a flowering plant. Medicine is made from the root, underground stem (rhizome), plus dried flower tips.

Heart disorders, such as heart failure & irregular pulse, are treated with lily of the valley. It's also used to treat kidney stones, UTIs, labor contractions that aren't strong enough, fluid retention (edema), epilepsy, strokes with paralysis, eye infections (conjunctivitis), as well as leprosy.

Lily of the valley should be kept in the dark, well-sealed containers.

Benefits

There is insufficient evidence to rate the efficacy of Kidney stones, Heart failure, Irregular heartbeat, Urinary tract infections, Epilepsy, Fluid retention, Paralysis, Weak contractions during labor, Strokes, Leprosy, Infection of the eye and other conditions.

Dosage and Preparation

- **Tincture:** 3g twice a day.
- **Liquid Extract:** 200 mg three times a day.
- **Dried Extract:** 75 mg twice a day.

Possible side effects/ drugs interaction

- When consumed by mouth, standardized lily of the valley extracts are POSSIBLY UNSAFE as with most people. In addition, Lily of the valley has been shown to have substantial negative effects on the heart and other systems. Although medical monitoring and supervision may lessen these side effects, usage is not advised for anybody.

- The lily of the valley herb is almost certainly dangerous. If you mistakenly ingest lily of the valley, get medical attention straight away. Nausea, vomiting, irregular heart rhythm, headache, reduced awareness and visual color changes, and responsiveness is possible adverse effects.

FLOR DE MANITA

Description of the herb

Flor de manita flower is found on trees across South and Central America. This tree is 50 feet, and its flowers usually have five petals with a curl at the tips, which is why it's known as the "hand flower tree" or sometimes "devil's hand tree." The Spanish term for "hand" is "mano," and Spanish-speaking nations will often add an "ita" to the end of phrases to indicate that something is tiny. This is how "flor de manita" got its name.

Benefits

Both the flowers and leaves are edible. The herb is used to flavor cocoa, and the leaves are wrapped around tamales to provide a sweet and smoky flavor. The tea, a natural diuretic, helps the kidneys eliminate extra fluids and decrease water retention (edema). The petals are also traditionally used to cure diarrhea because they contain flavonoids that calm and protect the intestines and decrease stomach pain and irritation.

Extracts from the petals of this herb have antibacterial, antiprotozoal, propulsive, vasorelaxant, and antisecretory properties.

- It helps to treat heart illness.

- It helps in curing epilepsy.

- It is beneficial for infectious diarrhea and is used as an anecdotic remedy.

Dosage and Preparation

Dr. Sebi's Blood Pressure tea helps the cardiovascular system by providing nutritional and regulatory support. It's made up of Flor de Manita (Chiranthodendron Pentadactylon), often known as the Mexican hand tree, with its vibrant red finger-like petals, in which alkaloids and cardiac glycosides are in abundance. For generations, Flor de Manita has preserved heart health, stomach discomfort, and cardiac abnormalities.

- Take two cups of distilled water in a pan and bring it to a boil.

- Add two flowers to it and simmer it for 15 minutes.

- Let the mixture cool to room temperature and filter.

To nurture a healthy heart and circulatory system, consume this rejuvenating blood pressure tea couple of times a day.

It's okay to eat on an empty stomach and between meals.

Possible side effects/ drugs interaction

The safety of utilizing this plant's products (internally or topically) during pregnancy and early lactation has yet to be determined.

If you are presently using anti-hypertensive or anti-epileptic drugs, consult your healthcare practitioner beforehand to avoid any potential herb-drug interaction.

NETTLE

Description of the herb

The stinging nettle, often known as nettle, is native to northern Europe and Asia. Urtica dioica is its scientific name. The plant has heart-shaped leaves, and flowers are yellow or pink. The stem is coated in small, stiff hairs that, when touched, produce harsh chemicals. From June through September, the plant grows in nitrogen-rich soil and can reach a height of two to four feet.

The nettle plant's leaves, stems, and roots could be crushed and turned into powders, tinctures, lotions, teas, and more. This herb has been utilized as a remedy for generations. Current science now backs up many of the potential health advantages of nettle tea.

Benefits

The leaves and roots of the stinging nettle contain a wide range of nutrients such as vitamins A, C, K and B, minerals, fats, and essential amino acids.

- It helps in flushing out harmful bacteria and cleanse the urinary tract. This can help patients with urinary problems such as benign prostatic hyperplasia (BPH). In males, BPH produces an enlarged prostate gland. This might result in urination discomfort or other issues.

- It aids in treating pain and aching muscles, particularly those caused by arthritis.

- The effects of nettle on blood glucose levels have been encouraging. It aids the pancreas in producing or releasing insulin, the hormone which regulates blood sugar levels.

- Polyphenols, which are plant compounds, are abundant in nettle. These potent chemicals help prevent and treat various inflammation-related illnesses like diabetes, cancer, obesity, and heart disease.

- The stinging nettle is considered to be a potential natural hay fever therapy. Hay fever is caused due to inflammation over the nose lining.

- Stinging nettle extracts have been shown to reduce inflammation, which can cause seasonal allergies.

- Excessive bleeding has been reported to be reduced by medicines containing stinging nettle extract, particularly after surgery.

- The antioxidant qualities of nettle protect the liver from toxins, inflammation and heavy metals.

- Applying stinging nettle lotions to wounds, especially burns, may help them recover faster.

Dosage and Preparation

The flowers and dried leaves make a wonderful herbal tea. The leaves, roots, and stems can be cooked to make soups, smoothies, stews and stir-frys. Avoid fresh leaves as their barbs could cause discomfort.

- Take two cups of distilled water and one cup of leaves in a pan.

- Bring it to boil.

- Let the mixture cool for 5 minutes and filter.

- If too bitter, add a bit of honey.

Possible side effects/ drugs interaction

- Stinging nettle, whether dry or cooked, is typically safe to eat. However, be cautious while handling fresh leaves since their hair-like barbs can cause skin irritation as they inject chemicals such as Acetylcholine, Histamine, Serotonin, Leukotriene, and Formic acid that can result in rashes, hives, bumps and itchiness.

- Rarely, patients may experience a severe allergic response that is life-threatening. These compounds, however, decrease when the leaves are treated. Thus eating dried or cooked stinging nettle does not cause tongue or stomach discomfort.

- Stinging nettle should not be consumed by pregnant women since it might produce uterine contractions that can increase the chance of miscarriage.

- Consult your doctor if you're using medicines such as blood thinners, blood pressure medication, Diuretics (water pills), Diabetes medication, and Lithium. These medicines may interact with stinging nettle. For example, the plant may amplify the effects of diuretics, increasing the risk of dehydration.

NOPAL CACTUS

Description of the herb

The nopal cactus, commonly known as prickly pear cactus, is endemic to Mexico's southwestern regions and the United States. When the plant is young, the flat cactus pads of the young plant can be eaten. However, the cactus becomes too difficult to consume as it grows older. Therefore, the nopal cactus is commonly used as a culinary component in some parts of Mexico. It usually grows to a height of 5.5 meters and is bushy. It has enormous yellow flowers with a diameter of 7.5 to 10 cm (3 to 4 inches), followed by white, reddish-purple or yellow fruits. It is normally planted as a fodder crop and for the fruit and edible paddles in warmer climates. The oil is made from hard seeds. The stems, particularly of spineless species, are utilized as emergency stock feed in droughts because they have high water content.

Benefits

Because of the cactus' numerous health advantages, it has a variety of therapeutic applications.

- To avoid getting a virus, the greatest defense is prevention. The antiviral activities of the Nopal cactus have been discovered in the preliminary study against the respiratory syncytial virus (RSV), herpes simplex virus (HSV), and HIV.

- Like other body cells, nerve cells can be damaged. This results in sensory loss and pain. This is something the nopal cactus can help with. This can help protect nerve cells from being damaged or losing their functionality.

- Antioxidants can help protect our cells from free radical damage. Antioxidants are present in the nopal cactus. Cactus can lower oxidative stress. Everyone, regardless of age or pre-existing problems, can benefit from antioxidants.

- For diabetics, controlling blood sugar may be a significant challenge. The nopal cactus might be useful as a supplement. Taking nopal cactus alongside other diabetic medicines can help control blood sugar levels.

- The nopal cactus may aid in treating enlarged prostates and may even be useful in treating prostate cancer. Moreover, it could accomplish this with fewer adverse effects than conventional prescription medicines.

- The nopal cactus may relieve hangover symptoms. When taken before drinking, nopal cactus extract greatly decreases the intensity of hangovers.

Dosage and Preparation

The health advantages of the nopal cactus can be achieved in various ways. Eating the cactus is the most obvious method, and it also provides the highest health advantages. Supplements come in various forms, including capsules, extracts, powder, and liquids.

The majority of supplements propose taking at least one dosage of 500-650 mg each day. Nopal cactus is used to make Alkaline Electric Prickly Pear juice. Use the below-mentioned recipe for preparing two servings.

- Remove the ends of 6 pears and slice off the skin keeping the pear upright.

- Put pear in the blender and add 1/3 cup agave and 1/3 cup lime juice in it.

- Blend for 30 seconds

- After straining via cheesecloth, put the juice in the blender.

- Blend in the water or ice until thoroughly combined. Enjoy!

Possible side effects/ drugs interaction

- Nopal cactus supplements can cause headache, nausea, bloating, diarrhea, or increased stool.

- There isn't enough credible information on whether or not nopal cactus supplements are safe for pregnant women or attempting to get pregnant; therefore, they should avoid them.

- If you are a diabetic, you should avoid ingesting nopal cactus or its supplements since it might cause blood sugar problems.

HOLY BASIL

Description of the herb

Holy basil (Ocimum tenuiflorum), commonly known as tulsi or tulasi, is a mint family (Lamiaceae) flowering plant. It has fragrant leaves. Holy basil is a plant that thrives throughout Southeast Asia and is native to the Indian subcontinent. The plant is commonly used in Ayurvedic and traditional medicine and is loved in Hinduism. In addition, it is commonly used as a herbal tea for treating a wide range of illnesses.

It is also used as a food ingredient, having a strong flavor that gets stronger as it cooks. It has a peppery taste and is evocative of clove, mint, and Italian basil (Ocimum basilicum). It is considered an agricultural plant in certain regions outside its natural range.

Holy basil is a tiny and short-lived perennial plant that grows up to 1 meter (3.3 feet) tall. The hairy stems have simply toothed, or whole leaves face each other along the stem. Depending on the type, the aromatic leaves are purple or green. The tiny purple or white flowers are grown in terminal spikes and have purple or green sepals. The fruit produced is called net, which produces many seeds.

Benefits

Holy basil is a tonic for the body, soul and mind. It can be used from its leaves to the seeds. Different components of the plant are suggested for treating various ailments. This plant contains vitamin A and C, calcium, zinc, iron, and chlorophyll.

- Fresh flowers of Holy Basil are beneficial for bronchitis.

- Malaria can be treated by combining the leaves and seeds with black pepper.

- For diarrhea, nausea, and vomiting, use the whole plant.

- Eczema can be treated with pills or ointment.

- For eye problems and stomach ulcers, use an alcohol solution.

- Insect bites can be treated using an essential oil produced from the leaves.

- Adaptogens are found in all segments of the holy basil plant. An adaptogen is a natural chemical that aids in stress adaptation and mental stability.

- Holy basil is rich in antioxidants and aids in the body's detoxification. It protects your body from harmful toxins. It may also help to prevent cancer by inhibiting malignant cell development.

- Its leaf extracts are considered to improve wound healing.

- All portions of this plant can help lower blood sugar levels.

- It aids people suffering from arthritis or fibromyalgia.

Dosage and Preparation

Holy basil may be used in various methods in your everyday life. For example, you may use it in cooking, as a supplement, or prepare a tea with it. Essential oil of Holy basil is available.

- Combine two teaspoons of finely chopped basil and 1/8 teaspoon of grated ginger in a small saucepan.

- Fill the pot halfway with boiling water.

- 5 minutes of steeping

- Using a fine strainer, strain the mixture.

- If you're using lime and honey, toss those in as well.

Drink this tea, especially before sleep, for its calming benefits.

Possible side effects/ drugs interaction

- When consumed for up to six weeks, holy basil appears harmless, but its long-term safety has yet to be determined.

- The safety of using holy basil while pregnant or nursing has yet to be determined. People attempting to conceive should avoid using holy basil since preliminary animal studies have shown that it might induce uterine contractions and reduce fertility.

- According to another animal research, holy basil may reduce the pace of regular blood clotting; therefore, it's best to cease using it at least two weeks before a scheduled operation and two weeks following any sort of surgery.

GINGER

Description of the herb

The fragrant, pungent rhizome (underground stem) of the perennial herb plant Ginger, presumably native to southeastern Asia, is used as a spice, food flavor, and medicine. Zingiber is its generic name, is taken from the Greek zingiberis, derived from a Sanskrit word Singapura, which refers to the spice.

Ginger has been used in China and India since the olden days. By the 1st century CE, merchants had brought it to the Mediterranean region. It was well-known in England by the 11th century. Soon after the invasion, the Spaniards carried it to Mexico and the West Indies. By 1547, it was being sold from Santiago to Spain.

The spice has a somewhat bitter taste: bread, sauces, curry foods, pickles, confections, and ginger ale. It is generally dried and powdered. Green ginger is a fresh rhizome that is used in cooking. By boiling the peeled rhizomes in syrup, they can be stored. Slices of ginger are often eaten between courses or meals.

Ginger's leafy stems reach a height of around a meter. The leaves are about 6 to 12 inches (15 to 30 cm) long, elongated, alternating in two vertical rows, and emerge from stem sheaths. The flowers are arranged in thick conelike spikes that are approximately 1 inch thick, 2 to 3 inches long, and made up of overlapping green lobes with yellow edges. A single tiny yellow-green and purple flower is enclosed by each bract.

Benefits

- Drugs used for treating HIV/AIDS cause nausea and vomiting (antiretroviral-induced nausea and vomiting). In HIV patients, taking ginger by mouth for 14 days, 30 minutes before each dosage of antiretroviral therapy, decreases the incidence of nausea and vomiting.

- It helps in cramps during menstruation (dysmenorrhea). Taking ginger orally during the first 3 to 4 days of menstruation might help to alleviate unpleasant periods. It appears to be comparable to mefenamic acid, ibuprofen, or Novafen in pain relief. Taking ginger alongside other medications, such as mefenamic acid, appears to be beneficial.

- In some patients with osteoarthritis, taking ginger might help them feel better.

- In some women, taking ginger orally during pregnancy decreases nausea and vomiting. However, it may act slowly or less effectively than certain anti-nausea medications.

Dosage and How to use it

- In a small saucepan, combine all 1 cup freshly squeezed Orange Juice, 1 tbsp minced ginger, minced, 2 tbsp Agave, 1 tbsp minced Red Onions, 1 tbsp minced Red Bell Pepper, 1/2 tsp Crushed Red Pepper and stir to combine.

- Bring to a boil, lower to low heat and cook for 10-15 minutes. To keep the sauce from burning, whisk it every few minutes.

- To thicken the sauce, pour it into a dish and set aside 10-15 minutes.

Your Alkaline Electric Orange Ginger Sauce is ready to serve!

Possible side effects/ drugs interaction

Ginger is probably safe to eat. However, heartburn, diarrhea, burping, and stomach pain are possible adverse effects. The danger of adverse effects rises when you take greater dosages of 5 g per day.

- Some people may have skin discomfort as a result of it.

- When consumed in meals, ginger is most likely harmless. When used by mouth as medication during pregnancy, it may be safe. Some doctors advise against using it close to the due date since it may raise the chance of bleeding. It appears, however, that it is safe to use for morning sickness without causing harm to the baby. Before taking ginger while pregnant, see your healthcare practitioner.

- Ginger may help to prevent blood clots. However, it may result in more bleeding during or after surgery. So don't use it at least two weeks before surgery.

ARNICA

Description of the herb

Arnica (genus Arnica) is a genus comprising 30 plant species belonging to the Asteraceae family, most of which are found in the mountains of northwest America. Arnica species are typically perennial plants that grow to a height of 10–70 cm (4–28 inches). The oppositely oriented simple leaves have serrated or smooth edges and often have glandular trichomes (hairs).

Achene fruits (simple dry fruit) with bristles for dissemination produce composite flower heads, typically yellow. Rhizomes are found in a variety of plants. Unfortunately, arnica is poisonous and can cause deadly poisoning if ingested orally, despite its popularity in homeopathy and traditional medicine.

A notable species, Mountain arnica (Arnica montana), is a perennial plant native to the central northern and European mountains. It produces an essential oil that was once used to cure bruises and sprains, and it's popular as a garden decorative. Narrowleaf arnica (A. Angustifolia) has orange-yellow flower heads measuring 5–7 cm (2–2.5 inches) wide.

Benefits

Arnica treats bruises, discomfort, myalgia (muscle soreness), and arthralgia (joint aches). Because the plant may be poisonous, it's usually used as a homeopathic remedy. However, just a little scientific data supports treating any medical problem.

- Arnica proponents have long claimed that the herb contains anti-inflammatory qualities, making it a viable and safe organic alternative to NSAIDs.

- Whether used topically or taken as an oral supplement, Arnica can help minimize bruising and swelling after surgery.

- Myalgia (muscle discomfort) can be caused by various medical problems or simply by overusing your muscles.

- It's used to treat myalgia caused by strenuous exercise. Although there is limited evidence to support its usage in sports supplements, arnica has long been used for this purpose.

Dosage and How to use it

- Collect a handful of arnica flowers.

- Allow 30-60 minutes for arnica flowers to dry in the sun or a warm, dry location.

- Add flowers in a clean mason jar (of any size).

- Add oil to the flowers to the top of the jar.

- Place in a cold, dark place for 4 weeks after sealing it with the lid.

- For the first week, shake the jar several times a day, then once a day for the next four weeks.

- Using a fine-mesh strainer or butter-muslin, strain off the flowers and store the oil in a sealed jar in a cold, dark place away from direct sunlight.

Possible side effects/ drugs interaction

Even when used in extremely diluted topical formulations, Arnica induces adverse effects in herbal medicines. Oral versions can have more significant adverse effects.

- Arnica may induce a minor allergic response in non-homeopathic formulations, especially in those who have a previous sensitivity to the plants in the Asteraceae family, such as ragweed, chrysanthemums, marigolds and daisies.

- When applied excessively or on damaged skin, arnica can cause temporary rises in blood pressure and pulse rate. In addition, broken skin allows for more active substance absorption, and it may cause localized stinging.

- Arnica may delay blood coagulation; thus, any non-homeopathic arnica medicines should be stopped two weeks before surgery to avoid postoperative bleeding.

- Suppose you are on anticoagulant (blood-thinning) medications. In that case, you should avoid arnica since the combination might raise your risk of bleeding and bruising.

- Arnica's safety during pregnancy is a subject of debate. Consult your healthcare practitioner before taking arnica in any form if you are pregnant or nursing.

DAMIANA

Description of the herb

Damiana is a shrub that grows in the wild. It belongs to Turneraceae, an aromatic plant, and the Turneraceae family. It has been used by herbalists since the time of the Aztecs. This herb is abundant in Mexico, Central America, and the West Indies, where it treats a variety of ailments.

The name of this herb is attributed to the Greeks, as per historians. It was once known as Daman or Damia, which means 'to subdue or tame.' They put their leaves in herbal smoking mixtures and liquors to soothe their anxieties. It also aided them in enhancing their sexual desires.

Benefits

Chemicals in Damiana have an effect on the nervous system and brain.

- It raises sexuality, improves sexual pleasure, lowers vaginal dryness, helps weight reduction, relieves headaches, depression, and congestion, elevates mood, and increases mental and physical strength.

- It lowers the gastric emptying rate, protects the liver, and aids weight loss.

- It relieves depression and helps in stimulating the digestive system.

Dosage and How to use it

Use this herb by grounding it into powder. Take it less than 200grams at a time.

- Put 1 cup water in a saucepan over high heat and bring it to a boil.

- Stir and add 2 teaspoons of dried damiana leaves after removing the saucepan from the heat.

- Allow the tea to infuse for 15 minutes after covering the saucepan.

- Pour the tea into a glass and add the honey and lime slices.

To revitalize the body, serve the damiana tea hot.

Possible side effects/ drugs interaction

When consumed by mouth at proportions usually found in meals, Damiana is likely safe. Likewise, when taken orally in medication dosages, Damiana is totally safe. However, major negative effects have been when used in extremely high amounts. For example, after consuming 200 grams of damiana herb, people have reported convulsions and other symptoms identical to strychnine poisoning or rabies.

- Damiana isn't safe to use while pregnant or breastfeeding because there isn't enough concrete data. So to be safe, avoid using it.

- Damiana may have an effect on blood sugar levels in diabetic patients. If you have diabetes and take Damiana, keep an eye out for low blood sugar (hypoglycemia) indicators and constantly monitor your blood sugar levels.

- Damiana appears to alter blood glucose levels; thus, it may affect blood glucose control pre and post-surgery. Therefore, Damiana should be stopped at least two weeks before a planned surgery.

HORSETAIL

Description of the herb

Since ancient Romans and Greeks, horsetail (Equisetum arvense) has been used as a herbal cure. It was originally used to cure tuberculosis and renal disorders, control bleeding, and cure ulcers and wounds. It is also known as Equisetum, derived from the Latin words Equus, which means "horse," and seta, which means "bristle."

Horsetail comes from massive, tree-like plants that flourished 400 million years ago in the Paleozoic epoch. Horsetail is a nonflowering weed widespread in Europe, Asia, the Middle East, and North America. It is a near relative of the fern. The plant is perennial (comes back every year) with hollow stems and asparagus-like shoots. Silica crystals that grow in the stems and branches of the plant look like feathery tails as they dry, giving the plant a scratching look. This explains why it was once used to clean metals, particularly pewter.

Benefits

- Horsetail has been used as a diuretic for centuries. One research examined how persons with uric acid kidney stones tended to use horsetail. Horsetail users had more diuresis than those who didn't (urine output). In addition, horsetail contains antioxidant qualities, according to other studies, and may suppress cancer cell proliferation.

- Horsetail comprises silicon, a mineral required for bone health; it's been considered a cure for osteoporosis (thinning bone). In one study, 122 Italian women were given dry horsetail extract or Osteosil calcium 270 mg twice daily. Horsetail supplementation enhanced bone density.

Dosage and How to use it

- Place 2 handfuls of herbs in a sieve over a kettle of boiling water and set aside (double boiler, etc.). The soft, heated herbs are wrapped in linen and put to an adenoma, cyst, ulcer or tumor.

- Bring 9-ounce leaves to a boil in 1 gallon of water. Cook for 5 minutes before straining. Toss into the bathwater.

Possible side effects/ drugs interaction

- Horsetail is not suggested for young children since it carries traces of nicotine.

- When used properly, horsetail treatments from Equisetum arvense are typically regarded safe. However, Equisetum palustre, a different type of horsetail, is harmful to horses. Never take that type of horsetail if you want to be safe. Make careful you get things from a reputable, well-established brand. Choose goods with proven potency or standardized extracts whenever possible.

- When you take horsetail by mouth, your body's vitamin B1 (thiamin) levels may drop. However, suppose you consume horsetail on a routine basis. In that case, you should also take a good multivitamin or a B complex supplement daily.

- Horsetail should not be used by anyone with heart or kidney problems, diabetes, or gout.

- Horsetail may lead thiamin levels to fall, so don't consume alcohol regularly when taking it.

- Horsetail may cause potassium to be flushed out of the body; hence it is not recommended for persons at risk of low potassium levels.

LINDEN

Description of the herb

Linden is commonly found in the Northern Hemisphere. Only a few of the approximately 30 species are out as beautiful and shade trees. It has heart-shaped and coarsely edged leaves. The flowers are fragrant, cream-colored, and little globular fruit is drooping from a short leafy bract. They are some of the most elegant of deciduous trees. The American linden, also known as whitewood or basswood, is a huge shade tree that can reach up to a height of 40 meters (130 feet) and produces wood for beehives, furniture, crafting, and excelsior. Linden honey is yellowish and has a particular flavor, and it is a favored bee tree. The European linden, sometimes known as small-leaf linden, is extensively planted as a roadside tree. The Redmond linden, an elegant pyramidal variety with a single straight trunk, is a hybrid Crimean linden that can grow to a height of 20 meters (66 ft).

Benefits

- Linden appears to minimize mucus production and alleviate anxiety.

- Linden is a type of tree. Medicine is made from dried petals, leaves, and wood.

- Colds, sore throats, stuffy nose breathing troubles (bronchitis), headaches, fevers, and coughing up mucus are all treated with linden leaf.

- Nervous tension, rapid heartbeat, insomnia, high blood pressure, heavy bleeding (hemorrhage), bladder control issues (incontinence), and muscular spasms are all treated with it.

- Linden leaf is also used to enhance urine output and produce sweat.

- Linden is applied directly to the skin for itchy skin, lower leg sores (ulcus), and joint pain caused by poor blood circulation.

Dosage and How to use it

- Put 1 tablespoon of linden flowers in a jug. Boil three cups of water and put it over the flowers.

- To keep the essential oils from escaping into the steam, cover it for 15 minutes of steeping.

- Pour the mixture into cups. To taste, adjust the sweetness.

Drink as much as you want. For centuries, linden tea has been known for its calming qualities.

Possible side effects/ drugs interaction

- The usage of linden regularly has been related to heart disease.

- Linden may have a diuretic or water pill-like effect. Taking linden could make it harder for the body to get rid of lithium. It might cause major side effects by increasing the amount of lithium in the body. It's possible that your lithium dosage needs to be adjusted.

- Do not consume during pregnancy or breastfeeding.

LAVENDER

Description of the herb

Lavender (genus Lavandula) is a genus of approximately thirty plant species in a family of mint plants. It is native to Mediterranean countries. The aromatic leaves and gorgeous flowers of lavender species make them popular in herb gardens. The plants are grown to smell various items for their essential oils. Lavender has traditionally been used in small sachets to scent closets and chests. Ancient Romans used it in their baths. It is often used to flavor sweets and beverages. In addition, lavender has a variety of herbal medicinal uses.

Benefits

- Lavender is a flowering plant. The lavender flower and oil are used to produce medication.

- Anxiety, tension, and insomnia are all treated with lavender. It's also used for depression, dementia, post-surgical pain, and other ailments. Still, there's no clear scientific evidence to back up many of these claims.

- Lavender is used as a flavoring in foods and beverages.

- Lavender is a fragrance ingredient in soaps, cosmetics, fragrances, potpourri, decorations, and pharmaceutical products.

- Lavender includes oil that has soothing properties and may help to relax some muscles. It also has antibacterial and antifungal properties.

- Taking lavender preparations appears to alleviate depression symptoms. While lavender seems to be less effective than the antidepressant imipramine, combining the two may provide additional benefits.

- Aromatherapy massages with lavender oil appear to be more effective than ordinary massages in reducing menstrual pain. Inhaling lavender oil during the first three days of menstruation also appears to help with stomach and backaches.

- Breathing lavender essential oil while taking pain relievers intravenously (through IV) can help lessen post-C-section pain. Breathing lavender for three minutes every six hours can help youngsters aged 6 to 12 years feel less pain after a tonsillectomy.

Dosage and How to use it

The most frequent way to consume lavender is to make tea from its buds. The oils and aromas of lavender buds are released by steeping them in tea.

- Bring 8 oz. Of water to boil

- Put 4 teaspoons of fresh lavender buds in a tea ball or sachet.

- In a teacup, combine the tea ball and the water.

- Allow for a 10-minute steeping time.

- Enjoy!

For a good night's sleep, try planting some in your garden and preparing yourself a cup before bedtime. If you cannot find fresh lavender buds, dried lavender buds will suffice.

Note: Lavender essential oil should never be used to brew tea. This has the potential to be exceedingly hazardous.

Possible side effects/ drugs interaction

- Lavender oil for aromatherapy massage does not appear to relieve cancer-related discomfort.

- Lavender can create constipation, headaches, and an increase in appetite if taken orally.

- When applied to the skin in medical proportions, lavender is usually safe. It may irritate you, but this is rare.

RED RASBERRY LEAF

Description of the herb

All of Canada and much of the United States are home to the American red raspberry (Rubus idaeus). In North America, there are different local kinds of red raspberries with specific distributions.

Raspberries grow best in the sun, but they can also be found in open woodlands. They typically grow around lake coastlines, creeksides, or along with edge habitats such as where the forest joins the field. If you reside in the city, you can also grow it along the side of a fence.

The berries of the red raspberry are easy to recognize. However, if you're selecting the leaves for medical purposes, you should do so before the flowers grow.

The leaves are 3-5 pinnately complex leaflets that grow alternately on the stalk. Often the middle leaflet has two or three lobes. The leaflets have a silvery underside.

The stem (or "cane") might be straight or curved. It is armed with firm, straight to slightly curved bristles. The tips of the canes do not need roots.

Benefits

- Red raspberry compounds have antioxidant properties and may aid in blood vessel relaxation. Depending on the amount and the muscles involved, they might also affect muscle contraction and relaxation. This is the concept behind the usage of red raspberry in labor and delivery.

- Vitamins and minerals abound in abundance in red raspberry leaves.

- Vitamin B, vitamin C, and minerals such as potassium, magnesium, phosphorus, zinc, and iron are found.

- Polyphenols are present in red raspberry leaves, such as tannins and flavonoids, which work as antioxidants in the body and can help protect cells from damage. In addition, small levels of ellagic acids are found in the leaves that have been demonstrated to neutralize carcinogens and even lead to cancer cell self-destruction.

- Red raspberry leaves have fragrance, a plant component that helps tighten and tone pelvic muscles, potentially reducing menstrual discomfort caused due to muscle spasms.

- Red raspberry leaf assists in strengthening uterine walls, shortening labor, and lessening the need for birthing interventions.

Dosage and How to use it

- Take 1 tbsp red raspberry leaves (or 1 teabag) and add 1 cup boiling water.

- Allow it to steep for 10-15 minutes.

- Drink the tea after straining it.

The red raspberry leaf tea flavor is comparable to black tea (without caffeine). So, if you enjoy tea, this simple red raspberry leaf tea is worth trying.

Possible side effects/ drugs interaction

It has laxative qualities, which may induce stool loosening in some persons. It also has a mild diuretic impact and can make you urinate more frequently.

SAGE

Description of the herb

Salvia officinalis, generally known as garden sage or common sage, is a fragrant mint family (Lamiaceae) plant. It is grown for its aromatic leaves. Sage is a Mediterranean herb that can be used fresh or dried to spice various meals, particularly poultry and pig stuffings and sausages. Certain kinds are also planted as ornamentals because of their lovely leaves and flowers. Sage also refers to several different species of the Salvia genus. Salvia officinalis, generally known as garden sage or common sage, is a fragrant mint family (Lamiaceae) plant. It is grown for its aromatic leaves. Sage is a Mediterranean herb that can be used fresh or dried to spice various meals, particularly poultry and pig stuffings and sausages. Certain kinds are also planted as ornamentals because of their lovely leaves and flowers. Sage also refers to several different species of the Salvia genus.

Sage is a plant that grows to 60 cm (2 ft). The oval leaves have a rough or wrinkled texture, with gray-green to pale green and variegated variants. The flowers are spiked and have tubular two-lipped corollas that attract a range of pollinators such as bees, hummingbirds, and butterflies. The flowers could be pink, purple, white, or red. The plant produces nutlet fruits.

Benefits

- Because of its powerful perfume and earthy flavor, sage is usually used in tiny doses.

- Sage is also utilized in spiritual sage burning or sweeping as a natural cleansing agent, insecticide, and ceremonial object.

- There are over 160 different polyphenols in sage that serve as antioxidants in the body.

- Sage is full of antioxidants, which have been linked to a variety of health advantages, including enhanced brain function and a reduced risk of cancer.

- Sage has antibacterial qualities, which may help fight germs that cause dental plaque to build.

- Sage can aid with menopause symptoms like hot flashes and irritability by reducing their intensity and frequency.

- While sage can reduce blood sugar levels by improving insulin sensitivity, a further human study is needed.

Dosage and How to use it

Sage tea has been used as a tonic for years because of its mildly stimulating effects. Sage was supposed to improve memory and enhance wisdom in medieval Europe. The main components of sage essential oil are thujone and borneol, up to 2.5 percent.

- Boil a pot of water in a kettle.

- Add 2 twigs of fresh sage.

- Fill a mug halfway with hot water. Allow for a 5-minute rest period.

- Allow for a 5-minute rest period. 1 slice lime, a tiny amount of honey (or agave). This step is necessary so that sage would not be too strong.

Drinking 1 cup (240 ml) of sage tea two times a day enhances antioxidant defense considerably.

Possible side effects/ drugs interaction

Sage is thought to be safe, with no known adverse effects.

However, thujone, a chemical in common sage, is a source of concern for certain people. In animal studies, high dosages of thujone have been demonstrated to be harmful to the brain. In contrast, there is no convincing evidence that thujone is harmful to people.

TAMARIND LEAF

Description of the herb

Tamarind leaves are tiny and oblong with curved corners, with 10 to 20 pairs of fern-like leaves ranging in length from 1 to 3 centimeters and width from 5 to 6 millimeters. The thick, feathery leaf is bright green on the top, while the underside is a dusty red-brown. Tamarind leaves are pinnately arranged and have the remarkable ability to fold at night. Although the tree is known to be evergreen, it may lose leaves for a short period. Tamarind leaves taste finest when they're fresh and soft before they've developed a fibrous texture. They have a sour and acidic taste.

Tamarind leaves, botanically known as Tamarindus indica, are harvested from one of the biggest trees in the tropics, reaching up to thirty meters in height with a twelve-meter-wide canopy. They are members of the Leguminosae family. These trees are known for their tangy fruits, used in preparing meals to add a flavourful bite. Tamarindo in Spanish, Tamarindo in the Philippines, Tamarandizio in Italian, Tamarin or Tamarinier in French, Ma-Charm in Thailand, and Ambli, Imli, in India. The leaves are a popular culinary item in Asia and Africa, where they are used in soups, curries, and stews.

Benefits

- The pulp of tamarind contains several phytonutrients that function as powerful dietary antioxidants and help in strengthening the body's natural immune system. Inflammatory effects of oxidative stress are reduced by antioxidants.

- Tamarind is high in polyphenols and flavonoids. It has been found to lower LDL cholesterol while increasing HDL cholesterol and reducing the risk of atherosclerosis. Dry pulp also has anti-hypertensive properties, lowering diastolic blood pressure.

- Fatty liver disease, also known as hepatosteatosis, rises globally. Tamarind fruit extract has been demonstrated to protect the liver by containing antioxidants called procyanidins, which protect the liver from free radical damage.

- Tamarind extract contains natural chemicals that can serve as a natural antibacterial against pathogenic germs. In addition, the antibacterial capabilities of a chemical known as lupeol have been discovered.

- Tamarind seed extracts have anti-inflammatory properties. In addition, it helps to enhance blood sugar management in diabetics.

Dosage and How to use it

- Tear out the needed quantity from a compacted block and soak in warm water for 10 minutes.

- Then combine it with water, strain it through a sieve, discard the pulp, and use the liquid.

- Mix 15ml tamarind with 4-6 tbsp warm water to concentrate tamarind.

Possible side effects/ drugs interaction

As a food, tamarind belongs to the legume family, which might trigger allergic reactions in certain people. If you have diabetes, you should take tamarind with care since it might drop blood sugar levels. When ingested in excessive numbers, it can also have a laxative effect.

YARROW

Description of the herb

Yarrow consists of 115 perennial plants in the Achillea genus of the Asteraceae family endemic to the North Temperate Zone. Their leaves are serrated and typically beautifully cut, and they can be fragrant. Small white, pink or yellow flowers are frequently arranged in flat-topped clusters.

Some species are grown as ornamentals in gardens. For example, Sneezewort (A. ptarmica) dried leaves are being used to manufacture sneezing powder. In contrast, yarrow or milfoil (A. millefolium) portions have been used for tea and snuff.

Benefits

For thousands of years, yarrow has been utilized for its possible health advantages. In reality, the genus name Achillea refers to the Greek warrior Achilles, who employed yarrow to cure the wounds of his warriors.

- Yarrow leaf extracts and ointments have been used to aid wound healing.

- Yarrow in animals has various digestive advantages, including treating ulcers and IBS symptoms.

- Flavonoids and alkaloids found in yarrow may help to alleviate sadness and anxiety symptoms.

- According to research, yarrow may help with epilepsy, multiple sclerosis, Alzheimer's disease, and Parkinson's disease symptoms.

- Although there is some evidence that yarrow might help with liver and skin inflammation, more study is needed.

Dosage and How to use it

- Simply place 1-2 teaspoons of dried yarrow flowers in a teapot.

- Simply place 1-2 teaspoons of dried yarrow flowers in a teapot.

- You may acquire a box of freshly dried yarrow at our Wild Store today if you wish to reward yourself.

Possible side effects/ drugs interaction

Yarrow is generally considered to be safe for most people. However, if you have a bleeding condition, are pregnant, nursing, have surgery, or are allergic to ragweed, you should avoid it.

YELLOW DOCK

Description of the herb

Yellow dock is a tiny, leafy plant that thrives worldwide. It is a member of the Polygonaceae family, which includes buckwheat. Its popular name is derived from its yellowish-brown roots. The roots are 8-12 inches (20-30 cm) long, 0.5 inches (1.27 cm) thick, meaty, and not forked. The stem can grow 1-3 feet tall (0.3-0.9 meters). Because of its long lance-shaped leaves that are somewhat ruffled along their margins, the yellow dock is also called a curly or curled dock. Its leaves are edible, and both the roots and leaves are utilized to make herbal treatments. Rhubarb and sorrel have a lot in common with yellow dock.

Benefits

- Yellow dock is most commonly used to treat digestive issues, liver illnesses, and skin conditions. Alterative, cholagogue, astringent, hepatic, laxative, and nourishing have all been used to characterize it.

- Anthraquinone glycosides, potent laxatives in greater dosages, are found in modest levels in the yellow dock. Yellow dock, on the other hand, is used as a mild laxative since it contains just trace levels of these compounds. Yellow dock is also known as a hepatic tonic since it is utilized to strengthen and restore liver function.

- Yellow dock is used to cure skin cuts, swelling, boils, rashes, burns, bleeding hemorrhoids, dog and bug bites, and wounds as an antiseptic and astringent. The usage of yellow dock as a skin remedy is illustrated by an ancient British charm that was sung when the dock was applied to skin irritations caused by stinging nettle: "Nettle out, dock in, dock removes the nettle sting."

- Internally, yellow dock treats psoriasis, acne, acne, poison ivy, and other rashes. It is typically used with other herbs, including red clover, cleavers, dandelion root, and burdock.

- Yellow dock is also used to treat problems with the liver and gallbladder. In addition, it is termed a cholagogue since it is supposed to boost bile and digestive fluid production.

- Vitamin C, calcium, iron, and phosphorus are all found in the yellow dock, making it healthy. It even has enough tannin to be used in leather tanning.

- Roots and leaves are utilized for external applications. For example, it's possible to pound the root and use it as a poultice. Old skin irritations are treated using fresh leaves and stems. By boiling the root in vinegar, an ointment is usually made.

Dosage and How to use it

Yellow dock's roots and leaves are both utilized in herbal medicines. Yellow dock is seldom used alone but in combination with other herbal treatments due to its moderate and widespread action. The roots are excavated between August and October in late summer and fall. Before drying, they are thoroughly cleaned and split lengthwise. The roots are crushed and used to make ointments, decoctions, tinctures or teas. The ground root should be kept cold and dry but not frozen.

- Boil 1-2 tsp (5-10 g) yellow dock root in 500 mL (2 cups) water for 10 minutes to make tea.
- Boiling 0.5 pounds of crushed root in a pint of sugar yields syrup.

Commercially accessible dried extracts of yellow dock are also available as tablets or capsules.

Possible side effects/ drugs interaction

- The yellow dock should not be used by pregnant or lactating women, babies, or children under six as no safe dosage has been found. In addition, the yellow dock should not be taken by anybody who has a persistent gastrointestinal ailment such as duodenal ulcers, spastic colitis, esophageal reflux, diverticulosis, or diverticulitis.

- The yellow dock should not be used by anybody who has had kidney stones before since the tannins and oxalates may worsen the problem.

CANAFISTULA

Description of the herb

Canafistula is a moderate-sized deciduous tree that grows to a height of around 9 meters. Compound leaves have 4-8 pairs of opposing leaflets. It bears golden-yellow flowers that hang in showering clusters up to 40 cm long. Thus, it has the nickname "golden shower tree." Butterflies and bees love the flowers, which come while the branches are naked and shortly before the new leaves sprout. Following the flowers, the tree produces two-foot-long, cylindrical, dark brown woody seed pods that stay on the tree all winter before falling to cover the ground. Each flower has five petals of similar shape and size and measures 4-7 cm in diameter. The fruit is a 30-60 cm long, 1.5-2.5 cm wide legume with a strong odor and many seeds. The tree's wood is robust and utilized in building construction.

Benefits

- Many Cassia species are employed in herbal medicine systems across the world. This specific plant family is well-known for its laxative properties. It is frequently used as a highly efficient mild laxative that's also safe for kids.

- Canafistula is also used to treat abdominal, liver, glandular, stomach, and throat tumors and burns, constipation, cancer, convulsions, delirium, dysuria, diarrhea, epilepsy, gravel, pimples hematuria, and epithelial tumors.

- The seeds are used for adenopathy, burning feelings, leprosy, skin illnesses, syphilis, and tubercular glands in Ayurvedic medicinal systems. In contrast, the root is used for adenopathy, burning pains, leprosy, skin disorders, syphilis, and tubercular glands. Erysipelas, rheumatism, malaria and ulcers are all treated with the leaves. The seeds are used as a laxative in Brazilian herbal medicine. At the same time, the leaves and/or bark treat pain and inflammation.

- Eating the fruit pulp might assist you in passing stools if you have clogs in your gut. In addition, it cures constipation and eases the passage. The fragile leaves can also be cooked and consumed like a leafy vegetable.

- Cassia fistula is used for its skin-soothing properties. Make a paste out of the fragile leaves and put it to infected areas, eczema, ringworm, or breakouts on the skin. This will provide you with relief and allow you to get rid of the skin problem in a short period.

- Chronic cough symptoms can be relieved by a preparation produced from the fruit pulp of the cassia fistula tree. Combine the fruit pulp and a few tablespoons of ghee in a bowl. For two weeks, drink this in the morning and at night. Your cough will go. Bronchitis sufferers might relieve their symptoms by mixing the fruit paste with plant-based milk.

Combine 5 g of fruit pulp, sugar, and water in a mixing bowl. This should be consumed after your daily meal.

Possible side effects/ drugs interaction

However, the leaves and bark can produce vomiting, nausea, stomach discomfort, and cramping in big dosages.

CHANCA PIEDRA

Description of the herb

Chanca Piedra is a tropical plant that thrives in tropical environments such as South America's jungles. Phyllanthus niruri is its scientific name. The plant may reach a height of approximately 2 feet (61 cm) and has thin, leaf-covered branches. Its seedpods, which develop into little green flowers, grow underneath the leaves, earning the moniker "seed-under-leaf."

Chanca piedra supplements are made from the entire plant, including the leaves, flowers and stems.

Benefits

- Chanca piedra is famous for its capacity to dissolve kidney stones; thus, I have been given the name "stone breaker."

- Because the plant is alkaline, it may aid in the prevention of acidic kidney stones. It's an over-the-counter, less-priced alternative to prescription potassium citrate, an alkalizing chemical often used to avoid acidic kidney stones. It may also assist you in urinating more frequently.

- In test-tube trials, chanca piedra extract could destroy the Helicobacter pylori bacteria that causes stomach ulcers. However, this does not imply that an oral supplement is helpful against stomach ulcers for humans.

- The antioxidants in chanca piedra in animals enhance fasting blood sugar levels and control blood sugar.

- The alkalizing qualities of chanca piedra may help prevent gallstones for the same reason they may aid with kidney stones. It's used to treat gallstones in several traditional medical methods.

- Gout flare-ups can develop when large uric acid accumulates in the blood. Chanca piedra may assist in bringing these levels back into balance and avoid gout episodes.

- Chanca piedra's antioxidant presence may aid enhance liver function and prevent the liver from cellular damage caused by free radicals, which are unstable chemicals that may cause harm when they pile up in high concentrations in the body.

- Hepatitis B appears to be helped by the plant.

- According to certain animal studies, chanca piedra may help relax blood arteries, potentially lowering blood pressure.

Dosage and How to use it

- Bring 3 cups of water to a boil on the stove to create chanca piedra tea.

- Place 1 tablespoon of chanca piedra tea leaves in a teapot or infuser.

- Allow for 15 minutes of steeping time after pouring boiling water over the tea leaves. After that, tea leaves should be strained and served hot.

To treat an urgent problem with kidney stones, drink 1 cup 2-3 times a day.

Possible side effects/ drugs interaction

Cancha Piedra may cause abdominal pain, painful urination, blood in the urine, and nausea.

CHICKWEED

Description of the herb

Chickweed refers to two types of small-leaved pink plants (Caryophyllaceae). Chickweed flowers are inconspicuous yet delicate, white, and star-shaped in both species.

The common chickweed (Stellaria media), sometimes known as stitchwort, is a native of Europe that has become widely naturalized. It generally grows to a height of 45 cm (18 inches), but it is a low-growing, spreading annual weed on cut lawns. It's a vegetable that may be eaten raw or cooked, and it's frequently used in salads. It may also be used as a canary meal.

Benefits

- Chickweed might aid with phlegm accumulation if you're feeling crummy.

- According to one study, using entire chickweed as a plaster over swollen regions or even shattered bones has anti-irritation, anti-inflammatory, and relaxing benefits.

- Another study found that when the entire plant is used to treat irritated skin, joints, and respiratory disorders like bronchitis, it helps reduce inflammation.

- Chickweed has antibacterial properties and may aid in healing wounds and illnesses. It has been used in traditional Chinese medicine for ages, notably for skin problems and dermatitis.

- Chickweed has been used for centuries to treat various ailments, including lowering inflammation and combating infections. It may also help you maintain your weight and function as an expectorant if you're unwell.

Dosage and How to use it

- Chickweed leaves may be steeped in hot water to form a tea that may help with pain relief, inflammation reduction, and relaxation.

- To create your own chickweed tea, combine 1 1/2 cups (300 g) of chickweed leaves with 3 cups (710 mL) water and simmer for 10 minutes over medium heat. Remove the leaves and savor. Consume a cup every 2–3 hours.

Possible side effects/ drugs interaction

- Excessive use of chickweed can result in nausea, stomach distress, diarrhea, and vomiting. Furthermore, the plant has a significant amount of saponins, which might cause gastrointestinal trouble in certain people.

- Chickweed has also been known to induce a rash when applied directly to the skin; however, this might be related to an allergy.

- Furthermore, there is little proof that chickweed is safe for children or pregnant or breastfeeding women; thus, these groups should avoid it to avoid negative consequences.

FEVERFEW

Description of the herb

Feverfew (Tanacetum parthenium L.) is a plant that originated in the Balkan Peninsula. It is currently found in Australia, China, Europe, Japan, and North Africa. The plant was first brought to the United States in the mid-nineteenth century. Across eastern Canada, Maryland, westward and Missouri, the plant thrives along roadsides, waste areas, fields, and the edges of wooded regions.

Benefits

- Feverfew is a plant traditionally used to cure fevers, rheumatoid arthritis, migraine headaches, stomach pains, toothaches, bug bites, infertility, and issues with menstruation and delivery.

- The feverfew plant has been used in traditional and folk medicine for centuries, particularly by Greek and early European herbalists. Psoriasis, asthma, allergies, tinnitus, dizziness, vomiting, and nausea have all been treated with feverfew. This plant includes a variety of natural compounds. Still, the active components are most likely one or more of the sesquiterpene lactones, such as parthenolide, that are known to be present.

- It has various medicinal characteristics, including anticancer, anti-inflammatory, antispasmodic, cardiotonic, emmenagogue, and worm enema. The plant is extensively cultivated in many parts of the world. Its prominence as a medicinal plant is developing rapidly as more and more evidence of its numerous therapeutic applications emerges.

- The herb has been used to heal several ailments throughout Central and South America. It is highly valued by the Kallaway Indians of the Andes Mountains for treating colic, renal discomfort, morning sickness, and stomach ache. An infusion of the plant is used in Costa Rica to help digestion, as a cardiotonic, a worm enema, and an emmenagogue. It's used as an antispasmodic and a tonic to control menstruation in Mexico. It is used to cure earaches in Venezuela.

- The leaves are eaten dried or fresh, with a daily intake of 2–3 leaves being normal. Before intake, the harshness is sometimes sweetened. For its powerful, long-lasting odor, feverfew has been planted around dwellings to purify the air. A tincture of its flowers is used as a balm for insect bites and insect repellent. In addition, it is being utilized as an antidote for opium overdose.

- Feverfew is also a powerful antioxidant, protecting the body from free radical damage.

- It helps relieve joint pain by avoiding the degradation of the bone lining. This decreases friction between the ends of two bones at the point where they combine to create a joint, perhaps providing long-term comfort for arthritis sufferers.

Dosage and How to use it

Boil the root for 30 minutes to an hour. Then, strain the tea and drink it twice a day. This will relieve joint pain.

Possible side effects/ drugs interaction

- There have been no significant negative effects associated with the usage of feverfew. However, nausea, digestive issues, and bloating are possible side effects.

- Chewing the raw leaves can cause mouth ulcers and discomfort.

- Feverfew can cause allergic responses in those allergic to ragweed and similar plants.

MIMOSA PUDICA

Description of the herb

Mimosa pudica is a prostrate creeper with reddish-brown cylindric stems and spiky leaves. When a Mimosa pudica plant is touched, the leaflets and pinnae fold swiftly, and the petiole attachment droops downward. The leaves droop at night and when revealed to rain or extreme heat. This reaction might be a defense against herbivorous insects, desiccation, or nutrient leaching.

Mimosa pudica develops a thick ground cover that prevents other species from reproducing. As a result, it has become a weed in many tropical places in corn, tomato, and soybean fields. It's especially difficult to weeding by hand, as the thorns can create severe wounds. In pastures, on the other hand, it is tolerated or appreciated as a feed plant.

Benefits

In the old period, Ayurveda, a holistic medical system in India, used this fern-like plant. Ayurvedic practitioners have utilized Mimosa pudica for various diseases, including mood problems and wound healing.

- The enzymes responsible for breaking down mucilage and other forms of fiber are lacking in your digestive tract. For example, Mimosa pudica mucilage passes all the way through your intestines, doing its cleansing action because it isn't digested.

- Mimosa pudica seed catches parasites in the gut and excretes them in the stool.

- Neurotransmitters, also known as nerve messengers, are produced in your gut and assist in regulating your mood. As a result, something like Mimosa pudica seed, which supports intestinal health, may be able to help you with your mental health.

- Mimosa pudica seed can help you get gut health and emotions back on track by focusing on gut restoration and parasite cleansing.

- Phytochemicals and vitamins having antioxidant effects are found in Mimosa pudica. Superoxide dismutase is present. This is a strong antioxidant also contained in the body's cells. Its levels, however, decrease as you become older.

- Mimosa pudica extract may be an effective treatment for sciatica.

- The bacteria that causes Lyme disease can hide in the liver. In addition, parasites including liver flukes, Ascaris lumbricoides, and other worms can also lurk in the liver/bile duct system. These organisms can cause inflammation by clogging the system. Mimosa pudica helps protect the liver from harm, particularly when overburdened with pollutants.

- The microscopic organisms make up the microbiome found throughout your body. Some of these are quite important for health and well-being. Unfortunately, others can damage you, particularly if they dominate the "good" microorganisms or upset the microbiome's compositional balance. Mimosa pudica can help defend against infection and disease caused by "bad" bacteria.

- The antibacterial effect of Mimosa pudica is assumed to be related to its high concentration of phytochemicals, flavonoids, tannins, alkaloids, and glycosides are among them.

- It's also common to apply a warm paste from the plant's leaves to pus-filled, inflamed skin, such as boils. It is claimed to aid in breaking the boil and the discharge of the pus. T

Dosage and How to use it

- Make a powder out of the leaves

- You can drink a teaspoon of root and leaf powder with water or plant-based milk three times daily.

Possible side effects/ drugs interaction

Pregnant or breastfeeding women should not consume it.

SANTA MARIA

Description of the herb

This cheerful blooming plant's vivid yellow or orange compact flowers make it easy to identify. Mexican marigold is a perennial that grows up to 30 inches tall in full light in the southern United States and Mexico. It's an annual in northern latitudes, and many people use it to put mosquitos away. It has a tarragon-like flavor, thus the moniker "Mexican tarragon."

Fresh leaves and flowers are used by herbalists.

Benefits

- Cough, colds, TB, asthma, and chronic bronchitis are all treated with it. It's also used to treat things like fever and dry mouth. In addition, it is used by some people to ease muscular spasms and remove phlegm.

- Santa herb is occasionally administered directly to the skin to treat bruises, cuts, sprains, bug bites, and joint discomfort.

- An extract of this plant is used as a flavor in meals and beverages.

- Santa is used in the pharmaceutical industry to disguise the harsh taste of certain medicines.

Dosage and How to use it

- A handful of flowers and leaves per 10 ounces of water is used to make Santa Maria's Person tea.

- Allow ten minutes for the tea to steep.

- Similarly, add two heaping teaspoons of pre-cut Santa Maria to 10 ounces of water when using pre-cut Santa Maria.

Possible side effects/ drugs interaction

- When consumed in proportions usually found in foods, this plant is LIKELY SAFE. However, there isn't enough credible evidence to tell whether it is safe in the doses found in medications or the potential adverse effects.

- There isn't enough credible information to say whether it is safe to consume while pregnant or nursing. To be safe, avoid using it.

WILD CHERRY BARK

Description of the herb

Although wild cherry and other types of cherry have been planted for many years for decorative purposes in Northern Ireland, it is not a very common tree.

Wild cherry is a large tree that grows in forests in alkaline soil. It tends to stay tiny since it is near the boundary of its native range. However, it grows quite a huge tree in warmer European nations and is commonly used for lumber. Though seeds (called stones) disseminate efficiently, it readily produces suckers (new trees emerging from their roots), making them comparable to aspen in this regard. The bark of a wild cherry tree is often reddish-brown and smooth. Horizontal bands may be present, which can peel off. Lenticels abound in the bark. These are tiny holes in the bark that allow cells beneath it to 'breathe.'

Benefits

- The wild cherry is a kind of plant. Medicine is made from its bark. Colds, bronchitis, whooping cough, and other lung issues are treated with wild cherry.

- It is also used in treating diarrhea, gout, pain, digestive disorders, and cancer.

- Because of its drying, sedative, expectorant, and cough-suppressing properties, it's also utilized in cough syrups.

- Wild cherry contains compounds that could decrease inflammation and have an astringent impact on the tissues.

Dosage and How to use it

- Coarsely grind the dried wild cherry bark.
- Put 1 teaspoon in a tea ball and steep it for 10 minutes in boiling water.
- To taste, adjust the sweetness.
- Drink 1 cup to relieve an unpleasant cough, up to 3x a day.

Possible side effects/ drugs interaction

- If you're pregnant or breastfeeding, it's probably not a good idea to eat the wild cherry. Prunasin, a toxin found in wild cherries, has been linked to birth abnormalities. There isn't enough information on the safety of using wild cherries when breastfeeding. To be on the safe side, avoid using it.

- Wild cherry bark is a powerful remedy that should only be taken for a limited time.

WORMWOOD

Description of the herb

Wormwood is a bitter or aromatic plant or shrub that belongs to the Artemisia genus of the Asteraceae family. It is found in many places of the world. Tiny, greenish-yellow flower heads are arranged in clusters on these plants. Green, greyish green, or silvery-white leaves are generally split and alternating along the stem.

The leaves of the most well-known species, common wormwood, have been utilized in medications and alcoholic drinks like absinthe. Common wormwood is a European native found in Canada and the United States. Another well-known species, tarragon, is used as a flavoring, while mugwort leaves are frequently used to flavor drinks.

Benefits

- Wormwood is a kind of plant. Medicine is made from above-ground plant components and oil.

- Wormwood is often used to treat various digestive issues, including appetite loss, stomach distress, gall bladder illness, and intestinal spasms. It is also used to cure fever, liver illness, depression, muscular discomfort, memory loss, and worm infections and produce perspiration and boost sexual desire. In addition, wormwood is used to treat Crohn's disease and IgA nephropathy, a kidney ailment.

- Wormwood oil is also used to treat digestive problems, stimulate imagination, and improve sexual desire.

- Some individuals apply wormwood simply to the skin for osteoarthritis (OA), wound healing, and bug bites. In addition, wormwood oil is a pain reliever that acts as a counterirritant.

- Wormwood oil is used to make soaps, cosmetics, and fragrances as a scent component. It's also used to kill insects.

-

Dosage and How to use it

Wormwood is most commonly consumed as a tea. Wormwood tea can be made with dried (not fresh) leaves.

- In one cup (250 mL) of boiling water, soak 1/2 to 1 teaspoon of dried wormwood leaves.

- Allow for five to ten minutes of steeping; the longer it steeps, the bitter the flavor becomes.

- To taste, add peppermint, lime juice or honey.

Possible side effects/ drugs interaction

- The chemical thujone found in wormwood oil stimulates the central nervous system. It can, however, result in seizures and other side effects.

- Wormwood is reasonably safe for people to utilize for two to four weeks. However, side effects can occur if you use it for four weeks or more and/or take more than the prescribed dose.

GOLDENSEAL

Description of the herb

Hydrastis Canadensis (Goldenseal) is a perennial herb endemic to eastern North America. Its leaves and roots have long been utilized in traditional medicine to treat various diseases, including infections and inflammation.

Goldenseal is now one of the most widely used herbal treatments globally. Colds, digestive disorders, hay fever, skin issues and sore gums are treated using herbal extracts, teas, or capsules derived from this plant.

Goldenseal is also found in feminine hygiene products, ear drops, flu and cold cures, eyewash formulations, allergy relief products, digestive aids, and laxatives, among other over-the-counter medications.

The herb is generally high in a group of alkaloid chemicals, with the greatest amounts of hydrastine, berberine, and canadine.

These alkaloids have antibacterial plus anti-inflammatory characteristics and are thought to be the primary cause for goldenseal's alleged health advantages.

Benefits

- The antibacterial and anti-inflammatory effects of goldenseal are well-known. As a result, it's commonly used to prevent or cure upper respiratory infections, as well as the common cold.

- It has been used to treat a lack of appetite, indigestion, skin conditions, sinus infections, painful/ heavy periods, and other digestive or inflammatory problems.

- Goldenseal is a famous natural remedy for the upper respiratory tract infections, such as the common cold.

- Goldenseal is frequently mixed with echinacea, including over-the-counter cold medicines or herbal coughs.

- Some people believe that goldenseal might aid in detoxifying the body from toxins and toxic chemicals.

- Goldenseal is a popular herbal therapy for urinary tract infections and yeast infections.

- Plants containing berberine, such as goldenseal, may benefit your skin.

- Goldenseal may aid in the prevention of tooth infections.

- Goldenseal extracts appear to be efficient against the C. jejuni bacteria, a common cause of gastroenteritis.

- The berberine within goldenseal has been shown in animal experiments to stimulate uterine contractions, which may help to induce labor.

- Individuals having type 2 diabetes may benefit from goldenseal.

Dosage and How to use it

- Goldenseal may also be made into a tea by dipping 2 teaspoons of your dry herb for 15 minutes into (240 mL) 1 cup of boiling water.

Dried root supplements ranging about 0.5–10 grams, three times per day.

Possible side effects/ drugs interaction

When used in the authorized doses for short periods, goldenseal is deemed safe.

- Nausea, vomiting and decreased liver function are all possible side effects

BOOK 10: <u>DR. SEBI'S BOOK OF REMEDIES</u>

DISCOVER THE SECRET COLLECTION OF DR. SEBI'S BEST HERBAL REMEDIES FOR COMMON AILMENTS AND CHRONIC CONDITIONS | HOW TO GROW, STORE AND PREPARE YOUR ALKALINE HEALING HERBS

Chapter 1: Acidic Body, Mucus Build-up and Diseases

What is Acidosis?

Consider an acid chemical for a second. What exactly does it do? Sulfuric acid, for example, is one of the most corrosive acids and will swiftly tear through skin, uncovering the layers beneath. It's one of the strongest and possibly hazardous acids ever discovered. If you get even a speck of it in your eyes, you'll receive significant burns and may lose your vision. Did you know that sulfur-containing amino acids found in animal proteins and wheat are both converted into sulfuric acid? Consider what an excess of acid may be doing inside your body—to your digestive system, to your cardiovascular system—if it can do that to your skin and eyes. Many of us have too much chronic acid, inflammation, and oxidation in our bodies, which is the same as rusting and decaying from the inside out. The buildup of toxins in the body, commonly known as acidosis, causes disease.

You'll want to pay close attention if you have low energy, pains and myalgia, digestive issues, acid reflux, inflammation, immune system issues or skin problems, or if you're having trouble losing those last few pounds, as we uncover the root cause of the chronic disease: over-acidity caused by poor choices in the way we eat, think, and move. Consuming sugar, cereals, excess animal proteins, dairy, artificial sweeteners, alcohol and GMO foods; quite so much tension; and chemical exposure and insecticides are a few examples of how the body is subjected to this type of trauma. Next, I'll explain why doing all of the "right things" for your health may not be working for you, and I'll give you a simple set of methods to help you turn your health around and reach your goals.

From Acid to Alkaline

While many of us are familiar with the word pH from other settings, such as the pH of a swimming pool, most of us are unaware of what it means when it comes to our bodies. The concentration of hydrogen ions in a substance or solution indicates how acidic or basic (alkaline) that substance is. pH stands for "potential of hydrogen," representing the concentration of hydrogen ions in a substance or solution indicates how acidic or basic (alkaline) that substance is. All medical physiology literature acknowledges the pH balance of the human bloodstream as one of the most important biochemical balances in all of human body chemistry.

"The control of hydrogen ion concentration is one of the most critical components of homeostasis," according to Guyton's Textbook of Medical Physiology. The pH scale goes from 0 to 14, with 0 being pure acid (imagine burning a hole in metal) and 14 being pure base—or totally alkaline (lime, for example, has a pH of 12.3 and is used to balance overly acidic soil). A pH of 7 is considered neutral. Higher values indicate that a substance is more alkaline in nature, with a larger ability to absorb hydrogen ions. The lower the value, the more acidic the environment is and the less opportunity for hydrogen ion absorption. When the human body's interior environment is somewhat alkaline, it flourishes

Similarly, when the body's environment gets toxic and acidic, it starts to have health issues. Everything in nature, in fact, is dependent on a perfect pH balance. The pH of the seas, for example, should be 8.2. Still, rising quantities of acidic carbon dioxide gas in the atmosphere have reduced it to 8.1. As a result, coral reefs off the coast of Australia, such as the Great Barrier Reef, are dying at unprecedented rates. Also, think about our soil. The minerals, nutrients, and alkalinity in our food have been degraded due to unnatural farming techniques like pesticide usage and genetic modification of our crops (GMOs).

Similarly, the use of synthetic fertilizers and rising quantities of acid rain have altered the structure of our soil, raising its pH. Plants perish when the pH range of soil is outside of 6–7. The human body, according to researchers, is reacting similarly to these bad conditions: we are getting more toxic and acidic, resulting in a dramatic increase in chronic illness rates. That simply goes to illustrate how critical pH is, but how many doctors are discussing it with you? The pH scale is logarithmic, which means it is exponential. For example, a material with a pH of 6 (carbonated water) is ten times more acidic than one with a pH of 7 (neutral), despite the difference being just 1.0 on the pH scale. A pH of 5 (black coffee) is ten times more acidic than a pH of 6 but a hundred times acidic than a pH of 7. (Neutral). And a pH of 4 (soda) is one thousand times more acidic than a pH of 3 (water). The pH of our bodies is critical because it regulates the rate at which our bodies' biological processes occur.

The pace of enzyme activity and the speed at which electricity travels through our bodies are affected by pH. The quality of your choices will, in the end, define the quality of your pH. To function effectively, different sections of your body require different pH values. For instance, the stomach pH should be between 1 and 3, the epidermis at 5.5, the large intestines around 8, saliva between 6.5 and 7.4, and pancreatic chemicals between 7.5 and 8.8. However, these values are on a scale. Contemporary dietary and lifestyle choices can cause pH levels to be more acidic than they should be, requiring the body's natural mechanisms to work considerably more to maintain optimal pH levels.

You may think of your pH as a thermostat. Isn't it true that if you're stuck on an iceberg, your body will have to work hard to keep a temperature of 98.6°F? Your body would shiver and use a tremendous amount of energy to generate heat, and your blood would flow from your hands and feet to your vital organs. Why? To keep you alive! However, your body would soon be unable to

Maintain this temperature regulation, and you would be forced to leave the iceberg to survive. The pH of your body is the same way. Consider this: if you monitor the pH in a pool and find that it isn't in the ideal range, you simply add chemicals to the pool water to bring it back into balance. Otherwise, it will devolve into a bacterial-infested quagmire. Diseases thrive in an overly acidic bodily environment. You must restore equilibrium if you want to get rid of all the nasty stuff in your system. Here's another illustration: What happens when there's still water in a stagnant pond? Mosquitoes. You can apply pesticides to kill mosquitoes, but they will return if the pond remains stagnant. The mosquitoes will go if the pond is cleaned out and given healthy, flowing water. You are in the same boat. If you wish to restore your health, you must eliminate the toxins accumulated over time and provide your body with the nutrients it has been denied. That's all there is to it.

Diet Can Be the Cause

Many people consume a mostly acidic diet. When I say "acidic," I'm referring to a diet that creates hazardous acid salts as a result of digestion, which the body must work hard to expel. In fact, the average American diet is 80 percent acidic when it should be 80 percent alkaline. Sugar, cereals, dairy, animal protein, colas, carbonated drinks, numerous teas, and coffee all metabolize as harmful acids when consumed. Lactic acid is produced when you ingest sugar, for example. The sugar fructose, maybe the worst of all, produces uric acid (which contributes to gout, kidney issues, and even type 2 diabetes). Sulfuric acid is produced when grains, specifically wheat, are consumed. Tannic acid is abundant in teas and coffee. Acetic and lactic acid is produced by unhealthy lipids. Phosphoric acid is abundant in colas, and carbonated water—one of the most surprising acidic suspects—will produce carbonic acid.

Sulfuric acid, phosphoric acid, and nitric acid are all hazardous acids that must be expelled quickly by your kidneys after eating steak. These acids are all exceedingly hazardous and will cause your pH to drop. These toxins are usually stored in adipose tissue, or fat cells, which function as buffers to protect your body from dangerous poisons. This will safeguard you in the near term. However, if the poisons are there for an extended length of time, they will erode your tissues and cause harm. Therefore, your body must work hard to clear them as rapidly as possible to avoid this. However, before your body can eliminate these acids, alkaline minerals must neutralize the toxins. This helps to keep them from causing more harm.

How Does Mucus Correlate to Disease?

Mucus is a gel-like substance secreted by the goblet cells of the human intestine. It is a protective barrier against bacteria and germs. It's excreted along with stool, but that's alarming if the stool has a greater mucus content. It signifies infection, inflammation and unhealthy gut. People with more mucus secretion usually have IBD, and this causes diarrhea or, at times, constipation. Not just

that, bloating and flatulence are also experienced by patients, and their lifestyle is greatly affected. In short, changes in mucus concentration are secondary to inflammation or disease.

The body's effort to remove acids causes an overabundance of mucus. Mucus, like cholesterol, is slippery and sticky, trapping acid and attempting to transport it out of the body. However, the mucus accumulates in the digestive tract over time, clogging the small and large intestines. Mucus is a vehicle for removing excess acids, and a cold is frequently nothing more than your body requiring you to stay in bed for a few days so it can clean house. Hippocrates was misquoted; in fact, he stated, "If you feed a cold, you must starve a fever."

To put it another way, if you have a cold, you should fast on water or juices to allow your body to rid itself of toxins. You will heal more quickly and completely if you do this. So the phrase "feed a cold, starve a fever" is incorrect.

Chapter 2: Harvesting, Dry, Preserving and Purchasing Herbs

Medicinal herb gardening typically starts with one of two questions: "What should I grow?" or "How do I know what to grow?" Then, "How can I make the most of the plants I already have?" Everyone enjoys a nice "top five" list of herbs to cultivate for optimal health. But you can guarantee that if every herbalist made a top-five list, it would be significantly different from one individual to the next. The fact is that the best herbs to cultivate for you will be determined by your health needs, growth

circumstances, and which plants you resonate with the most. You'll get so much more out of your own medicine garden if you interact with the plants in this way.

It's critical to demand high-quality, preferably organically cultivated herbs. Although these herbs are a few pennies more expensive, they are considerably better for our medications and, in the end, our world. Always have at least 2 ounces of the herbs you want to use on hand. Also, don't utilize endangered or threatened herbs in the wild, whether they're from this nation or another. When utilizing herbs today, it's vital that everyone takes responsibility for their origins and grows and harvests them. Many medicinal plants can attract pollinators and offer lovely colors to your home's landscaping, in addition to treating minor diseases in your household.

Focus on perennial plants to reduce the amount of gardening work you have to do each year. Echinacea, bee balm, catnip, and lavender are wonderful perennials to consider. If you suffer from migraines, feverfew should be included in your perennial herb garden. Prepare a growing space for your medicinal plants before bringing them home to ensure they stay healthy. Follow the planting directions to the letter, and

keep a watch on them for the first week after transplanting, as they may require additional water or shade until they settle in.

Planting, Care, and Maintenance

Herbs are the least picky of all the plants you can grow. Most of the plants in this book flourish in a lush, vegetable-worthy garden bed with rich, well-drained soil, consistent watering, and plenty of sunlight. However, they'll commonly put up with drier, poorer soils, partial shade, and other less desirable situations. Herbs will meet

you where you are, but by learning about each plant's preferred environment and caring for your soil ecology, you may make them happier. This method takes time, but it's not complicated or costly.

My husband and I bought a house near a state park thirteen years ago. For decades, the previous owner grew medicinal plants for personal use. Weeds abound (the sheep sorrel! the crabgrass!), acidic and sandy soil, hungry fauna, a short season, and restricted sun owing to the massive pine trees that ring the land have all been obstacles. It's been a delight to watch the soil structure — and the plants — improve over time by mulching, depositing manure (from friends' horses and my poultry), and gradually expanding the land with new beds each year. We never saw earthworms over those first several years. The herbs are thrilled that our garden beds are rich with excellent earth and crawling buddies.

Finding the Best Site for Your Plants:

Observation is the first step toward a good garden. Throughout the season, keep an eye on your property. Keep an eye on which plants grow there. (What's the difference between horsetail and jewelweed? There's a puddle there.) Where does the sunburn the earth, and where are the shady spots? In the winter, where does snow accumulate? What is the first site where it melts and vanishes? If you have a slope, you may expect drier, sandier, or rockier soil at the top and moist, rich soil at the bottom. Although various plants need different soil types — somewhat sandy, humus-rich — most plants will grow in well-drained, organic-rich soil. If you want to add amendments like lime, greensand, or blood meal, you should do a soil test to acquire a baseline; otherwise, you'll be flying blind and wasting money on goods you don't need. Contact your local extension office or organic land care organization for testing firms and recommendations.

Finally, keep an eye out for microclimates. Buildings, fences, and stone walls create cool shade or reflected light and heat microclimates. They also provide wind, light frost, and animal traffic protection. Make a note of your north-facing (dark), south-facing (sunny), and east/west-facing (part shade) locations. Consider growing the same plant in three different areas and seeing which flourishes the best.

Building Your Bed

You may follow my lead and construct beds utilizing the lazy lasagna gardening method regardless of your soil type. Choose the location and size of your garden

bed, as well as whether you'll frame it with wood, brick, stones, or other materials, or just edge it using a lawn edging tool. You'll need a proper bed for harvesting. Planting, Maintenance, and Care Herbs are the least picky of all the plants you can grow. Most of the plants in this book flourish in a lush, vegetable-worthy garden bed with rich, well-drained soil, consistent watering, and plenty of sunlight. However, they'll commonly put up with drier, poorer soils, partial shade, and other less desirable situations. Herbs will meet you where you are, but by learning about each plant's preferred environment and caring for your soil ecology, you may make them happier. This method takes time, but it is neither complicated nor costly.

Today is the day for planting! If possible, pick a drizzly spring day with rain in the forecast, or water your plants regularly after they've been planted. Hot, bright weather dries up young plants rapidly and destroys them and maintains them regularly — such as culinary herbs — don't make the bed too broad, as you'll want to be able to work it without walking in it. A breadth of three to four feet is generally sufficient. Build your bed in the fall, if

possible, so you can plant in the spring. This will allow the soil to settle and beneficial bacteria to take over.

However, if you're short on time, you may create and plant your beds on the same day.

• **Loosen the soil (optional):** Break up dense dirt with a broad fork without overworking it. This stage is optional, but it produces higher-quality soil penetrating deeper into the earth.

• **Cardboard or newspaper base:** Lay flattened cardboard boxes (not really organic due to glue but incredibly effective and cheaply accessible) or several layers of damp black-and-white newspaper over the area. This smothers grass and most weeds, and after the bed has established, it ultimately decomposes into the soil.

• **Edge or frame it:** Cut a perimeter around your bed using your edger tool, or place/build your bed frame. If a stone isn't an option, untreated pine planks are simple and inexpensive, lasting 5 to 10 years in our yard. Use 2 inches thick and 6 to 8-inch broad planks. Cedar is more expensive, but it lasts longer. (Pressure-treated wood lasts longer, but it leeches toxins into the soil.)

• **Fill it:** Begin with a thick covering of leaves or straw, as well as twigs and short branches (for drainage). Then mix in some loam and compost. If you have enough room and material, continue stacking in this manner until the bed is completely covered. For the top layer, use compost coated with leaf mulch. Over time, the dirt will settle.

• **Plant it:** Pull aside the mulch and dig a hole slightly larger than the plant when you're ready to plant your seedlings. Remove the plant from its pot gently, and if the roots are entangled, unwind them. Fill in the hole with dirt and carefully push down the earth around the plant, flush with the soil line. Make a tiny depression in the soil to assist catch water if needed (or raise it up a bit in waterlogged areas). Water well and mulch the area. Keep an eye on newly planted seedlings and water them as needed until they establish themselves. Plant when there is a chance of mild rain, if feasible (as opposed to the hot sun).

Most annuals and delicate perennials should be planted after the threat of frost have gone. Tender perennials are herbs that can only survive in warm areas all year and will frequently die if exposed to frost. If feasible, "harden off" young seedlings by exposing them to the elements for longer periods, or at the very least, wait until a week of moderate weather is predicted before planting.

Getting Supplies

Buy organic compost and loam by the truckload or square yard from landscape supply shops, or scavenge loam from another part of your yard (like the location where you've been throwing grass cuttings and leaves for years). You can get well-aged manure from your own animals or from nearby farms. Although horse dung contains more weed seeds, it is frequently accessible. As part of our soil improvement initiative, we introduced a small flock of hens to our property, and they've been fantastic. In the fall and winter, we cover the beds with coop shavings before covering them with leaf mulch. (Avoid harvesting crops in these beds for 90 to 120 days following treatment for safety reasons.) Grass clippings, garden garbage, and kitchen waste may all be composted.

Mulch

Mulch is a good buddy of yours! It inhibits weed growth, retains moisture, increases organic matter, improves drainage, feeds earthworms, and increases microbial and fungal variety in your soil. Yes, it may attract slugs and ticks and impede self-seeding herb activity, but the advantages exceed the dangers. Pine needles, wood

chips, newspaper, straw, grass clippings, sawdust, wool, leaves – leaves are by far my favorite — are all good options. Run them through a shredder or drive over them with the mower if it's possible. This prevents the leaves from suffocating the soil, speeds up their decomposition to enrich the soil, and permits perennials to emerge. Our lawn mower collects leaves in the bag, which we either throw in a mound or straight on the garden beds in the fall. Extra bags are obtained from friends and pupils. Ensure they're from yards that haven't been sprayed and have invasive seeds like bittersweet berries.

Excessive quantities of oak, hemlock, or chestnut leaves should be avoided. Wood chips are beneficial to forest plants and trees. Still, they take longer to decompose and temporarily deplete soil nitrogen (sprinkle some organic fertilizer or blood meal onto the area to offset the nitrogen loss). Every few years, when the road employees cut around the power lines, we get a truckload of free wood chips, which are great for my shrub and tree beds along the forest's border, as well as garden walking walkways.

Harvesting

Many rookie herbalists become anxious, unsure of what to do or when when when it comes to harvesting time. It's quite simple! Harvest, on the other hand, when the plant appears, smells, and tastes powerful, tasty, healthy, and vibrant. When it's "happy," in other words, aromatic herbs that are gathered early in the day have a higher taste. Harvest herbs after the dew have evaporated if you're going to dry them (and check the forecast if you're counting on warm, sunny weather for the dehydration process). Pick flowers as soon as they bloom. Roots and barks can be harvested in the spring or fall. That's the ideal situation, but you'll have to work it into your schedule. If that means you're out late at night with a headlamp excavating a root in mid-June or leaping at a frost warning, so be it!

Preserving Herbs - Drying

Now that you've gathered your herbs, it's time to put them to use! You may utilize those fresh herbs right away in a treatment mix like a tincture, or you can dry or store them for later use. If you haven't already, go over your plant material and eliminate anything that's buggy, dead, hitchhiking (living bugs, other plants), or otherwise unwanted before proceeding to the next stage.

Drying

Dry herbs may be used to make tea, cook, and make year-round remedies. It's inexpensive and simple to dry herbs, especially if you're unsure when or how you'll utilize them. In ideal storage circumstances, most dried herbs, flowers, and fruits last at least a year (page 30), with roots, bark, and mushrooms lasting much longer. They usually last a long time; most of what you buy online and in stores is already one to three years old. You may use dried herbs as long as they still look, smell, and taste well.

On the other hand, dried herbs may take up a lot of cupboard and closet space. Most herbs may be used fresh or dried, with a few exceptions. When dried, milky oat seed, St. John's wort, and motherwort are almost worthless; therefore, use them fresh whenever possible. Dried skullcap, lime balm, echinacea, California poppy, valerian, and rosemary can be used in recipes. Still, they won't be as powerful or effective as new versions. The dried herbs passionflower, calendula, lime verbena, limegrass, and linden are attractive. Still, they lose their strength faster than other dry herbs (in about 3 to 8 months). When drying these herbs, use particular caution.

Should I Wash My Herbs?

We seldom wash herbs, except for roots. This is because introducing water to dried herbs and various herbal medicines increases the danger of deterioration (glycerites, honey). Simply select reasonably free plants of dirt, pollen, animal dung, and contaminants, and reject any potentially hazardous items. If your plants are muddy, wash them with a hose before harvesting, then let them air dry before harvesting. If you have herbs that need to be washed, use cold water and a salad spinner to rinse them, then gently towel dry them before continuing with your processing. If you can remove the dirt with a clean, dry brush or cloth instead, do so. Coldwater should be used to cleanse the roots.

Drying Methods

Every herbalist will recommend a different "optimal" method for preparing dried herbs. Convenience, resources, space, environment, and the plant (and section) you're drying will all influence the best way for you. Drying flowers, roots, and berries in a single layer are recommended. Leave aerial portions on the stem; utilize complete flowers; full fruit or cut into smaller pieces; sliced mushrooms; and chopped roots. Once dried, certain mushrooms and roots are tough to slice. Your aim is to have plants that are completely crisp and dry. Any leftover moisture might ferment or destroy the plant in storage, especially problematic for flower heads and berries. Remove your plant as soon as it has dried to prepare and store it. If herbs are left out too long, they get dusty and less powerful.

Air-Drying

Herbs are dried in bundles by the rafters or over the woodstove in the renowned herbal kitchen. Tie a few stems together with thread or an elastic band, hang them from pegs, or lay them flat on screens, preferably out of direct sunlight in a well-ventilated, dry environment. It

takes a few days to a week or longer to air-dry leaves and blooms, as well as cut roots (if the air is dry enough). Use it to dry juicy herbs that become black when dried, such as basil and comfrey. If your air is dry, air-drying is a good option. If there's a lot of humidity, herbs won't get crisp-dry at room temperature. Start by air-drying the plants to remove most moisture before crisping them with a low-heat method.

Low-Heat Drying

Increase the heat and ventilation when the humidity rises to help your plants dry out. Depending on the plant and ambient humidity, most herbs' ideal maximum drying temperature is 95 to 110°F (35 to 43°C) (higher for fruit, roots, and mushrooms). Low-heat techniques dry herbs fast, resulting in higher-quality dried herbs than those that are air-dried for days or weeks. Every 6 to 24 hours, check on your plants and shift them about if certain sections are drying quicker than others. Commercial herb farmers employ drying sheds, shade cloth-covered hoop buildings, or tobacco trailers to dry herbs.

Storing Dried Herbs

The quality of your herbs is degraded by heat, light, air, and moisture. Dry herbs and shelf-stable treatments should be kept cold, dark, and dry, such as in a pantry or cupboard. The finest jars to use are glass jars with tight-fitting lids. Use a Mason jar vacuum sealer to extend the shelf life of herbs that won't be used for several months. This method isn't feasible if you plan to open the jar frequently.

Freezing

Freeze plants, especially culinary herbs like basil, chives, and limegrass stems, lose their flavor after drying. You may accomplish this in various ways, depending on the herb and how you wish to utilize it. Always identify your items, so you know what you're dealing with and how long they've been sitting around. Keep them as airtight as possible in thick, freezer-safe bags or containers. To avoid freezer burn, they should be consumed within a few months to a year.

Ice Cubes

In recipes, freeze chopped or puréed herbs in ice cube trays. Place chopped herbs in a tray and cover with water, broth, juice, or any other acceptable liquid,

depending on how you intend to utilize the herbs. Place the frozen cubes in a labeled bag or container. Any herb will suffice. This ingredient benefits smoothies, soups, sauces, and flowery ice cubes. Herbs can also be juiced or made into a slurry in water and then frozen. Tea and herb broths that have been concentrated freeze well.

Frozen Paste

Susan Belsinger, a culinary herbalist, taught me that oil seals in the taste and preserves herbs from degeneration in the freezer. Purée fresh greens in your favorite oil (olive oil, or something mild for baked goods). Fill a ziplock bag halfway with water, flatten it, and push out as much air as you can. Freeze in a balanced state. Then you can quickly extract a block of frozen herb oil from the freezer to use in soups, stews, sauces, and baked goods. Lime balm (for cake), basil (for pesto), cilantro (for salsa), curry paste, and parsley are all good choices.

Herb Butter

In melted butter, fold in finely chopped herbs. Shape, freeze, and store to use in cooking or on bread later. This herb benefits from chives, parsley, chervil, lime balm, and savory and sweet mixes.

Vacuum Seal

Chives and limegrass stalks, in particular, may be frozen in a bag or container and kept fresh for a long time. If you have an excess of herbs, vacuum sealing them will keep them fresher for longer, which works well for parsley but not so well for cilantro and basil (use immediately upon opening the bag). Because the cell walls of these delicate herbs break down in the freezer, making them mushy, they're best used in prepared foods.

Chapter 3: Alkaline Herbal Remedies for Common Ailments

Basic recipes, modest cooking utensils, and a well-stocked pharmacy of herbs can be used to cure common diseases. You'll discover a large range of beneficial cures here, whether you were stung by a bee while tending your tomatoes or hit by a flying baseball at your child's Little League game.

ACNE

When they become infected, Sebaceous glands produce painful pimples that are red and inflamed. While this is a disorder that mostly affects teenagers, it may also impact adults. Herbal medicines can help you look and feel better whether your acne is limited to your face or has extended to your chest, back, or other body regions.

REMEDY

Calendula Toner

<u>For making a half cup</u>

This basic toner contains calendula, which soothes irritation. It also has witch hazel that kills germs while relaxing your skin. This toner will last for at least a year if maintained in a cold, dark area.

- Two tablespoons calendula oil

- One third cup witch hazel

1. Combine the contents in a dark-colored glass container and gently shake. Apply 5 or 6 drops to your freshly cleaned face or any areas of concern with a cotton cosmetic pad. As required, add a bit more or less. Use twice a day till the acne clears up. If you want a chilly feeling, keep the bottle in the refrigerator.

Agrimony-Chamomile Gel

<u>For making a two-third cup</u>

Redness and irritation are reduced when agrimony and chamomile are mixed with aloe Vera gel. The gel should be kept in the refrigerator. It can stay fresh for up to two weeks if kept in an airtight container.

- Two teaspoons dried agrimony

- Two teaspoons dried chamomile

- Half cup water

- One fourth cup aloe Vera gel

1. Combine the agrimony and chamomile with the water in a saucepan. Over high heat, bring the mixture to a boil, then decrease the heat to low. Reduce the mixture by half, remove it from the heat and set it aside to cool completely.

2. Soak a piece of cheesecloth in water and lay it over the funnel's mouth. Pour the contents into a glass bowl using the funnel. Squeeze the liquid out of the herbs with the cheesecloth until there is no more liquid.

3. Blend the aloe vera gel into the liquid using a whisk. Fill a sterile glass jar halfway with the final gel. Refrigerate the container with the lid securely closed.

4. Apply a tiny coating to all afflicted areas using a cotton cosmetic pad twice daily.

Precautions

If you use blood thinners or are sensitive to plants in the ragweed family, leave out the chamomile.

ALLERGIES

Allergies are immunological reactions to a common material such as cat dander, pollen, or dust that are abnormal. Food, beverages, and the environment contain allergens, making it impossible to avoid them entirely. However, herbal medicines are significantly milder than conventional treatments, which block your body's immunological reaction to allergens that impact you.

REMEDY

Feverfew-Peppermint Tincture

For making two cups

During an allergic attack, feverfew and peppermint open up the airways. If you can't have feverfew, create this tincture using only peppermint. The tincture will last up to 7 years in a cold, dark spot.

- Two ounces dried feverfew
- Six ounces dried peppermint
- Two cups unflavored
- Eighty-proof vodka

1. Combine the feverfew and peppermint in a sterilized pint jar.
2. Fill the jar all the way to the top with vodka.
3. Close the jar firmly and give it a good shake. Then, for 6 to 8 weeks, keep it in a cold, dark cabinet and shake it several times a week.
4. Soak a piece of cheesecloth in water and lay it over the funnel's mouth. Pour the tincture into another sterilized pint jar using the funnel. Remove the moisture from the herbs by wringing them out. Transfer the final tincture to dark-colored glass bottles after discarding the wasted herbs.
5. When allergy symptoms flare up, use 5 drops orally. If the flavor is too strong for you, dilute it with water or juice and consume it.

Precautions

If you are sensitive to ragweed, do not take feverfew. In addition, Feverfew should not be used during pregnancy.

ALOPECIA

It is typical to lose roughly 150 hairs every day, but certain pressures on the body might cause this number to rise. Alopecia is the medical term for hereditary hair loss. It affects males significantly more than women and is a common symptom of aging, beginning with a receding at the temples or forehead and progressing over time (though rarely ending in total baldness). Hair loss can also be caused by severe sickness, high fever, pregnancy and childbirth, shock, stress, skin damage (from burns, infection, radiation, or chemical harm), skin cancer, chemotherapy, vitamin A excess, hypothyroidism, and syphilis. Baldness, also known as alopecia, is the loss of all or some hair on the scalp. The condition may be transient or permanent. Pattern baldness is the most frequent kind of alopecia. This genetic characteristic affects more men than women due to the male hormone testosterone. Male pattern baldness progresses until only a sliver of hair grows back on the back and sides of the head. In the United States, up to 86 percent of males will develop some kind of pattern baldness.

Baldness in women frequently progresses until barely a sliver of hair remains over the head. An imbalance of sex hormones may play a role in premature baldness. Typhoid fever, the flu, pneumonia, or stress can cause sudden transient hair loss. Severe nutritional deficiencies, TB, cancer, and thyroid or pituitary gland diseases can cause hair loss over time. Exposure to nuclear radiation or X-rays and the internal use of some anticancer medications can induce temporary baldness.

REMEDY

Sage Tea

When sage tea is consumed and administered topically, it promotes hair growth.

- Two teaspoons dried sage or five or six fresh leaves

- One cup (235 ml) boiling water

- Juice of half lime

- Honey to taste

1. For at least 5 minutes in hot water, steep the sage.
2. Remove the sage leaves and mix with the lime juice and honey before drinking.

*Nettle tea aids in the cleansing of the system and promotes hair development.

ANXIETY

Anxiety is a fearful or apprehensive reaction to a threat or danger. It is a good, natural response since it permits the body to prepare itself (through adrenaline) to deal with the threat. However, anxiety can take over a person, resulting in anxiety neurosis. The individual is then considered to be in an anxious state. This might be chronic

anxiety, which is characterized by a continual sense of worry and is often linked to depression, or an acute anxiety attack. The person is abruptly overcome by panic and emotions of dread. When we are confronted with a terrifying or dangerous scenario, our bodies activate the "fight or flight" reaction, in which adrenaline floods the system and the body prepares for action. Physiological bewilderment, often known as a panic attack, occurs when no action is taken, and nervous energy is not expelled.

Dizziness, vision disturbances, clammy hands, racing heart, parched lips, and excessive breathing are all possible symptoms. Up to 70% of patients who suffer from panic attacks see up to ten doctors before receiving a proper diagnosis. Women tend to be affected twice as much as males regarding anxiety. In addition, there is evidence that certain persons are biochemically predisposed to panic episodes. According to the National Center for Health Statistics, anxiety disorder medications are among the top 20 most commonly prescribed pharmaceuticals. Research by the Royal College of Psychiatrists in the United Kingdom estimated that more than 9 million Britons might experience excessive worry and worries at some time in

Their life. Many psychiatric problems, such as phobias, panic attacks, obsessive-compulsive disorders, and post-traumatic stress disorder, include anxiety as a component.

REMEDY

Skullcap Tea

Equal parts of:

- Skullcap

- Linden Flowers

- Sage

1. Equal quantities of dried skullcap, linden blossoms, and sage leaf should be combined. Keep in a dark, airtight container.

2. Make a cup of boiling water with 1 teaspoon of the mixture and 1 teaspoon of the mixture. Drink one cup before exams or three cups every day while studying.

Precaution

Commercial remedies were discovered to include deadly germander a few years ago. Always get your herbs and herbal remedies from a trusted source.

ASTHMA

This chronic disease is characterized by inflammation throughout the lungs and restricted bronchial tubes. Asthma episodes may be terrifying, so some people have panic attacks when breathing becomes difficult.

REMEDY

Ginkgo-Thyme Tea

<u>For making one cup</u>

Ginkgo biloba and thyme widen your airways and relax your chest muscles, allowing you to breathe more easily. If you don't like the taste of this tea, you may improve it by adding a teaspoon of honey or dried peppermint to the mix.

- One cup boiling water

- One teaspoon dried Ginkgo Biloba

- One teaspoon dried thyme

1. Fill a large cup halfway with boiling water. Allow the tea to steep for 10 minutes after adding the dry herbs and covering the mug.

2. Relax and inhale the steam while gently drinking the tea. Repeat this process up to four times a day.

Precautions

If you're taking a monoamine oxidase inhibitor (MAOI) for depression, don't take it. Ginkgo biloba can take blood thinners to work better, so consult your doctor before taking it.

Peppermint-Rosemary Vapor Treatment

<u>For making one treatment</u>

Rosemary leaves contain important histamine-blocking oil, while peppermint helps expand your airways and aid breathing. Suppose you don't have any fresh herbs on hand. In that case, two drops of peppermint essential oil and four drops of rosemary essential oil can be substituted.

- Four cups steaming-hot water (not boiling)

- Half cup crushed fresh peppermint leaves

- Half cup finely chopped fresh rosemary leaves

1. Combine all of the ingredients in a large, shallow bowl. Place the bowl on a table and comfortably take a seat in front of it. Cover your head and the bowl with a large cloth. Inhale the fumes released by the plants.

2. As required, get some fresh air and cover your eyes if the fumes are too powerful. Continue to treat the water until it has cooled.

3. When asthma symptoms begin, repeat as required. This therapy is mild enough that you can use it as frequently as you like.

Precautions

If you are epileptic, stay away from rosemary. Stronger oils, such as rosemary, fennel, sage, eucalyptus, hyssop, camphor, and spike lavender, have been known to produce seizures.

ANEMIA

The lack of hemoglobin in the red blood cells, which is the molecule that transports oxygen, is called anemia. Iron deficiency, which can be caused by trauma, surgery, delivery, severe monthly bleeding, a poor diet, or a failure to absorb iron from meals, is the commonest cause of anemia. Anemia can also be caused by excessive red blood cell breakdown (hemolytic anemia), vitamin B12 deficiency (pernicious anemia), and gecausenetic illnesses such as sickle cell anemia and thalassemia. Women account for 20% of all victims, while children account for 50%. Iron deficiency anemia is the most prevalent kind of anemia caused by continuous blood loss, not just that, a shortage of iron in the diet, decreased iron absorption from the gut, or an increased requirement for iron, such as during pregnancy. Iron is a necessary component of hemoglobin, which, in chemical interaction with its iron atoms, transports oxygen to the tissues.

Pernicious anemia is a chronic hereditary condition in which the stomach fails to generate a component necessary for the absorption of vitamin B12, which is required to mature adult red blood cells. In addition, the lack of bone marrow cells to produce mature red cells causes aplastic anemia. Toxic substances (benzene) or radiation are the most common causes.

REMEDY

Chinese Angelica Root

1. Cut the stems into one in. (2.5cm) lengths and cook until tender in sugar water. Strain. Simmer for an hour in a sugar syrup (2 cups [500g] sugar in 1 cup [250ml] water).

2. Allow drying after straining. Dust with powdered sugar and keep in an airtight container.

3. Every few hours, apply a 2in. (5cm) strip.

*Alfalfa, dandelion root, nettles, watercress, and yellow dock are rich in iron.

AGING

Wrinkles are a ubiquitous indicator of age and are significantly easier to avoid than remove. Herbs, like cosmetics, won't suddenly eliminate your crow's feet and fine wrinkles; they can, however, help you obtain naturally smoother skin.

REMEDY

Calendula Toner

For making a half cup

This soothing toner hydrates and refreshes your skin profoundly. Calendula encourages new skin cells, resulting in a smoother complexion. When kept refrigerated, this toner can last up to a year.

- One third cup witch hazel

- Two tablespoons calendula oil

- Shake the contents together carefully in a dark-colored glass container. Apply 5 or 6 drops to your freshly cleansed face with a cotton cosmetic pad.

- As required, add a bit more or less. Repeat this process twice a day. Consider completing one treatment while getting ready for the day and the other while getting ready for bed.

1. Shake the contents together carefully in a dark-colored glass container. Then, apply 5 or 6 drops to your freshly cleansed face with a cotton cosmetic pad.

2. As required, add a bit more or less. Repeat this process twice a day. Consider completing one treatment while getting ready for the day and the other while getting ready for bed.

Aloe Gel Facial

For making one treatment

Aloe Vera gel hydrates the skin and replenishes dehydrated cells, minimizing fine lines and wrinkles. The second phase of this therapy, using coconut oil, helps the skin shed dead, dull cells faster, resulting in a smoother-looking complexion.

- One tablespoon aloe Vera gel

- One teaspoon coconut oil

1. After you've cleaned your face, apply the aloe Vera gel. Allow it to soak before applying the coconut oil. Using warm water, dampen a face towel.

2. Relax and cover your face with the handkerchief. Remove it after 2 minutes of being in place. Next, rinse your face with warm (not hot) water to remove any extra coconut oil.

3. Repeat four times per week.

BACK PAIN

While overwork or injury is the most common cause of back pain, it can also be caused by inactivity, muscular spasms, or inflammation. Rest as much as possible to let your body heal, and visit your doctor if the pain is severe or accompanied by numbness, tingling, or incontinence.

REMEDY

Passionflower–Blue Vervain Tea

Passionflower and blue vervain both calm the nervous system and relieve muscular pain. This is a wonderfully calming combination, so use it when you have an opportunity to relax.

For making one cup

- One cup boiling water

- One teaspoon dried passionflower

- One teaspoon dried blue vervain

1. Fill a large cup halfway with boiling water. Cover the mug with the dried herbs and steep the tea for 10 minutes.

2. Slowly sip the tea while you relax. Repetition is allowed up to two times each day.

Precautions

Passionflower and blue vervain should not be used during pregnancy. Also, if you have prostate issues or baldness, stay away from passionflower.

Ginger-Peppermint Salve

<u>For making one cup</u>

Potent elements in ginger and peppermint permeate the skin, causing a warming feeling that aids muscular relaxation. When stored in a cold, dark area, this salve will last for up to a year.

- One cup light olive oil

- One-ounce dried ginger root, chopped

- One ounce dried peppermint, crushed

- One ounce beeswax

1. Combine the olive oil, ginger, and peppermint in a slow cooker.

2. Set the slow cooker to the lowest heat setting, cover it, and let the herbs sit in the oil for 3 to 5 hours.

3. Allow the infused oil to cool after turning off the heat. In the base of a double boiler, bring about an inch of water to a simmer. Reduce the heat to a low setting.

4. Over the top part of the double boiler, drape a piece of cheesecloth. Pour the infused oil into the cheesecloth, then wring and twist it until no more oil comes out. Next, remove the cheesecloth and herbs that have been used.

5. Place the double boiler on the base and add the beeswax to the infused oil. Warm gently over low heat. Remove the pan from the heat after the beeswax has completely melted.

6. Pour the contents into clean, dry jars or tins as soon as possible, and set aside to cool fully before capping.

7. Treatment can be repeated up to four times per day.

Precautions

If you're on blood thinners, have gallbladder illness, or have a bleeding issue, don't use ginger.

BRONCHITIS

Bronchitis develops when the bronchial linings become inflamed due to irritation, infection, or allergies. A heavy, rasping cough is also a common symptom of the illness. When paired with increased fluid intake and lots of rest, Herbal therapies have been shown to help reduce and eliminate bronchitis symptoms.

REMEDY

Rosemary–Licorice Root Vapor for treating Bronchitis

<u>For making enough to treat once</u>

Rosemary and licorice roots expand the airways, increase circulation, and relieve the pain and inflammation associated with bronchitis.

- Five cups water

- Half cup fresh rosemary leaves

- One-fourth cup chopped dried licorice root

1. Combine the water and the dried licorice root in a saucepan. Bring the mixture to a boil, lower the heat to a low setting.

2. Cook for 10 minutes on low heat. Combine the water, licorice root, and rosemary leaves in a small dish. Cover your head and the bowl with a large cloth. Inhale the fumes released by the plants.

3. As required, get some fresh air and cover your eyes if the fumes are too powerful. Continue to treat the water until it has cooled. Then, as required, repeat the process. This therapy is mild enough that you can use it as frequently as you like.

Precautions

If you are epileptic, hypertensive, diabetic or have renal difficulties or cardiac disease, you should not use this therapy.

Goldenseal-Hyssop Syrup

<u>For making about two cups</u>

Hydrastine and berberine are two powerful antiviral and antibacterial compounds found in goldenseal. Hyssop relieves bronchial spasms and helps eliminate lung congestion while also providing a relaxing, soothing

effect. This syrup can also be used to treat a common cold. When refrigerated, it will last up to 6 months.

- One ounce dried hyssop

- Two cups water

- Half ounce dried goldenseal root, chopped

- One cup honey

1. Combine the goldenseal and hyssop with the water in a saucepan. Reduce the liquid by half by bringing it to a low simmer and partially covering it with a lid.

2. Fill a glass measuring cup halfway with the contents of the saucepan, then strain the mixture through a soaked piece of cheesecloth into the saucepan, wringing the fabric until no more liquid comes out.

3. Warm the mixture over low heat with the honey, stirring regularly until the temperature reaches 105°F to 110°F.

4. Fill a sterilized jar or bottle with the syrup and keep it in the refrigerator. Take 1 tablespoon three to five times a day, orally, until your symptoms go away.

Precautions

If you're pregnant or nursing, don't use it. If you have epilepsy or high blood pressure, avoid using this product. In addition, diarrhea and heartburn can be aggravated by goldenseal. Children under the age of 12 should take 1 teaspoon twice a day, two to three times a day.

BURN

Minor burns, such as those experienced during cooking, can be treated using herbal medicines. However, any burn that seems deep includes charred skin or covers a wide body area should be treated quickly.

REMEDY

Chickweed-Mullein Compress

For making one treatment

Mullein's antibacterial and anti-inflammatory effects assist in keeping burns from becoming infected, while it's cooling and astringent characteristics aid in relieving pain. Chickweed adds to the cooling effect and aids in the healing process.

- Two teaspoons finely chopped chickweed

- One teaspoon finely chopped fresh mullein leaf

1. Cover the burn and surrounding region with the freshly cut plant stuff and a soft towel. Allow 10 to 15 minutes for the poultice to dry.

2. Use every 2 to 3 hours, or as needed, until the discomfort is gone.

Fresh Aloe Vera Gel

For making one treatment:

Antibacterial chemicals in aloe Vera gel help prevent burns from becoming infected, and it also has anti-inflammatory properties. In addition, because aloe promotes collagen synthesis, the skin regenerates more quickly after mild burns. While fresh aloe gel from the plant is best, bottled aloe gel can suffice in a pinch.

1. Aloe vera is a kind of plant. Using the tip of an aloe vera leaf, cut a 1-inch slice. The rest of the leaf should be left on the plant to continue to grow.

2. Slit the leaf open with a sharp knife. Scoop the gel from the center of the loaf with your fingertips or a cotton cosmetic pad and apply it to the burn and the surrounding area. While your burn heals, repeat once or twice a day.

COLD

Coughing, sneezing, and a sore throat are just some of the symptoms of a common cold. Begin therapy as soon as symptoms occur to shorten the length of your cold.

REMEDY

Thyme Tea

For making one cup

Thyme is an antitussive, or cough suppressor, that relieves coughing immediately. It also serves as an expectorant, which helps relieve congestion from the lungs. It also helps ease the agony of a sore throat and the body aches of a cold. Add a spoonful of honey to the tea if you like a sweeter flavor.

- One cup boiling water

- Two teaspoons dried thyme

1. Fill a large cup halfway with boiling water. Allow the tea to steep for 10 minutes after adding the thyme and covering the mug. Relax and inhale the steam while gently drinking the tea.
2. Repetition is allowed up to six times per day.

Herbal Cold Syrup with Comfrey, Mullein, and Raspberry Leaf

For making two cups

Coughs and sore throats are relieved by comfrey. In contrast, mullein, thyme, and raspberry leaf relieve fever, body pains, and lung irritation. If you're missing one or two of the herbs in this recipe, don't panic; they're all healthful and can help you get rid of your cold symptoms. When refrigerated, this syrup can last up to 6 months.

- Half ounce dried comfrey

- Half ounce dried raspberry leaf

- Half ounce dried mullein

- Two cups water

- Half ounce dried thyme

- One cup honey

1. Combine the herbs and water in a saucepan. Reduce the liquid by half by bringing it to a low simmer and partially covering it with a lid.

2. Fill a glass measuring cup halfway with the contents of the saucepan, then strain the mixture through a soaked piece of cheesecloth into the saucepan, wringing the fabric until no more liquid comes out.

3. Warm the mixture over low heat with the honey, stirring regularly until the temperature reaches 105°F to 110°F. Fill a sterilized jar or bottle with the syrup and keep it in the refrigerator.

4. Take 1 tablespoon three or four times a day, orally, until your symptoms go away. Children under the age of 12 should take 1 teaspoon twice or three times a day.

Precautions

Fresh raspberry leaves might cause nausea, so never use them if they aren't entirely dry.

COUGH

Coughing is a natural way for the body to get rid of irritants and extra mucus from the lungs and airways. However, if an uncomfortable itch in your throat persists, it might develop into a dry, hacking, and ineffective cough. While you treat the underlying problem, herbal therapies can help calm sore throat tissues.

REMEDY

Fennel-Hyssop Tea

<u>For making one cup</u>

Fennel helps coughs become more productive by loosening mucus. So if you're suffering from throat irritation and a non-productive cough, this tea will bring immediate relief.

- One cup boiling water

- One teaspoon of fennel seeds

- One teaspoon dried hyssop

1. Fill a large cup halfway with boiling water. Let the tea steep for ten minutes after adding the herbs and covering the mug.

2. Calm down and inhale the steam while gently drinking the tea.

3. Repeat this process four to 4 times a day.

Precautions

Don't consume hyssop during pregnancy or if you are epileptic.

Licorice-Thyme Syrup

For making about two cups

Licorice root is an anti-inflammatory that soothes sensitive tissue in the throat rapidly. At the same time, thyme is an expectorant that clears the lungs. Thyme is also an antitussive, which helps relieve coughing spasms. When kept refrigerated, this cough syrup lasts for 6 months. Licorice root is an anti-inflammatory that soothes sensitive tissue in the throat rapidly. At the same time, thyme is an expectorant that clears the lungs. Thyme is also an antitussive, which helps relieve coughing spasms. When kept refrigerated, this cough syrup lasts for 6 months.

- One ounce licorice root, chopped

- One ounce thyme

- Two cups water

- One cup honey

1. Combine the licorice root, thyme, and water in a saucepan. Reduce the liquid by half by bringing it to a low simmer and partially covering it with a lid.

2. Fill a glass measuring cup halfway with the contents of the saucepan, then strain the mixture through a soaked piece of cheesecloth into the saucepan, wringing the fabric until no more liquid comes out.

3. Warm the mixture over low heat with the honey, stirring regularly until the temperature reaches 105°F to 110°F.

4. Fill a sterilized jar or bottle with the syrup and keep it in the refrigerator.

5. Take 1 tablespoon three or four times a day, orally, until your symptoms go away. Children under the age of 12 should take 1 teaspoon twice or three times a day.

Precautions

Avoid licorice if you have high blood pressure, diabetes, renal difficulties, or heart disease.

CONSTIPATION

Constipation is characterized by abdominal discomfort and difficult bowel motions. Herbs are significantly less harsh on your system than harsh pharmaceutical laxatives and give great relief. Increase your fiber intake, drink plenty of water, and increase your physical activity to help things go along faster.

REMEDY

Aloe Vera Juice

For making about three cups

Aloe vera juice aids digestion and cleanses the gastrointestinal tract. It's ideal for treating persistent constipation because of this. Aloe juice should be taken within three days of making it.

- One fresh 3-to 4-inch aloe leaf from the inner portion of the plant

- Three cups fresh juice, water, or coconut water

1. Hold the aloe leaf over the sink upside down so that the resin drains away from the cut. Cut the leaf in half lengthwise once the glue has stopped leaking, and carefully scoop out the gel from the interior.

2. Fill a blender halfway with liquid and add the gel. Blend until smooth, then chill before serving.

3. Drink 1 cup every day and keep the leftovers in a firmly closed container or jar in the refrigerator.

Precautions

If you're pregnant or nursing, avoid taking aloe internally.

Dandelion-Chickweed Syrup

For making about two cups

Dandelion and chickweed are both mild laxatives that relieve constipation without harsh medications. Both of these plants may be found in your own backyard; just be sure they haven't

been polluted with herbicides or chemical fertilizers. When refrigerated, this syrup can last up to 6 months.

- One ounce dandelion root, chopped

- One ounce fresh or dried chickweed

- Two cups water

- One cup honey

1. Combine the dandelion root, chickweed, and water in a saucepan. Reduce the liquid by half by bringing it to a low simmer and partially covering it with a lid. Fill a glass measuring cup halfway with the contents of the saucepan, then strain the mixture through a soaked piece of cheesecloth into the saucepan, wringing the fabric until no more liquid comes out.

2. Warm the mixture over low heat with the honey, stirring regularly until the temperature reaches 105°F to 110°F.

3. Fill a sterilized jar or bottle with the syrup and keep it in the refrigerator. Take 1 tablespoon three or four times a day, orally, until your symptoms go away. Children under the age of 12 should take 1 teaspoon twice or three times a day.

CELLULITE

Cellulite is distinguished by its orange peel appearance caused by fat accumulations beneath the skin. The thickened fat cells, fluids, and poisons cause an uneven look. It is significantly more common in women than in males, and it is assumed to be linked to female hormones. Poor circulation, alcohol, processed carbohydrates, and caffeine are all potential triggers since they contribute to the build-up of toxins in the body. Many physicians do not regard cellulite as a medical problem. However, environmental or nutritional toxins are frequently deposited as persistent, ugly fat. Exercising, cleaning your teeth, massaging your skin, and eating as many organic and less processed foods as possible may all help.

REMEDY

1. Take a cleaning drink with herbs like marigold and massage with juniper-infused oil.

2. Fresh ginger promotes circulation in the body; regularly consume an infusion or chew fresh ginger to treat the ailment.

3. Chewing juniper berries can help prevent and cure cellulite by purifying and detoxifying the body.

CRAMPS

The soreness and spasms accompanying cramped muscles can keep you awake at night and prevent moving properly. Herbs can help you relax and rest so that your body can recuperate. Consult your doctor if you get cramps or spasms regularly, as cramps and spasms might indicate an underlying medical issue.

REMEDY

Rosemary Liniment

For making a half cup

Rosemary increases circulation and has pain-relieving components. When you add rosemary essential oil to this

easy cure, it becomes much more powerful. It will keep for up to 7 years if kept in the refrigerator.

- Two tablespoons rosemary tincture

- One-third cup unflavored 80-proof vodka

- Twenty drops of rosemary essential oil (optional)

1. In a dark-colored glass jar, gently combine the components. Then, apply 5 to 10 drops to the confined region using a cotton cosmetic pad.

2. Add a little more or less as needed. If you suffer cramps or muscle spasms, repeat every hour.

Precautions

Don't consume rosemary if you are epileptic.

Ginger Salve

For making about one cup

Ginger promotes blood flow and has a warming impact that penetrates deep into the skin. Because of its anti-inflammatory and pain-relieving characteristics, it's a simple yet efficient way to treat muscular cramps.

- Two ounces dry or freeze-dried gingerroot, chopped

- One cup light olive oil

- One ounce beeswax

1. Combine the ginger and olive oil in a slow cooker. Set the slow cooker to the lowest heat setting, cover it, and soak the ginger in the oil for 3 to 5 hours.

2. Allow the infused oil to cool after turning off the heat. In the base of a double boiler, bring about an inch of water to a simmer. Reduce the heat to a low setting.

3. Cover the top of the double boiler with cheesecloth. Pour the infused oil into the cheesecloth, then wring and twist it until no more oil comes out. Next, remove the cheesecloth and herbs that have been used.

4. Place the double boiler on the base and add the beeswax to the infused oil. Warm gently over low heat. Remove the pan from the heat after the beeswax has completely melted.

5. Fill clean, dry jars or tins halfway with the salve and set aside to cool fully before capping. Massage a dime-size quantity into the tight region using your fingertips. When cramping is an issue, use a little more or less as needed, and repeat.

DIARRHEA

Food indiscretion frequently induces Diarrhea, although it can develop due to sickness. It's usually accompanied by slight stomach discomfort, and it goes away once the offending chemical has been expelled. Because diarrhea can induce dehydration, make sure to drink enough water. If your diarrhea is lengthy or regular, or if blood or mucus is present, get medical help.

REMEDY

Agrimony Tea

For making one cup

Agrimony is a mild astringent that helps halt diarrhea by reducing irritation in the digestive tract. It has a lovely citrus taste that most people enjoy. Consider preparing an additional cup of agrimony tea to use as a soothing gargle if you're suffering from diarrhea as a flu symptom and also have a sore throat.

- One cup boiling water
- Two teaspoons dried agrimony

1. Fill a large cup halfway with boiling water. Allow the tea to steep for 10 minutes after adding the dried agrimony.
2. Slowly sip the tea while you relax. While diarrhea is a concern, repeat up to four times each day.

Catnip–Raspberry Leaf Decoction

For making one quart

Mild astringents like catnip and raspberry leaf can help halt diarrhea. This is a fantastic cure if your diarrhea is accompanied by stomach cramps, as raspberry leaves can assist smooth muscle tissue in relaxing. When refrigerated in a properly closed container, this decoction can keep for 2 days. If you don't like the natural flavor of the herbs, a small amount of honey can be added.

- Eight cups water
- Two tablespoons dried catnip
- Two tablespoons dried raspberry leaf

1. Combine all of the ingredients in a saucepan. Bring the water to a boil over high heat, then turn it down to a low temperature. Simmer the herbs until the liquid has been reduced by half.

2. Allow the decoction to cool to the point where it is safe to consume. Then, enjoy a cup while it's still warm, or refrigerate it in a sealed bottle or jar.

Precautions

Fresh raspberry leaves might cause nausea, so never use them if they aren't entirely dry. Catnip can produce a lot of relaxation, so don't drive or operate machinery until you've figured out how it affects you.

EARACHE

When the sensory nerve endings in the eardrum respond to pressure, it causes an earache. At the first indication of discomfort, use natural medicines. If the discomfort intensifies or does not go away, see your doctor since a serious ear infection can spread and cause irreversible hearing loss.

REMEDY

Blue Vervain Infusion and Poultice

For making one treatment

Blue vervain aids in pain relief and circulation. The heated poultice comforts the ear region immediately from the outside. At the same time, when consumed, the infusion relieves the throat pain that might accompany an earache. Because the infusion has a bitter flavor, you may sweeten it.

- Two teaspoons dried blue vervain

- One cup boiling water

1. Place the blue vervain in a tea infuser in a mug, then pour in the boiling water. Allow 10 minutes for the infusion to steep. Remove the infuser from the water and set it aside to cool until it is still warm but manageable.

2. Transfer the blue vervain to a 4-inch square of cheesecloth and fold it in half. While sipping the tea carefully, press the poultice against your ear. Wrap the poultice in a damp cloth and microwave it for 5 to 10 seconds to revive it for next usage.

3. Repeat the procedure up to three times each day until your earache is disappeared.

550

FATIGUE

Work, education, and having a family might leave you feeling absolutely exhausted. Even a fun-filled trip might leave you exhausted and depleted of energy. Herbs are considerably gentler in their support than caffeinated beverages or sugary foods. So the next time you feel like you've struck a brick wall, try one of these suggestions.

REMEDY

Feverfew Tincture

For making about two cups

Feverfew can relieve the tension and worry that commonly comes with exhaustion, as well as the bodily aches and headaches that come with it. When stored in a cold, dark area, this tincture will keep its strength for up to 7 years.

- Eight ounces feverfew

- Two cups unflavored 80-proof vodka

1. Place the feverfew in a pint jar that has been sterilized. Fill the jar with vodka, filling it all the way to the top and fully covering the herbs. Close the jar firmly and give it a good shake. For 6 to 8 weeks, keep it in a cold, dark cabinet and shake it several times a week.

2. If any alcohol evaporates, fill up the jar with vodka until it's completely full. Then, soak a piece of cheesecloth in water and lay it over the funnel's mouth.

3. Pour the tincture into another sterilized pint jar using the funnel. Remove the feverfew's liquid by wringing it out. Transfer the final tincture to dark-colored glass bottles after discarding the wasted herbs.

4. While weariness is an issue, mix 10 drops of tincture into a glass of water or juice and consume it two or three times each day.

Precautions

Avoid using feverfew if you are pregnant or sensitive to plants in the ragweed family.

Licorice-Rosemary Syrup

For making about two cups

Licorice promotes adrenal gland function and can help you feel more energized, while rosemary is a great anti-fatigue tonic. Honey is a natural energy enhancer with a slew of health advantages. When maintained in the refrigerator, the syrup will last for 6 months. If you don't have time to create it, take a licorice extract supplement and diffuse rosemary essential oil in the area where you spend the most time.

- One ounce dried licorice root, chopped

- One ounce dried rosemary leaves, chopped

- Two cups water

- One cup honey

1. Combine the herbs and water in a saucepan. Reduce the liquid by half by bringing it to a low simmer and partially covering it with a lid.

2. Fill a glass measuring cup halfway with the contents of the saucepan, then strain the mixture through a soaked piece of cheesecloth into the saucepan, wringing the fabric until no more liquid comes out.

3. Warm the mixture over low heat with the honey, stirring regularly until the temperature reaches 105°F to 110°F. Fill a sterilized jar or bottle with the syrup and keep it in the refrigerator.

4. Take 1 tablespoon three times a day orally till your symptoms go away.

Precautions

Avoid taking licorice root if you have high blood pressure, diabetes, renal difficulties, or heart disease. If you have epilepsy, avoid using rosemary.

FEVER

Fever is the body's natural defense against illness, so if you can, give it a chance to fight. Herbs known as febrifuges (fever-reducers) might assist if your fever persists or worsens. If your kid has a fever, be extremely cautious about seeking medical help. Any fever of 100.4°F or higher in a baby under four months requires immediate medical attention. If your kid has a temperature of 104°F or greater, you should consult a doctor right once.

REMEDY

Feverfew Syrup

For making about two cups

Feverfew gets its name from the fact that it works as a febrifuge. This syrup is moderate and tasty enough for youngsters to consume. It may be kept refrigerated for up to 6 months.

- Two ounces dried feverfew
- Two cups water
- One cup honey

1. Combine the feverfew and water in a saucepan. Reduce the liquid by half by bringing it to a low simmer and partially covering it with a lid.
2. Pour the contents of the saucepan into a glass measuring cup, then pour the mixture back into the saucepan through a soaked piece of cheesecloth, wringing the liquid out of the cheesecloth.
3. Warm the mixture over low heat with the honey, stirring regularly until the temperature reaches 105°F to 110°F.
4. Fill a sterilized jar or bottle with the syrup and keep it in the refrigerator.
5. Take 1 tablespoon three times a day orally till your symptoms go away. Take 1 teaspoon three times a day for children under 12.

Precautions

If you're pregnant or sensitive to ragweed, don't take feverfew.

Blue Vervain–Raspberry Leaf Tincture

For making about two cups

Blue vervain and raspberry leaf are both powerful

febrifuges that lower fever gradually. When stored in a cold, dark area, this tincture will last up to 6 years.

- Four ounces dried blue vervain

- Four ounces dried raspberry leaf

- Two cups unflavored 80-proof vodka

1. Combine the herbs in a pint jar that has been sterilized. Fill the jar with vodka, filling it all the way to the top and fully covering the herbs. Close the jar firmly and give it a good shake.

2. For 6 to 8 weeks, keep it in a cold, dark cabinet and shake it several times a week. If any alcohol evaporates, fill up the jar with vodka until it's completely full.

3. Soak a piece of cheesecloth in water and lay it over the funnel's mouth. Pour the tincture into another sterilized pint jar using the funnel. Squeeze the liquid out of the herbs with the cheesecloth until there is no more liquid. Remove the roots and pour the tincture into dark-colored glass vials.

4. Orally, take 10 drops two or three times each day. If the flavor is too strong for you, dilute it with water or juice and consume it.

Precautions

Blue vervain should not be used during pregnancy. Fresh raspberry leaves might cause nausea, so never use them if they aren't entirely dry.

HAIR LOSS

Hair loss is commonly thought to be a male-only problem; however, it may also affect women. Thinning hair can be caused by various factors, including over styling, stress, and even vitamin deficiencies. Herbs won't help if your hair loss is caused by a hereditary condition. Still, they can encourage hair growth in many other cases.

REMEDY

Ginger Scalp Treatment

For making a half cup

Ginger stimulates hair follicles by increasing circulation in the scalp. When maintained in the refrigerator, this treatment will last for up to two months.

- Two ounces fresh ginger root, chopped

- One fourth cup sesame oil

1. Combine the ginger and sesame oil in a slow cooker. Set the slow cooker to the lowest heat setting, cover it, and let the herbs sit in the oil for 3 to 5 hours. Allow the infused oil to cool after turning off the heat. Over a basin, drape a piece of cheesecloth. Wring the cheesecloth until no more oil comes out after pouring in the infused oil. Throw away the ginger that has gone bad.

2. Allow the infused sesame oil to cool fully before closing it in a clean, dry container or jar. Before shampooing your hair, apply 1 tablespoon to the scalp. It should be massaged in.

3. Allow 30 minutes for the treatment to take effect before shampooing and conditioning your hair as usual. Then, three to four times each week, repeat.

Precautions

If you're on blood thinners, have gallbladder illness, or have a bleeding issue, don't use ginger.

Ginkgo-Rosemary Tonic

Ginkgo and rosemary, along with witch hazel, stimulate hair follicles by increasing circulation in the scalp. Rosemary improves your look and self-esteem by adding luster and strength to your remaining hair. When refrigerated, this tonic will last up to 6 months.

<u>For making about one cup</u>

- Half ounce dried Ginkgo Biloba

- Half ounce dried rosemary leaves

- Two tablespoons fractionated coconut oil

- One cup witch hazel

1. Combine the herbs and fractionated coconut oil in a slow cooker. Set the slow cooker to the lowest heat setting, cover it, and let the herbs sit in the oil for 3 to 5 hours.

2. Allow the infused oil to cool after turning off the heat. Over a basin, drape a piece of cheesecloth. Pour the infused oil into the cheesecloth, then wring and twist it until no more oil comes out.

3. Remove the cheesecloth and herbs that have been used. Combine the witch hazel and the infused oil in a dark-colored glass container with a spray cap. To thoroughly combine, give it a little shake. Apply a gentle mist of 1 or 2 spritzes to areas where hair loss is a concern after washing and conditioning your hair, adding more if necessary.

4. With your fingertips, massage the scalp. Then, once or twice a day, repeat.

Precautions

If you're using a monoamine oxidase inhibitor (MAOI) for depression, don't take Ginkgo Biloba. Ginkgo biloba can help blood thinners work better; see your doctor before taking it. If you have epilepsy, avoid using rosemary.

HANGOVER

Overindulgence happens, but it doesn't mean you have to suffer the consequences. While employing additional remedies to promote the detoxification process, try remedies that target each of your concerns—headache, nausea, and exhaustion.

REMEDY

Feverfew-Hops Tea

For making one cup

Feverfew relieves a headache while hops relax you. This tea is strong enough to assist you in falling asleep so that your body can recuperate more quickly.

- One cup boiling water

- One teaspoon dried feverfew

- One teaspoon of dried hops

1. Fill a large cup halfway with boiling water. Allow the tea to steep for 10 minutes after adding the dry herbs and covering the mug.

2. Slowly sip the tea while you relax. Repetition is allowed up to three times each day.

Precaution

If you are pregnant or sensitive to ragweed, avoid using feverfew.

Milk Thistle Tincture

<u>For making around two cups</u>

Milk thistle detoxifies the body while supporting the liver. This cure will not make you feel better right away, but it will help your system cope. It will keep for up to 6 years if stored in a cold, dark area.

- 8 ounces dried milk thistle

- 2 cups unflavored 80-proof vodka

1. Place the milk thistle in a pint jar that has been sterilized. Fill the jar with vodka, filling it all the way to the top and fully covering the herbs. Close the jar firmly and give it a good shake. For 6 to 8 weeks, keep it in a cold, dark cabinet and shake it several times a week. If any alcohol evaporates, fill up the jar with vodka until it's completely full.

2. Soak a piece of cheesecloth in water and lay it over the funnel's mouth. Pour the tincture into another sterilized pint jar using the funnel. Squeeze the liquid out of the herbs with the cheesecloth until there is no more liquid. Transfer the final tincture to dark-colored glass bottles after discarding the wasted herbs.

3. After overindulging, use 10 drops orally two or three times a day for 7 to 10 days. If the flavor is too strong for you, combine it with some water or juice and consume it. If you don't want to drink alcohol, mix the tincture into a cup of hot tea. Within 5 minutes, the alcohol will have evaporated.

Precautions

Milk thistle might produce moderate diarrhea if taken in excess. If this happens, reduce the amount or frequency.

HEADACHE

Headaches are commonly caused by stress or muscular tension. Still, they can also be caused by coffee withdrawal, eyestrain, or high blood pressure. If your headaches are regular or chronic, see your doctor since they might be a sign of something more serious.

REMEDY

Blue Vervain–Catnip Tea

For making one cup

Blue vervain and catnip work together to promote relaxation, enhance circulation, and relieve tension. In addition, this mix is great for headaches caused by stress.

- 1 cup boiling water
- 1 teaspoon dried blue vervain
- 1 teaspoon dried catnip

1. Fill a large cup halfway with boiling water. Allow the tea to steep for 10 minutes after adding the dry herbs and covering the mug.

2. Slowly sip the tea while you relax. Repetition is allowed up to three times each day.

Precaution

During pregnancy, avoid using blue vervain or catnip.

Skullcap Tincture

Skullcap is a moderate sedative with anti-neuropathic properties. A skullcap is a viable option if you suffer from migraines and cannot use feverfew. This tincture gives immediate relief. Skullcap is also available in capsule form if convenient for you. This tincture will keep for up to 6 years if kept in a cold, dark area.

- Eight ounces skullcap

- Two cups unflavored 80-proof vodka

1. Place the skullcap in a pint jar that has been sterilized. Fill the jar with vodka, filling it all the way to the top and fully covering the herbs. Close the jar firmly and give it a good shake. For 6 to 8 weeks, keep it in a cold, dark cabinet and shake it several times a week. If any alcohol evaporates, fill up the jar with vodka until it's completely full.

2. Soak a piece of cheesecloth in water and lay it over the funnel's mouth. Pour the tincture into another sterilized pint jar using the funnel. Squeeze the liquid out of the herbs with the cheesecloth until there is no more liquid.

3. Transfer the final tincture to dark-colored glass bottles after discarding the wasted herbs. Take 1 teaspoon orally two or three times a day when you have a headache. If the flavor is too strong for you, combine it with some water or juice and consume it.

Precautions

Skullcap should not be consumed when pregnant.

IBS

Irritable bowel syndrome (also known as the spastic colon) is a common condition characterized by recurring stomach discomfort, intermittent diarrhea, and constipation. In addition, worry, stress, or food intolerance may cause a disruption in the large intestine's muscular action, which can be induced by anxiety, stress, or food intolerance.

- Women suffer from IBS in significantly greater numbers than males.
- IBS affects 10–20% of the population, and it accounts for up to 50% of all health cases seen by gastroenterologists.
- The great majority of patients are women, with the young and middle-aged particularly vulnerable.

<u>REMEDY</u>

1. The relaxing impact of slippery elm may be felt all the way down the intestines. Herbal teas with antispasmodic properties, such as chamomile, peppermint, and balm, can help you relax.

2. Fresh ginger can be chewed to help ease spasms.

HIGH BLOOD PRESSURE

High blood pressure, often known as hypertension, can lead to early cognitive impairment, heart disease, renal failure, and stroke if left untreated. Natural techniques to promote healing include losing weight, exercising, and meditating. However, if you can't lower your blood pressure on your own after two months, visit a doctor right away.

REMEDY

Angelica Infusion

For making one quart

Angelica includes chemicals like calcium channel blockers (drugs that relax and expand blood

arteries, affecting arterial wall muscles), commonly lowering blood pressure. This infusion is a tad bitter, but it may be sweetened or combined with juice if desired. It will keep for three days in the refrigerator.

- Four teaspoons dried angelica

- Four cups boiling water

- Four teaspoons fresh lime juice

1. Combine the dried angelica and boiling water in a teapot. Allow the infusion to steep for 10 minutes before adding the lime juice to the saucepan.

2. Relax and carefully sip a cup of the infusion. You may keep the remaining in the fridge and drink it over many days, either warmed or over ice.

Precautions

If you're pregnant or using anticoagulants, avoid taking angelica.

Dandelion-Lavender Tincture

<u>For making about two cups</u>

Dandelions are high in potassium, which helps manage salt levels and reduce blood pressure naturally. The aroma and oils of lavender calm and regulate the nervous system.

- Four ounces dried dandelion root, finely chopped

- Four ounces dried lavender leaves, chopped

- Four cups unflavored 80-proof vodka

1. Combine the herbs in a pint jar that has been sterilized. Fill the jar with vodka, filling it all the way to the top and fully covering the herbs. Close the jar firmly and give it a good shake. For 6 to 8 weeks, keep it in a cold, dark cabinet and shake it several times a week. If any alcohol evaporates, fill up the jar with vodka until it's completely full.

2. Soak a piece of cheesecloth in water and lay it over the funnel's mouth. Pour the tincture into another sterilized pint jar using the funnel. Squeeze the liquid out of the herbs with the cheesecloth until there is no more liquid. Transfer the final tincture to dark-colored glass bottles after discarding the wasted herbs.

3. Orally, take 10 drops two or three times each day. If the flavor is too strong for you, combine it with some water or juice and consume it. Continue to make healthy lifestyle changes and take steps to lower your blood pressure.

Precautions

This tincture should not be used for more than two months. Excessive dandelions usage might result in dangerously low blood pressure. In addition, excessive quantities of lavender taken by mouth might cause constipation, headaches, and an increase in appetite. If you have any negative side effects, contact your doctor right once.

INSOMNIA

Insomnia is caused by factors, including anxiety, caffeine, and stress. Overexposure to devices, particularly in the hour leading up tonight, is another key factor. When utilizing herbal sleep aids, be careful to consider these variables.

REMEDY

Valerian Tea with Hops and Passionflower

For making cup

Valerian hops and passionflower create a relaxing combination that relieves stress and anxiety while encouraging deep, peaceful sleep.

- One cup boiling water

- One teaspoon chopped dried valerian root

- Half teaspoon crushed dried hops

- Half teaspoon dried passionflower

1. Fill a large cup halfway with boiling water. Allow the tea to steep for 10 minutes after adding the dry herbs and covering the mug.

2. Slowly sip the tea while you relax. Repeat each night before going to bed if you're having trouble sleeping.

Precautions

Prepubescent youngsters of any gender should not be given hops. If you have prostate issues or baldness, you should avoid using passionflower. Also, do not use it if you are pregnant.

Chamomile-Catnip Syrup

Although chamomile and catnip are extremely calming herbs, this mixture is gentle enough for youngsters to use when experiencing periodic sleepiness. This syrup can last up to 6 months when kept in the refrigerator.

For making two cups

- One ounce dried chamomile

- One ounce dried catnip

- Two cups water

- One cup honey

1. Combine the chamomile, catnip, and water in a saucepan. Reduce the liquid by half by bringing it to a low simmer and partially covering it with a lid. Fill a glass measuring cup halfway with the contents of the saucepan, then strain the mixture through a soaked piece of cheesecloth into the saucepan, wringing the fabric until no more liquid comes out.

2. Warm the mixture over low heat with the honey, stirring regularly until the temperature reaches 105°F to 110°F. Fill a sterilized jar or bottle with the syrup and keep it in the refrigerator. 30 minutes before bedtime, take 1 tablespoon orally. 30 minutes before bedtime, children under the age of 12 should take 1 teaspoon.

Precautions

Catnip should not be used during pregnancy. Also, avoid using chamomile if you are sensitive to ragweed plants or prescription blood thinners.

MENSTRUAL PROBLEMS

Dysmenorrhea (painful menstruation), menorrhagia (heavy menstrual flow), and amenorrhea are the most prevalent menstrual issues (no menstrual bleeding). There is either an elevated level of or sensitivity to prostaglandin. This hormone-like substance causes uterine contractions in primary dysmenorrhea. Endometriosis, fibroids, a pelvic infection, stress, or a thyroid issue can all induce secondary dysmenorrhea (abnormal menstrual cramps) three years after menstruation begins. Sharp pain or a dull discomfort in the lower abdomen and lower back, headaches, sweating, and diarrhea are all signs of both. Vomiting and fainting may occur in extreme situations. Menorrhagia is defined as excessive menstrual bleeding that interferes with daily activities. Fibroids,

polyps, pelvic infection, endometriosis, hypothyroidism, blood-clotting issues, stress, or the use of an IUD or injectable contraception can all contribute to the condition. Menstruation does not begin before the age of 18 and is referred to as primary amenorrhea. Low body weight or genetics are the most common causes. Menstruation ceases for more than six months due to pregnancy, weight reduction, beginning oral contraceptives, severe shock, stress, anemia, thyroid condition, or a fibroid.

REMEDY

1. Menstrual cramps can be relieved by chewing on cramp bark. Also, a lady's mantle is an astringent that can help with heavy menstrual flow. As needed, take three times daily.

2. Yarrow can aid with menstrual irregularities.

3. Raspberry leaves can aid in the regulation of an overabundance of blood flow.

4. Drinking thyme tea in the morning and evening might help manage the excessive flow.

5. Angelica root can aid in the promotion of menstruation that has been delayed.

6. During menstruation, drink catnip tea every evening and morning to relieve discomfort.

NAUSEA AND VOMITING

Nausea and vomiting are signs of various conditions, including gastroenteritis, inner ear infection, migraine, excessive food or alcohol consumption, hiatus hernia, pancreatitis, indigestion, food poisoning, gallstones, or liver disease. Hormonal changes like pregnancy and menstruation, travel, and specific odors and sights might also trigger them. Nausea might be accompanied by dizziness and a sense of faintness. Vomiting is frequently preceded by nausea, with sweat, increased salivation, and a lowering of the pulse rate. It's most likely that a continual sense of nausea with no vomiting, but a headache and stomach discomfort, is caused by stress or worry.

REMEDY

1. Warming the stomach and relieving cold nausea can be achieved by drinking ginger tea or chewing a piece of crystallized ginger. This can be used to relieve nausea during pregnancy or when traveling.

2. If you have persistent nausea, it might signify that you have a problem with your liver. Seek medical help.

SINUSITIS

Sinusitis is an inflammatory condition that affects the sinuses, air-filled chambers in the bones around the nose. The lining of the sinuses expands, as a result, obstructing the route that drains them. A build-up of mucus discharge occurs, resulting in severe discomfort and pressure. Sinusitis is most commonly caused by a viral

Illness, such as a cold. Still, it can also be caused by pollution or cigarette use. An allergy or bacterium injected through the nasal passages can cause inflammation of the sinuses, resulting in infection with discomfort and soreness. Chronic sinusitis can be caused by either kind or a mix of the two. A cold can cause maxillary sinusitis, or swimming in polluted water can induce it. A molar tooth extraction may occasionally disrupt the maxillary sinus floor, allowing germs to enter and cause illness. Localized headache, surface discomfort, and, on rare occasions, swelling of the eyelids are all indications of frontal and ethmoid sinusitis. Because of its closeness to the optic nerves, sphenoid sinusitis can produce impaired vision.

REMEDY

1. Elderflower is beneficial for sinusitis and catarrh. To alleviate symptoms and promote recovery, drink an infusion as needed.

2. During an acute episode, drink a golden seal infusion every two hours.

STRESS

Each person can handle a varied level of stress in their life. Although some appear to have limitless reserves to keep going, others succumb. While a certain amount of stress may be stimulating, continuous stress can be harmful to both the mind and the body. The majority of us associate stress with stressful circumstances and anxiety. In truth, there are many different types of stress. Environmental pressures include pollution, noise, housing issues, cold, or overheating; bodily stresses include diseases, injuries, and an inadequate diet; mental tensions include relationship issues, financial constraints, grief, and employment challenges.

These factors influence the body, leading it to respond to hazardous or demanding conditions by undergoing a sequence of fast physiological changes known as "adaptive reactions." Hormones are pumped into the circulation during the initial stage of stress. As a result, the heart beats faster, the lungs take in more oxygen to power the muscles, blood sugar levels rise to provide more energy, digestion slows, and sweat rises. The body begins to heal the damage created by the first stage of stress in the second stage. The stress symptoms disappear as the stressful circumstance is resolved. However, tiredness will set in if the condition persists, and the body's energy will be depleted. This stage may last until important organs are compromised, illness or death may occur.

Among the signs and symptoms are: an increase in stress-related chemicals such as adrenaline, noradrenaline, and corticosteroids may result in the following: Nausea, tight muscles, and increased breathing and heart rate. Stress is considered to cause sleeplessness, depression, high blood pressure, hair loss, allergies, ulcers, heart disease, digestive disorders, menstruation issues, palpitations, impotence, and premature ejaculation in the long run. Psychological stress is caused by dangers that are either experienced or expected. Stress can be acute, a reaction to a life-threatening circumstance, or persistent, as in a person's unpleasant living condition. The bodily mechanics are the same in both cases. Chronic physical sickness nearly invariably has substantial psychological consequences.

On the other hand, long-term psychological stress frequently results in severe alterations. Medical researchers classify people's conduct into two categories based on how they react to stress. People with type-A personalities react to stress by being more aggressive, competitive, and putting self-imposed pressure on themselves to get things done. Increased risks of heart attack and other ailments have been related to Type-A behavior. Type-B people may have the same serious goals as type-A people, but they are more patient, easygoing, and calm. Stress plays a significant role in disorders whose physical symptoms are caused or exacerbated by mental or emotional issues. Stress-related diseases account for 50–80% of all illnesses, yet stress isn't always the root reason.

1. Balm, lavender, chamomile, passiflora, and oats are herbs that promote relaxation and work as nervous system tonics. So when you're in a stressful situation, drink them as an infusion as often as you need.

2. Ginseng is a great "adaptogenic" plant, meaning it may help you feel better when you're fatigued and relax when you're stressed. It also energizes and strengthens the immune system. During stressful circumstances, some therapists advocate taking a daily dosage.

URINARY TRACT INFECTIONS AND CYSTITIS

Cystitis is a bladder and urinary system infection. Symptoms include painful, burning urination; a persistent need to pee but an inability to do so; poor energy; and, in rare cases, fever. If the infection affects the kidneys, it can be deadly, so be cautious and treat it as soon as possible.

In most cases, cystitis and urinary tract infections (UTIs) may be treated at home. Begin therapy as soon as you notice the first signs: a minor burning sensation when peeing or an incomplete bladder emptying. The illness should clear up in a day or two if you follow even a few of these tips.

Slow down and get some rest since your body is fighting an illness.

REMEDY

- Two parts cleavers

- Two parts fresh or dried cranberries

- Two parts uva ursi

- One part buchu (optional; use if the infection is severe)

- One part chickweed

- One part marshmallow root

1. Combine the herbs and make an infusion.

2. Drink 2 cups every day

Chapter 4: Remedies for Common Childhood Problems

BEDWETTING

Bedwetting isn't considered a concern until your child reaches the age of five. Many youngsters, particularly males, are reluctant to understand that they must get up to use the restroom at night, but this has nothing to do with their mental or physical health. It may take longer for a kid to become night dry if they sleep a lot, but most

youngsters are dry by the age of two or three. Stress, such as relocating, changing schools, or family fighting, can trigger bedwetting in children who have previously established a pattern of dry nights. In addition, immature nerves and muscles governing bladder function may affect children who have never been dry at night. Diabetes, urinary infection, dietary deficiencies, and food allergies are other medical factors.

REMEDY

1. To ease an irritable bladder and encourage bladder control, drink St. John's wort and horsetail teas, sweetened with honey throughout the day.

2. Vervain and lime balm relax and soothe if bedwetting is caused by an emotional upset or disturbance.

CRADLE CAP

Cradle cap (seborrheic eczema) is characterized by a thick encrusted covering of skin on the baby's scalp during the first three months of life. Cradle cap affects over 90% of all newborns at some time during their first several months. Yellow scales will appear in places, particularly on

the top of the skull. The cradle cap can persist for up to three years in extreme circumstances. Cradle cap is when the seborrheic glands become hyperactive, similar to dandruff. It is frequently connected with seborrheic dermatitis, a skin ailment characterized by red, scaly regions on the forehead and brows, among other locations.

REMEDY

1. After bathing, rinse the scalp with a meadowsweet infusion, which is anti-inflammatory and relieves irritation.

2. Burdock may also be used to rinse your baby's hair after washing it.

3. Butternut can be given internally to promote healing (1 drop, three times a day, mixed in water).

THRUSH

Thrush is highly frequent among those with a weak or weakened immune system. It most commonly affects children's mouths and diaper areas, where it manifests as an itchy red rash with a white top.

REMEDY

1. Keep in mind that the dose for youngsters should be reduced. Instead of requiring the patient to swallow a dose, rinse the baby's mouth or dab drops into the afflicted region.

2. Try using a vaporizer in the child's room for aromatherapy. You may also apply diluted Rescue remedy lotion to the afflicted region.

TEETHING

Your baby's first teeth will most likely develop around six months of age, and teeth may not come through until two or three years of age. Most newborns suffer some pain, ranging from moderate to severe, accompanied by dribbling, loose feces, and sleeping issues. A red patch on one cheek is a common sign.

REMEDY

1. Inflamed gums can be soothed with marshmallow root syrup. Several tablespoons can be added to your baby's regular meals.

2. To relax and soothe, provide chamomile or fennel infusions.

COLIC

Colic is defined as seemingly constant frenzied sobbing that occurs simultaneously every day or night. The baby's legs are brought up to his tummy, and he looks to be in excruciating discomfort. Excessive sobbing leads the infant to swallow air, aggravating the situation and causing stomach bloating. Colic can be caused by bowel contractions, an allergy to anything in the formula (if bottle-fed), the mother's diet (if breast-fed), or just too much air being swallowed in during frequent episodes of sobbing. Three-month colic is the most frequent type of colic, usually in the evening. It lasts anywhere from a few minutes to several hours. Burping or placing the infant over the knee or shoulder has minimal effect in most cases.

REMEDY

1. Because tension aggravates colic, soothing herbs are frequently recommended in the bath or steeped, chilled somewhat, and taken by the bottle.

2. The most beneficial herbs include chamomile, lime balm, and lime flowers.

3. A warm bath with a dill, fennel, marshmallow, or lime balm infusion helps calm a fussy infant.

DIAPER RASH

Contact with pee or feces causes diaper rash because the skin produces less protective oil and provides a less effective barrier to additional irritation. Irritating compounds in feces, not fully washing soap or detergent out of diapers, and chemicals in disposable diapers can also cause it. In regions touched by diapers, the baby's buttocks, thighs, and genitals become painful, red, spotty, and weepy. In addition, the foreskin in boys can become irritated, making urinating difficult. If the infant has been given antibiotics or the breast milk contains antibiotics, or if the mother has oral or vaginal thrush, the rash may become secondarily infected with the Candida fungus.

REMEDY

1. The acidity of the urine will be reduced with Buchu. To soothe and minimize irritation, apply marigold ointment to the diaper region.

2. Wash the diaper region with marigold, rosemary, or elderflower infusions.

3. Before putting on a new diaper, apply powdered goldenseal to a clean diaper region. To lower the acidity of the urine, give your infant lots of calming beverages, such as diluted chamomile tea.

WORMS

Worm infestations in the digestive system are very prevalent, especially in young children, who generally get them at school. Worms can be observed near the anus or in the feces, and they cause inflammation in the intestine or rectum where they adhere. Humans can be parasitized by various worms ranging from microscopic to several meters long. Most infestations are infrequent in the United Kingdom and the United States, except for threadworms. Threadworms, which are small white thread-like worms that infest the rectum, are not hazardous, although they can make sleeping difficult. They produce itching around the anus and minor colicky belly pain on occasion. Worms can be contracted by eating raw or undercooked diseased meat, coming into touch with worm larvae-infested soil or water, or inadvertently ingesting worm eggs from infected feces-infested soil.

REMEDY

- Cayenne pepper and senna can be used together; the former stuns the worms while the latter facilitates their expulsion. Finally, mix in a little live yogurt to avoid upsetting the digestive tract.

- Worms will be stunned by Wormwood tea.

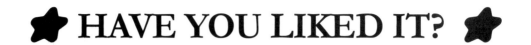

⭐ HAVE YOU LIKED IT? ⭐

To provide the best quality cases to customers, **I would love to hear your thoughts and opinions on this collection.**

TO DO SO, I WOULD ENCOURAGE YOU TO <u>LEAVE A HONEST REVIEW ON AMAZON.</u>

Your comment will ultimately aid me in continually improving my current and future books. I genuinely hope that your experience with my product was positive and memorable!

The best way to do it? Upload a brief video with you talking about the **#1** thing you liked the most about this book.

Is it too much for you? Not a problem at all! A simply written review is still an amazing thing!

<u>THANK YOU IN ADVANCE FOR YOUR VALUABLE FEEDBACK.</u> THIS WILL HELP ME A LOT AS A SELF-PUBLISHED AUTHOR!